The Comprehensive Physicians' Guide to the Management of PANS and PANDAS

The Comprehensive Physicians' Guide to the Management of PANS and PANDAS

An Evidence-Based Approach to Diagnosis, Testing, and Effective Treatment

Dr. Scott Antoine

With Dr. Ellen Antoine

Forefront
BOOKS

Published by Forefront Books.
Distributed by Simon & Schuster.

Library of Congress Control Number: 2023921132

Print ISBN: 978-1-63763-269-7
E-book ISBN: 978-1-63763-270-3

Cover Design by Bruce Gore, Gore Studio, Inc.
Interior Design by Bill Kersey, KerseyGraphics

This book is dedicated to

Dr. Ellen Antoine, who figured out what was wrong with
our daughter and how to help her while holding our family
together during a mighty storm. She is the best physician and
the best person I have ever known. I love you immensely;

our daughter, Emma, and her siblings, Jacob, Dylan,
Nick, and Kyle, who endured this challenge with her.
You are our life, and we are so proud of you;

Nan and Herb Tesser, who drove countless miles
and helped our family at every opportunity;

Sharon Tesser Frizzell Myers, who was always the
voice of reason and a shoulder on which to cry;

the physicians and other healthcare professionals reading this
textbook who will help return lost children to their parents;

the children and parents currently fighting against PANS and
PANDAS—may you have enduring hope and complete healing.

CONTENTS

FOREWORD

(ELISA SONG, MD)

Katelyn was moving out of state the summer after 3rd grade. I remember seeing her in my office for her last well check – a spunky, bright, chatty, athletic nine-year-old girl who loved math, hip-hop, gymnastics, and lacrosse. And mostly, she loved hanging out with her friends. What she didn't share at that visit with me or mom, was that she was starting to have urges to touch certain things in particular ways.

Three years later, her family moved back, and reached out because they were at a loss as to how to help her. Katelyn's urges in third grade to touch things had ramped up along with her anxieties. She started catastrophizing about bad things happening to her family. She was doing competitive gymnastics, and started developing extreme anticipation anxiety and OCD around meets—she would spend hours tumbling and touching things around the house, turning lights on and off, not wanting to step over lines. It was exhausting for her to do. It was exhausting for her family to watch.

Along with her anxiety and OCD came an element of chaos that was difficult for her parents and her to describe. She had always been organized at school and at home, and now there was a constant state of disorganization— in her room, backpack, binders, etc. She forgot to put her name on things and forgot things she had learned before—even her rock-solid math facts she knew like the back of her hand.

They noted that the year before in the spring of fifth grade, everything worsened. Her anxiety and OCD went through the roof. She could barely leave the house. And she was starting to hurt herself. Her parents reluctantly started her on an SSRI antidepressant medication—they couldn't have her suicidal ideation and self-injurious behavior worsen. It didn't help as much as they had hoped, and before throwing a dart to see which psychiatric medication to try next, they wanted to explore any integrative and functional medicine options that might help. Something just didn't feel right. Katelyn was not the child she had been, and they wanted to find out why.

When I saw twelve-year-old Katelyn in my office, I hardly recognized her. She could barely make eye contact or hold a conversation. When I asked her a question, she would look at me as though she were terrified, pupils dilated, staring at me like a deer in headlights. I could tell her brain was working hard to just understand the simple questions I was asking. Her voice was quavering and soft, with a nasal, baby-like quality that I hadn't noticed when she was nine. Her hands were shaky, and she had bruises all over her shins. Mom had forgotten to mention that over the past year, Katelyn had gone from being a competitive, coordinated gymnast, to being clumsy, uncoordinated, unable to remember her routines, and being totally accident-prone—hence, the bruises. Her poor performance in gymnastics seemed trivial compared to everything else Katelyn was going through.

As we combed through her history, one key detail stood out to me—something that I might have overlooked in years past had I not known what PANS/PANDAS was. During spring break of her fifth-grade year, Katelyn had gone to Disney with her friend's family. She recalled being happy and relaxed when she was there and wished that she could go back to how she used to be. During that trip, she had a fever and sore throat that was presumed viral. Her fever and sore throat resolved, but it was about a week after coming home that her anxieties and OCD started to ramp up. And then the cutting began.

An extensive lab workup revealed zinc and vitamin D deficiencies, suboptimal thyroid functioning, gluten and egg sensitivities, and most importantly—elevated antistreptolysin O (ASO) and anti-DNase B Strep antibodies. Some of the most elevated I'd ever seen. We started Katelyn on supplements to support her

nutrient deficiencies and immune function, and a trial of antibiotics.

A short six weeks later when I saw Katelyn back in the office—she was "back!" Her eyes were bright and her voice was strong as she answered my questions with the same happy spirit I remembered from three years before. Her OCD and anxiety were nearly gone. Her clumsiness was totally gone, although she decided to step back from competitive gymnastics because of the stress. She was organized, and her executive functioning skills were re-emerging. Her mood was great, and she felt so much better physically and emotionally. Both Katelyn and her parents noted that it was like a "night and day" difference. They went back to her psychiatrist to share the great news and to see if she could wean off of her SSRI as she stabilized. And the first thing her psychiatrist said, **"There's no such thing as PANDAS."**

I wish I could say that Katelyn was the first and only child with PANS/PANDAS to be told this. Sadly, even as a pediatrician practicing literally down the street from the Stanford Immune Behavioral Health (formerly PANS) Clinic, there are too many pediatricians, psychiatrists, and pediatric practitioners who do not believe in PANS/PANDAS. And even for those who do believe, the PANS Clinic is virtually impossible to get into, and they don't know who else to refer their patients to.

What physicians on the front lines need is a place to start so that their patients don't become the 7 in 10 who had to see three or more doctors before getting the right diagnosis (PANDAS Network Survey 2018). You can't recommend the right treatments if you don't have the right diagnosis.

In 2018, nearly half of parents said that "Our journey was met with medical professionals who meant well but were unable to help our child." Over half said that "Our journey was met with doubting medical professionals who made us feel like we were crazy."

If you're reading this book, I know that you are one of the medical professionals who knows that PANS/PANDAS is real. And you are one of the medical professionals who wants to understand how to help the children in your practice—but you're not necessarily sure where to start or how. Or you're unclear what else can be done besides sometimes unattainable treatments like IVIG. You want an evidence-based guide to sort out the noise and offer effective treatment options so that your patients don't go down the Dr. Google rabbit hole.

Enter Drs. Scott and Ellen Antoine. My dear friends, colleagues, functional medicine and PANS/PANDAS physician experts, parent warriors, and patient advocates. Through their personal story, they learned by any means necessary how to help their daughter with crippling PANS symptoms, despite being told multiple times by respected physician colleagues that there was no such thing. Scott and Ellen pieced together the diagnostic and treatment plan for their daughter based upon the principles of their already proven Fully Functional® process that now paves the way for other physicians to do the same for their patients. No more fumbling around trying to piece together the latest clinical research. No more feeling alone in your quest to support your patients who are not receiving the support they need from specialists, therapists, or schools.

The Comprehensive Physicians' Guide to The Management of PANS and PANDAS is the physician's guidebook that I wish I had fifteen years ago, as I was navigating my way through the research and trying to translate this into practical, clinically relevant and actionable diagnostic and therapeutic plans for the patients sitting in front of me. Dr. Scott Antoine wrote this book so that you don't have to fumble or feel alone.

In this essential guidebook for physicians, you will learn:

- An evidence-based, integrative and functional medicine approach to PANS/PANDAS
- The key elements in making a diagnosis of PANS/PANDAS
- How to identify the key infectious and inflammatory triggers of PANS/PANDAS - and what to do about them
- What laboratory and radiologic tests to order, based on your clinical history and physical exam
- How to manage the symptoms of PANS/PANDAS with evidence-based supplements and therapeutics (and why SSRIs and other psychiatric medications often fail)
- Ways to resolve immune dysregulation (including strategies to get IVIG covered for your patients)
- 1200+ references to share with colleagues and parents who may need more "evidence"

The Appendices are worth their weight in gold as a go-to reference guide for the practicing physician—from exact test code numbers for LabCorp and Quest, medication and supplement dosages by age, and what to do during a PANS/PANDAS flare.

This book is written by a doctor for doctors to understand how to bring the art and science

> "Learn from yesterday, live for today, hope for tomorrow. The important thing is not to stop questioning." -Albert Einstein

of evidence-based medicine back to the treatment of children with what otherwise could be a devastating series of ineffective psychiatric medications and therapies and life-altering stress and grief for entire families. This will be your roadmap to navigate this journey with your patients for years to come so that your patients, and you, can move forward with hope and healing.

May you never stop questioning the power of the art and science of medicine to help your patients thrive.

Sincerely,
Elisa Song, MD, MPP

WHY I WROTE THIS TEXTBOOK AND HOW IT CAN HELP PHYSICIANS

The story behind why I wrote this book begins with our own family's story. It's the story of a mighty struggle and a victory that changed us forever.

It was a Friday night in the fall of 2013. Friday nights were the best. All seven of us (me; my wife, Ellen; Jacob; Dylan; Emma; Nick; and Kyle) would make dinner together. Friday dinners were usually extra fun since we would always have a theme, like "make your own pizza" or "make your own ice cream sundae." After dinner, we would find a family movie to watch on the TV over the fireplace. Once the movie was over, the sleepy clan was escorted upstairs to drift off to sleep and usher in the weekend.

This particular Friday night was a bit different. Emma, who was twelve at the time, seemed moody. She was usually carefree and upbeat. Something had suddenly changed from just a few days before. After dinner, just before we were about to start the movie, Emma came to us visibly upset. She said, "I'm scared that God does not think I'm a good person." We were completely shocked. We had several discussions that night. It seemed that whatever Ellen and I said, we failed to reassure her. Then she broke down crying. After praying with her, she seemed a bit better and was able

to watch the movie. We thought this was just "teenage stuff" and were not overly concerned. She had difficulty getting to sleep that night (which was unusual) and came into our room several times to ask if the doors to the house were locked.

We did not notice much over the next few days. All the kids went off to school. Emma went to soccer practice. She was spending more time with us, watching TV in our bedroom before she went to bed. As the week went on, it became more and more difficult to get her to her own bed to sleep. The crying episodes and talk about God continued. Though it was not unusual to discuss spiritual topics in our home, since we are people of faith, this was different. There was an insistence, an urgency in Emma's voice. Things were getting progressively worse.

About three weeks later, we noticed that Emma's hands were very red. She had open cracks on all her knuckles. About the time we noticed this, we also noticed that she was washing her hands—a lot. She was washing them at least once per hour and really scrubbing them. She was also using a lot of soap. Soon after this, she started taking two or three showers a day lasting 20–30 minutes each. Within a month we were rationing soap for showers and locking up all of the soap and shampoo in a hall closet we had fitted with a padlock.

The crying fits and questions continued. Emma then started saying she heard a "good voice" telling her to do the good things God wanted her to, and she heard a "bad voice" telling her to do bad things. She also began to lose control of her bladder. Although she had no burning or other signs of urinary tract infection, she began to lose bladder control several times a day, which resulted in the need for an extra-long shower.

Her behavior became increasingly defiant. What started out as a cry for help turned into distrust of what we were telling her. She could not understand why we were telling her she was clean after she had just finished a shower, because she still felt very dirty. Soon she was unable to eat any meat that we prepared because she convinced herself that it was raw and would make her sick.

Nighttime became a battleground. She would not stay in her room; she always had "just one more" question. These questions were about whether the food she consumed was cooked or whether there was dog poop on her bed clothes or whether her hands were clean. The questions went on, rapid-fire, for increasing periods of time. Soon we started limiting the time she could ask them. After we limited the number of questions she could ask, she would stand in the hallway in front of her room screaming, insisting on answers for all of the rest of her questions immediately. At the height of her illness, she kicked our locked bedroom door off its hinges.

Twice. All sixty-five pounds of her. It was like our daughter was gone.

Ellen and I had both been physicians for almost twenty years at this point, so our medical minds were not idle. But we had no plausible explanation for Emma's symptoms. We had never seen anything like it. She had no headaches. No fever. Her neurological exam was normal. It just didn't make sense.

Unsure how to proceed, we hit the books. Late one night, Ellen discovered some literature from physicians at the National Institute of Mental Health on something called "PANDAS." PANDAS stands for Pediatric Autoimmune Neuropsychiatric Disorder Associated with Streptococcal infections. Ellen read five or six peer-reviewed, professional articles on PANDAS from the pediatric mental health literature. Children with PANDAS develop very specific symptoms following a *Strep* infection: severe neuropsychiatric symptoms such as food refusal, obsessive-compulsive disorder (OCD), sleep disturbance, anxiety, defiant behavior, tics, and trouble with bladder control.

Once Ellen showed me the articles, I knew she had found the diagnosis. Emma had every single symptom of this disorder. Now that we had a direction, we needed help.

The very first call Ellen made was to Emma's pediatrician. She left a message that we thought Emma had PANDAS and that we needed help. We knew that some lab testing might be needed and hoped that she could help us get the testing and the treatment Emma needed. We never received a call back. At the time, we did not understand why her doctor did not return the call. Now that we have been involved in many of these cases, I can say that this is not a rare occurrence. Many parents with children fighting PANS (Pediatric

Acute-onset Neuropsychiatric Syndrome) and PANDAS are met with disbelief from their physicians. Next, I called a pediatric infectious disease physician from our local children's hospital and told him what was going on with Emma and asked if he could help us with PANDAS.

"I just don't believe PANDAS exists," he said. "I can't help you." He hung up the phone.

As our patients can attest, Ellen and I never give up looking for answers for them. And we certainly weren't going to give up on our own daughter. We soon began an exhaustive search for answers in the medical literature and searched for a physician colleague to help us. Luckily, Ellen remembered hearing a lecture by a physician from New York City who took care of children with complex medical conditions. She found his name and, soon after, she was on a plane with Emma headed to see him.

The physician walked in the room for Emma's initial evaluation, took one look at her and told Ellen, "You are correct, this is definitely PANDAS." We had been able to order some lab work before the visit. Emma's *Strep* antibody titers were elevated, which helped support the diagnosis. He prescribed some antibiotics but said, based on how sick she was, that he felt she needed intravenous immunoglobulin (IVIG).

We felt a bit better at this point because we finally had hope in the form of antibiotics and IVIG. Once Emma and Ellen got home, I called a pediatric neurologist at our local children's hospital who prescribed IVIG to children with other neurologic disorders. I started from the beginning and explained Emma's symptoms, which were getting worse by the day. I reviewed her lab results with him and asked about IVIG.

"Look," he said in an annoyed tone, "it sounds like your daughter just needs to be on antipsychotic medication and needs to be locked up in a mental hospital."

I simply replied, "Thank you" and hung up the phone. Not our daughter.

Then began a quest that gave a whole new meaning to the phrase *never give up*. We continued to search the world's medical literature and did countless hours of web searches. We called colleagues. Ultimately, we found a physician in a neighboring state who treats children with PANS and PANDAS. He also ordered IVIG for children who were severely affected, like Emma. We had an initial phone consultation, and he reviewed her labs and agreed that she needed IVIG therapy because of how sick she was. We were grateful that we were going to get what Emma needed, and thought it would not be a problem...until we tried to get approval from our insurance for IVIG treatment.

IVIG treatments cost around $20,000 for a two-day infusion. As a result, most insurers have very restrictive policies concerning IVIG. One common reason for denial of authorization given by insurance companies is that PANDAS and PANS don't exist, and that this is an "experimental treatment." If the IVIG is ordered for PANDAS, it results in an automatic denial of coverage (as in our case). At this point there are only two choices: parents must pay out of pocket, or they don't get IVIG for their desperately ill child.

We knew we had to make this happen, so Ellen got on the phone (multiple times over a six-hour period). Through tears and frustration, she convinced the physician working for the insurance company to approve the IVIG during a peer-to-peer consultation. Fortunately, she had the clinical experience caring for patients and could, in essence, "speak the same language" as the physician reviewer. He ultimately found some criteria under which to approve the IVIG infusion. This would not have turned out the same if we were non-physician parents appealing the denial.

I took Emma on a four-hour road trip to receive IVIG over two days. Once we finished the second day, we got in the car and drove four hours back to our home just north of Indianapolis, Indiana.

Then it happened.

It was as if the curtain had been lifted. Four days after IVIG—yes, four days—her symptoms disappeared. She was back. We cried. We prayed a prayer of thanksgiving to God. It was as if the light went on and she returned to us. She was sorry for the defiance (and for kicking the door off the hinges). She was happy again. No more voices. Her hands began to heal over the next few weeks.

Having a child who is sick is heartbreaking. But what is worse is having a child who is sick and having no hope. We held on to hope throughout Emma's illness. But it was hard, so hard. One of the worst parts of this whole ordeal was the fact that, even as physicians, we were stuck in a medical system that did not believe in PANS and PANDAS (despite extensive peer-reviewed literature from the National Institute of Mental Health and numerous academic centers).

After our ordeal, I knew I had found my purpose. We dedicated our practice to making sure that no family ever has to go through what we went through.

⬡⬡

This is a book *by physicians for physicians*.

We live in an age of disposable information and questionable sources. The material in this book was not assembled by scouring the internet for the most popular health and wellness blogs, but by thoughtful review of the primary sources from the peer-reviewed literature. It is composed of evidence from both the basic science and clinical literature.

This information was then combined with over thirty years of clinical experience caring for the sickest patients both in and out of the hospital. The result is the textbook you now hold in your hands. It is a work forged through a multitude of clinical encounters and has been developed for physicians while keeping both the patients and their families in mind.

This book was written to bring back some of the art of medicine to physicians caring for a group of children and families who really need it. PANS and PANDAS are complex disorders that can't be tackled with just antibiotics, steroids, and IVIG, although each of those things has their place. These disorders demand a rich, multifaceted response that ventures into the world of integrative medicine to find misunderstood (or forgotten) infections, toxins, and novel treatment approaches. There is currently no recognized standard of care for PANS and PANDAS. This may be because these disorders are still not widely recognized as being real; or it could be because the best medical care is not algorithmic but personalized. The standard of care for my daughter in the depths of her illness would have been psychiatric medications and hospitalization. But the very best physicians sometimes need to stray away from the standard of care just long enough to save a child. And we're so glad they did.

We feel privileged to have been able to add to this work and synthesize a new framework from which to move forward.

In this textbook, you will find rock-solid scientific evidence for the existence and pathophysiology of PANS and PANDAS, as well as the testing and novel treatment interventions we have successfully used in our practice. There is much to be gained by reading the book from cover to cover, but each chapter is self-contained; you will find some redundancy of published references between chapters to save the trouble of jumping around. At the end of the book, in the appendices, you will find helpful resources, such as labs that we typically order, doses of medications and supplements we commonly use, a sample PANS/PANDAS flare protocol, useful information to share with parents, sample IVIG orders, and much more.

I'd like to welcome you to this work. The patients and their families need you.

NOTE: *This textbook is for physicians and is intended to help them understand PANS and PANDAS through our unique clinical experience with these disorders. The information in this text is for educational use only and is not intended to be medical advice. Patients should always consult their personal physician before starting any new medications or supplements, or before implementing any lifestyle changes. Physicians must make decisions about patient care based on the history they procure, the physical examination findings, and the diagnostic data they obtain from their patients. They must also base treatment decisions upon their own medical experience and understanding of the disease process they are treating. The statements made about products and services have not been evaluated by the US Food and Drug Administration. This book and the information within it are not intended to diagnose, treat, cure, or prevent any condition or disease.*

DIAGNOSING PANS AND PANDAS

The good physician treats the disease;
the great physician treats the patient who has the disease.
~ SIR WILLIAM OSLER

KEY POINTS

▸ PANS and PANDAS are forms of autoimmune encephalitis
▸ PANDAS is a type of PANS
▸ PANS and PANDAS are clinical diagnoses
▸ Classic criteria establish the diagnosis of PANS and PANDAS
▸ The onset may be gradual in some cases
▸ Symptoms are typically severe
▸ PANS and PANDAS can only be diagnosed when the symptoms are not better explained by another neurologic or medical disorder

SOME QUICK DEFINITIONS

PANDAS is Pediatric Autoimmune Neuropsychiatric Disorder Associated with Strep (infection). PANS is Pediatric Acute-onset Neuropsychiatric Syndrome.

The concept of PANDAS was first defined in 1997. In PANDAS, an autoimmune attack on the brain occurs following an infection (either skin or throat) with a specific strain of group A β-hemolytic *Strep* (GABHS). PANS is the broader term, which includes not only cases following *Strep* infections but also cases following other infections, toxins, or even stress. So PANDAS is actually a type of PANS. A working definition of PANS was first introduced in 2012. A comprehensive discussion of the history and the compelling science behind PANS and PANDAS follows in Chapter 2.

> **Early investigators opined that some cases of mental illness in adults may represent missed cases of PANS or PANDAS as children.**

SOME NEEDED BACKGROUND

We are trained as physicians to look for specific details provided in the history and physical examination and subsequent testing. In a patient with appendicitis, for example, we would expect (at least according to what we have been taught) to find pain in the right lower quadrant, fever, and elevated white blood cell count with a left shift. As you likely know, many patients with appendicitis present that way, but we have seen patients with acute appendicitis arrive at the hospital without an elevated white blood cell count or fever, and only vague, non-localized pain in their abdomen. Some patients with an acute MI don't have chest pain. People are complex. Applying diagnostic criteria rigidly can cause us to miss potentially serious illness. PANS and PANDAS are no different.

The classic criteria presented below are based upon the most recent update, but we have had more than a few patients present with most of the signs and symptoms of PANS and PANDAS without actually meeting all the strict diagnostic criteria. The bottom line is, if your patient has more than two or three of the findings in any of these groups of symptoms, there is a problem. They may not technically meet the criteria for PANS or PANDAS, but the information in this textbook is still helpful, because other neuropsychiatric disorders in children share some of the same root causes as PANS and PANDAS and have responded very well to our approach.

You may notice that this chapter on the diagnosis of PANS and PANDAS does not contain a detailed discussion of laboratory or radiology testing. This was purposeful since PANS and PANDAS are clinically diagnosed; they do not require any specific lab or radiology testing to establish the diagnosis. Labs and radiology tests can be helpful, however, to rule out other diseases and to give you, the physician, an initial direction to begin to help the patient. Laboratory and radiology testing are discussed extensively in Chapter 7.

Although many parents call our office in hopes of finally getting a diagnosis of PANS or PANDAS, the diagnosis itself doesn't matter—healing does.

THE CLASSIC DIAGNOSTIC CRITERIA FOR PANS[1]

Refer to the section following the summary for specific details on each symptom.

Requirement 1: abrupt, dramatic onset of obsessive-compulsive disorder *and/or* severely restricted food intake

AND

Requirement 2: presence of symptoms from at least two of the following seven categories (similarly severe and of abrupt onset):

1. Anxiety
2. Emotional lability (rapidly changing moods) or depression
3. Irritability, aggression, and/or severely oppositional behaviors
4. Behavioral (developmental) regression
5. Deterioration in school performance
6. Sensory or motor abnormalities (new sensitivity to clothes, smells, loud sounds; facial, voice, or hand tics; clumsiness)
7. Somatic signs and symptoms (urinary issues or sleep disturbance)

AND

Requirement 3: not better explained by a known neurologic or medical disorder

Breaking down each step of the diagnosis

Age of onset - Although the original PANDAS criteria[2] stated that the age of onset was between three and thirteen, we now know that PANS or PANDAS may start after puberty. In our practice, we have seen older teens and even adults develop symptoms identical to those seen in PANS and PANDAS. In adults with similar symptoms, we don't use the terms *PANS* or *PANDAS* but refer to these patients as having *autoimmune encephalitis*. Early investigators opined that some cases of mental illness in adults may represent missed cases of PANS or PANDAS as children. The average age of onset in PANS and PANDAS is 7.5 years. Boys outnumber girls by a ratio of 2:1. Children at the younger end of the spectrum present a special challenge since they cannot vocalize what they are thinking. Terms in the medical literature commonly used to describe the magnitude of the initial symptoms are "ferocious" and "foudroyant."

Sudden onset - Large parental and physician surveys[3] show that 88% of cases are sudden onset (symptoms ramping up within three days). In other cases, a more gradual onset is noted. When questioned, even parents with a child who

> It is best to think of restrictive eating in PANS and PANDAS as a type of OCD.

has had a very rapid onset sometimes report that some milder symptoms were present in the weeks to months before the more concerning symptoms suddenly appeared.

OCD - These children usually have unwanted, intrusive thoughts and compulsions. These behaviors often involve rituals such as a required bedtime routine which, if violated, results in a huge tantrum. Other traditional manifestations of OCD are seen, such as counting things and having to do things a certain number of times. Obsessive religious thoughts (and negative self-worth tied to them) may occur. Children may express a concern that they will hurt someone or poison them. In this case, it is the fear of having the thought that is distressing for the child (and concerning for the parents).

Magical thinking is seen, such as a child believing that if they don't perform a certain action or ritual, a family member will get sick or die. Sexual thoughts toward siblings, parents, or teachers may occur. This is particularly disturbing for parents, who may assume the child has been the victim of abuse.

Children with PANS and PANDAS may enter what we refer to as the "continuous question mode" where they repeatedly ask for reassurance ("Is the door locked?" "Is the meat cooked?") hundreds of times daily. Children may tell the parent that if they just answer one last time it will make them feel better. Unfortunately, answering fuels the fire of the OCD, resulting in even more questions. The OCD portion of PANS and PANDAS is one of the most uncomfortable and heartbreaking aspects of these disorders.

> **Extremely defiant behavior may just be an expression of severe anxiety and OCD.**

Restrictive eating - This criterion does not refer to children who are picky eaters or have a small decrease in appetite. Children with restrictive eating are often concerned they will choke on foods. They also may suddenly object to certain textures or flavors of foods (which they may have liked before the illness). These children are sometimes diagnosed with ARFID (avoidant restrictive food intake disorder),[4] which is a psychiatric diagnosis listed in the *DSM-5*. Although these children may meet the criteria for this disorder, it is an incomplete description, as they also have the sudden onset of other symptoms as noted previously. It is best to think of restrictive eating in PANS and PANDAS as a type of OCD. If oral intake is significantly impacted, weight loss and dehydration may be seen. In extreme cases, children may need to be hospitalized for IV fluids or artificial nutrition. If concerns for an actual physical blockage or obstruction are present, a consultation with a gastroenterologist or ENT physician is necessary for an appropriate workup.

Anxiety - The sudden onset of anxiety is reported in 96% of cases.[3] Separation anxiety is very common. Parents may find that the child will plead with them not to leave for work. Older children may repeatedly call or text the parent when they are gone. Unfulfilled OCD rituals are a common cause of extreme anxiety for the child. As with OCD, reasoning with the child is not effective when the child is experiencing a severe flare.

Emotional lability or depression - One parent related a story about watching a movie with her family when her child suddenly stood up and threw an entire bowl of popcorn and began to scream with no apparent trigger. Depressive symptoms can also be seen. The child may express suicidal thoughts to the parent and threaten self-harm, such as taking their seat belt off in the car or threatening to jump out when the car is moving. This behavior may require emergent psychiatric evaluation.

Irritability, aggression, or severe oppositional (defiant) behaviors - We often tell parents that extremely defiant behavior may just be an expression of severe anxiety and OCD. Extreme fear may cause the child to become aggressive or uncooperative.

Aggressive behavior may be directed toward siblings, friends, and (less often) parents. Defiant behavior in school may lead to disciplinary action against the child, though the behavior is actually caused by a medical condition (PANS and PANDAS). For this reason, we recommend parents get involved early at their child's school and insist upon getting an individualized education plan (IEP) in place. More information on IEPs and other school support may be found in Appendix D.

Following the great flu pandemic in 1918, post-viral encephalitis with a clinical picture very similar to PANS appeared. In 1926, an article by Bond and Partridge[5] commented on the behavioral changes seen in these children as follows:

> One would prefer a physical trouble which would produce outspoken feeble-mindedness with its limited range of harmful effects to this encephalitis which may produce an intellectual, tormented, and cruel monster out of a gentle girl or boy.

Behavioral (developmental) regression - This can appear as baby talk or playing with toys generally used by younger children (a teenager beginning to fingerpaint again). Emotional immaturity fits here as well. This can cause problems in social situations with peers.

Deterioration in school performance - Decreased comprehension and attentional issues abound in these children. They are often diagnosed with ADHD and medicated with stimulants, which may make anxiety worse. Computational ability may be lost, leading to issues with math. Margin drift is often seen when paragraphs are written by hand on a page. The left margin may gradually drift farther and farther to the right down the written page. Decreased ability to copy simple pictures may occur. In severe cases, handwriting can deteriorate into a jumbled mess with no word spacing and no distinction between capital and lowercase letters. Early establishment of an Individualized Education Plan (IEP) is essential to protect the child's rights at school and prevent disciplinary action from the school for behavioral changes caused by these medical conditions. See Appendix D.

> Parents have to choose their battles, and clothing choices are not worthy battles in this fight.

Sensory or motor abnormalities - Some of the symptoms in this category have to do with increased sensitivity to sensory stimuli such as temperature change, immersion in water, tight-fitting clothing, loud sounds, or strong smells (perfume, car exhaust, cooking food), which may cause the child to become very uncomfortable. This often leads to behavioral problems.

Intolerance of certain food textures or strong smells may be confused with food refusal for other reasons, such as fear of choking. These children may throw a fit when parents are trying to get them dressed. This can be the initial presentation of PANS or PANDAS, as a child may wake up and refuse to put on socks or pants. Unable to express what they are feeling, they often use the phrase "it's not right!" when this occurs. Clothing refusal can prevent the child from attending school or going outside.

Overreaction to sensory stimuli can be a source of great conflict between parents and children with PANS and PANDAS. We often tell parents that, to these children, putting on socks feels like having ice water poured down your back. Letting the child dictate which comfortable clothes they wear or what sounds and smells they are exposed to goes a long way toward calming them down. Parents have to choose their battles, and clothing choices are not worthy battles in this fight. Decreased ability to tolerate siblings can often be traced to the simple fact that children are loud. A rarely seen subtype of sensory abnormalities is children who suddenly become sensory seekers. These children will want to climb, run, or go very fast on their bicycle. Protecting them from injuries is important.

Tics also fall into this category. Motor tics consist of small jerking movements of hands or fingers, scrunching up the nose, squinting, or repetitive blinking. Vocal tics usually consist of throat clearing, coughing, or sniffing. Rarely, vocal tics are manifested by the repetition of a specific word. This is one differentiation between PANS and PANDAS and Tourette syndrome (TS), where different words and phrases are more common.

The medical community and Tourette syndrome organizations have stated that Tourette syndrome has no immunologic basis. However, in position statements by these organizations, they acknowledge that TS patients often have OCD and anxiety along with tics.[6] The same position statement also notes that TS occurs as a result of genetic predisposition and environmental factors.

> **Sleep disturbances are the norm.**

We believe that, over time, infection and environmental toxins along with immune dysregulation will be recognized as the underlying root causes of TS, just like they are in PANS and PANDAS. Once that happens, TS and PANS and PANDAS will be viewed not as distinct and unrelated disorders but as points along a continuum of neuroinflammation and autoimmunity. It is important to note that tics seen in patients with PANS and PANDAS are usually small in caliber. Larger, flailing-type movements of a whole extremity or violent movements of the head and neck are not common with PANS and PANDAS and may point to the diagnosis of Sydenham chorea, which requires IVIG, long-term prophylactic antibiotics, and an evaluation for the cardiac complications of acute rheumatic fever.

Children suffering from PANS or PANDAS may also exhibit increased clumsiness and lose the ability to ride a bicycle, do gymnastics, or throw a ball accurately. Increased falls or dropping things may be seen. Protection from harm during these activities is very important.

Somatic signs and symptoms - This category usually refers to issues with sleeping and urinary changes.

Sleep disturbances are the norm. These children may experience difficulty falling asleep or may have early waking. Agitation and anxiety commonly increase at night. New or worsened fear of the dark is also common. Screaming at night may disturb others trying to sleep. Many times, these children don't want to sleep alone, but want to sleep with their parents. Although they sometimes may want to sleep in their parents' bed, more often than not they want a parent (usually the mom) to sleep in their bed with them. Sleep helps remove toxins from the brain and has a neuroprotective effect.[7] Sleep deprivation thus adds insult to injury. If stimulants are prescribed for attentional issues in these children, sleep may be adversely affected even further. In both children and adults, sedatives to induce sleep are not a good solution since they inhibit much needed REM sleep.[8]

Urinary changes are very common. Incontinence can be seen during the day with new nocturnal enuresis in a child who had previously been dry at night. Many of these children will have greatly increased urgency when they do have to urinate. They will be going about their day at school or home when they suddenly have extreme urgency to urinate. If a bathroom is not readily available, this can result in urinary incontinence. This may be particularly disturbing to children who have some OCD associated with contamination. Many parents will initially write these symptoms off and explain them by saying the child gets involved in activities and forgets to go to the bathroom until it's too late. Careful attention to this pattern, though, will reveal that it is a sensory issue unrelated to the will or activity level of the child. Obviously, dysuria, fever, or abdominal pain associated with these symptoms should prompt an evaluation for a UTI.

Not better explained by a known neurologic or medical disorder - This phrase is a vital part of the criteria and should *never* be overlooked.

We have a saying in medicine: " . . . until proven otherwise." Part of medical professionalism is ruling out an MI first before concluding that a patient's chest pain is due to a less serious diagnosis such as indigestion or anxiety. Failure to keep these additional diagnoses in mind can cause a physician to miss an alternative diagnosis requiring different treatment.

The same is true with otherwise healthy children (and adults) with a sudden neuropsychiatric complaint. A careful history and physical examination is essential to exclude the possibility that this behavioral change is caused by a structural brain problem or CNS infection, like meningitis. If still unsure after the history and physical examination, additional testing may be required to rule them out. This might involve laboratory testing, an MRI of the brain, or referral to the emergency department for more urgent testing if indicated. As previously noted, gastroenterology consultation may be required in the case of children with swallowing complaints to rule out the possibility of some blockage in the structures of the neck or esophagus.

CHAPTER 1 REFERENCES

1. Swedo SE, Leckman JF, Rose NR. From research subgroup to clinical syndrome: modifying the PANDAS criteria to describe PANS (pediatric acute-onset neuropsychiatric syndrome). *Pediatr Therapeut.* 2012;2:113:1–8

2. Swedo SE, Leonard HL, Mittleman BB, et al. Identification of children with pediatric autoimmune neuropsychiatric disorders associated with streptococcal infections by a marker associated with rheumatic fever. *American Journal of Psychiatry.* 1997;154(1):110–112

3. Calaprice D, Tona J, Parker-Athill EC, et al. A survey of pediatric acute-onset neuropsychiatric syndrome characteristics and course. *Journal of Child and Adolescent Psychopharmacology*. 2017;27(7):607–618

4. www.webmd.com/mental-health/eating-disorders/what-is-arfid, accessed 10/11/2021

5. Bond ED, Partridge GE. Post-encephalitic behavior disorders in boys and their management in hospital. *Am J Psychiatry*. 1926;6: 25–103

6. www.tourette.org/research-medical/pandas-pans-and-tourette-syndrome-disorder, accessed 10/1/2021

7. Eugene AR, Masiak J. The neuroprotective aspects of sleep. *MEDtube Sci*. 2015;3(1):35–40

8. Watson CJ, Baghdoyan HA, Lydic R. Neuropharmacology of sleep and wakefulness. *Sleep Med Clin*. 2010;5(4):513–528

THE SCIENCE AND HISTORY BEHIND PANS AND PANDAS

Nearly every great discovery in science has come as the result of providing a new question rather than a new answer.
~ **PAUL A. MEGLITSCH**

KEY POINTS

▸ The immune system is responsible for monitoring and reacting to foreign substances it deems harmful or noxious
▸ Autoimmunity is defined as a loss of self-tolerance which results in tissue damage
▸ Autoimmunity occurs as a result of molecular mimicry where pathogen-associated molecular patterns similar to human tissues trigger an immune response
▸ PANS and PANDAS are evidence-based concepts
▸ Many different infectious organisms have been shown to trigger neuropsychiatric symptoms
▸ Environmental factors can also trigger neuropsychiatric symptoms

To fully understand the discovery and pathophysiology of PANS and PANDAS, you have to start with the immune system.

When properly functioning, the immune system must:

1. Maintain barriers that prevent easy, unsupervised entry of foreign molecules into the body (skin, mucosa, tears, mucus)
2. Distinguish self from non-self molecules inside the body
3. Identify pathogens or other substances that may be harmful to the body
4. Mount an appropriate, proportional immune response to these pathogens and substances as needed while limiting host tissue damage

Cells of the immune system (including macrophages, monocytes, B lymphocytes, and dendritic cells) and epithelial cells have pattern recognition receptors (PRRs) on their surface. Toll-like receptors (TLRs) and NOD-like receptors (NLRs) are two examples of these PRRs. These receptors recognize unique proteins on the surface of pathogens called pathogen-associated molecular

> **Before the autoimmune process begins, there is always a triggering event.**

patterns (PAMPs). Activation of the PRRs initiates the innate and adaptive immune responses.

The innate immune response includes inflammatory signaling molecules (cytokines), which are part of the inflammatory response. Although

we tend to think of inflammation as a bad thing, the inflammatory response signals other parts of the immune system to come and respond to infections or toxins. Complement fixation, natural killer (NK) cells, and phagocytes are also part of the innate immune response.

The adaptive immune response relies mainly on different populations of T-cells and B-cells. This response takes longer to mount. There are various types of T-cells and each has a different job, including T regulatory cells, which monitor and regulate the immune response and T helper cells. B-cells mainly produce antibodies. The type of immune response that occurs depends upon the type or class of antibody. The main classes of antibodies in humans that we can measure and are concerned with are IgG, IgM, IgE, and IgA. Proper amounts of each are required for a normal immune response. Over 50% of children with PANS and PANDAS have immunoglobulin deficiencies, such as IgA deficiency, IgM deficiency, and IgG total and subclass deficiencies.[1] These deficiencies are a testament to the immune dysregulation we see in PANS and PANDAS.

An immunodeficiency occurs when any component of the immune response (innate or adaptive) is missing or dysfunctional. Autoimmunity occurs when the immune response is directed against the person's own bodily tissues and tissue damage occurs.

Why autoimmunity occurs

We have known for many years that autoimmune diseases have a genetic component. But before the autoimmune process begins, there is always a triggering event. The most well-studied triggering event shown to initiate autoimmunity is the concept of molecular mimicry. Molecular mimicry occurs when portions of the cell membranes of organisms (like PAMPs) resemble human tissues. When the immune system launches a defense against the invading organism, it mistakenly attacks the body's own tissues and causes damage.

The concept of molecular mimicry as a trigger of autoimmunity has been confirmed in the medical literature, including the rheumatology literature, for many years.[2–5] In fact, one publication that suggested a link between infection and autoimmunity was published in 1964.[6]

The health or impairment of the beneficial microorganisms of the gut microbiome also contributes to the onset of autoimmunity.[7,8] The vast majority of our patients have evidence of increased intestinal permeability on testing. Often called "leaky gut" in nonmedical circles, increased intestinal permeability is involved in several types of autoimmunity.[9,10] In the past, the concept of increased intestinal permeability was debated, but now even large medical centers[11] and peer-reviewed gastroenterology journals[12] have recognized the condition and its link to autoimmunity. The literature validating the concept of increased intestinal permeability and its role in various diseases is presented in Chapter 7.

One well-known autoimmune condition directly linked to molecular mimicry is rheumatic fever. Rheumatic fever may occur weeks to months after a *Strep* infection and is defined by an autoimmune attack on the skin, heart, and brain. When the condition involves the brain, it can cause Sydenham chorea. Sydenham chorea is a movement disorder which results in tics involving the face, arms, and legs. It also causes an abnormal gait.

PANDAS ENTERS THE PICTURE

In the early 1990s, a group of researchers, led by Dr. Susan Swedo, at the National Institute of Mental Health (NIMH) began to collect data on children who developed neuropsychiatric disorders (OCD and tics) following infections. They found that, in some children, there was evidence that anti-neuronal antibodies developed, which attacked the brain by the process of molecular

> **The concept of molecular mimicry as a trigger of autoimmunity has been confirmed in the medical literature, including the rheumatology literature, for many years.**

mimicry. In 1994, they published a commentary[13] in the journal *Pediatrics*, which discussed their findings and the link between group A *Strep* infections and the production of these antibodies. This commentary was based upon earlier work published in several professional medical journals.[14–16] The connection between anti-neuronal antibodies and Sydenham chorea was actually known as far back as 1976.[17]

In 1997, Dr. Swedo and her colleagues published the first article to describe the syndrome they named PANDAS.[18]

They described the criteria required to meet the definition of PANDAS as follows:
- onset of OCD or tic disorder
- onset age three to puberty

- episodic course of symptoms (reoccurring)
- evidence of previous *Strep* infection just before onset of symptoms
- neurologic criteria (hyperactivity and tics)

In 1998, an article[19] was published that described the first fifty patients studied who met this new criteria set. These fifty patients had 144 PANDAS episodes, which came and went during the study period. The authors also noted that these patients demonstrated emotional lability (rapidly changing moods), separation anxiety, nighttime fears or rituals, memory/school performance issues, and oppositional (defiant) behaviors.

Since there was an association with *Strep* bacteria, the initial treatment approaches focused on antibiotic therapy. One study[20] demonstrated that immediate resolution was seen with antibiotic therapy in children meeting the PANDAS criteria. In this study, OCD symptoms recurred in half the children when they were reinfected with *Strep*.

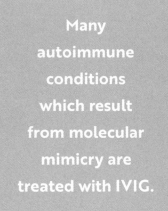

Many autoimmune conditions which result from molecular mimicry are treated with IVIG.

Many autoimmune conditions which result from molecular mimicry are treated with IVIG. Although we are not sure exactly how IVIG helps in autoimmune conditions, it is thought to possibly "reset" the immune system. Since PANDAS was also shown to be an autoimmune condition resulting from molecular mimicry, several trials of IVIG were undertaken. In 1999, a study in the *Lancet* demonstrated that IVIG and therapeutic plasma exchange (plasmapheresis) are effective in PANDAS.[21] Additional studies since that time have confirmed that

IVIG is beneficial in PANS and PANDAS. These follow-up studies are presented in Chapter 13.

In 2000, an NIMH study compared MRI studies of the brains of thirty-four children with PANDAS and eighty-two healthy children with no prior history of PANDAS. The comparison showed that the caudate, the putamen, and the globus pallidus were significantly larger in children with PANDAS than in the normal group.[22] Enlargements in these regions are also seen in patients with Sydenham chorea.

A small but fascinating study[23] was done with children getting IVIG for PANDAS. Serum antibodies from children with PANDAS and a control group of healthy children were injected into mice. Next, sections of the brain from these mice were examined to look for binding to specific cholinergic striatal interneurons. These neurons have been implicated in tic disorders. PANDAS serum antibodies showed 80% binding to these neurons while the serum antibodies from healthy children showed less than 50% binding. After IVIG was administered to the PANDAS group, serum antibodies were collected again and injected into the mice. Examination then showed that the increased binding had resolved. This study further supported the legitimacy of PANDAS as a diagnosis and of IVIG as a treatment option. An example of IVIG orders, helpful tips for getting IVIG approved, and a sample appeal letter for IVIG can be found in Appendix E.

The controversy begins

In the mid 2000s, as the literature evidence for PANDAS began to grow, controversy erupted. Many in the medical community expressed doubts that PANDAS was a real clinical entity. This occurred for several reasons.

First, it was a diagnosis established by clinical criteria alone. There was no blood test or radiology study that "proved PANDAS." This was a surprising objection since every established psychiatric disorder is currently diagnosed solely on clinical grounds.

Second, and maybe most importantly, PANDAS requires us all to look at mental illness in an entirely new way. As we look at the list of *DSM-5* psychiatric disorders, we recognize many of these symptoms in children with PANS or PANDAS. And we know, from the many articles published supportive of PANDAS (and PANS) that there is a biologic basis for the changes seen in these children. In an excellent peer-reviewed article[24] from 2015, researchers suggested that some cases of mental illness in adults could represent missed cases of PANS when they were children. This confirms what we have seen in our practice.

If we expand our thinking as a medical community, we will discover that mental illness does not just occur by chance or through genetics. Just like PANDAS and PANS, most mental illness requires some genetic predisposition and a specific trigger for the phenotype to express itself. By following our Fully Functional process, many of these patients have discovered that they can live an entirely different life, a life that they could not have imagined.

> PANDAS requires us all to look at mental illness in an entirely new way.

THE CONCEPT OF PANS AND PANDAS IS EVIDENCE-BASED MEDICINE

One final reason often given for opposition to PANS and PANDAS diagnoses is that there are no large studies with thousands of patients showing a response to one specific treatment or drug. For this reason, many doctors hold that these diagnoses or the treatments used are not "evidence-based medicine."

Evidence-based medicine (or EBM) was first proposed as a method of medical decision-making in 1991.[25] To paraphrase, the original article basically said that, if we as physicians are to advance medical knowledge, we should know how to quickly retrieve the latest medical literature in real time to help us make decisions rather than just rely on textbooks, expert lecturers, or more senior physicians. The article also suggested that we should understand statistics and risk calculations to determine whether the information we found could apply to the patient in front of us. This is a good idea of course—relying solely on opinion in science without rigorous testing can result in outdated (or even harmful) traditions which don't help patients.

Two additional articles subsequently appeared in 1996 and 2002 that attempted to clarify the true definition of EBM.[26,27] They both suggested that the process of practicing EBM could not solely rely on published studies from the medical literature. To do so would make physicians "slaves to the literature" by demanding that they do nothing without a specific published study to support their decisions. In fact, the articles clarified that EBM must consider the best available published evidence along with the clinical expertise of the physician, and the preferences of the patient. All three of these factors together, they argue, give the best outcomes. They also point out that physicians often make decisions in

> EBM must consider the best available published evidence along with the clinical expertise of the physician, and the preferences of the patient.

emergency cases with little published evidence. In essence, if there is no published evidence available, physicians should rely on their clinical experience and judgment coupled with patient preference, rather than doing nothing to help the patient.

Unfortunately, these two clarifying articles are not widely known, and it has become cemented in the collective psyche of many of our physician colleagues (especially in academic centers) that to prescribe medications or advocate for new and unusual diagnoses without a written article supporting your actions makes you no better than a modern-day witch doctor.

As a result, patients with conditions viewed as new or unusual, like PANS and PANDAS, have been left to suffer. Often, our patients' parents have heard from a physician that PANDAS is not real, that their child just has behavioral problems,

or worse yet, that their child's problems are the result of poor parenting.

Also, to complicate matters, PANDAS may present differently in different children. Some children get much better with antibiotics alone. Some need steroids, and some don't get better until they have IVIG. For these reasons, it can be difficult to gather a group that is similar enough in symptoms and responses to one type of medication to do a large traditional study. Insistence on waiting for large, double-blind, placebo-controlled studies before trying anything new for a sick patient results in a lot of untreated patients.

WHAT IF *STREP* IS NOT THE CAUSE?
PANS is defined

Throughout the late 1990s and early 2000s, clinical and academic investigations to understand PANDAS continued around the world. One problematic factor, though, was that there was a large group of children who had all of the characteristics of those with PANDAS, but in whom no evidence of prior or current *Strep* infection could be found. Some also presented after puberty. As a result, these groups were not being treated. It could have been that these patients had had *Strep* previously and this was simply a delayed presentation of PANDAS. However, in some of these patients, other active infections were noted. Treatment of these infections (such as *Mycoplasma*) with specific antibiotics improved symptoms, just as β-lactam antibiotics help with PANDAS.

In 2012, a scientific paper was published based upon the experience of six physicians who had treated more than four hundred children.[28] The study underscored the fact that some patients had other infectious etiologies besides

Strep. They also reported that these other infections and even psychosocial stress may act as a trigger for the symptoms. For these reasons, the authors coined the term PANS for Pediatric Acute-onset Neuropsychiatric Syndrome.

The connection, then, between PANDAS and PANS is this: PANS is the overall term, which includes PANDAS (if caused by *Strep*) and also includes episodes caused by other infections and stress. We would add toxins and toxicants to this list as well, as explained in Chapter 5. For the sake of future research and treatment, the physicians in the group formulated diagnostic criteria still in use today. These diagnostic criteria are defined in Chapter 1.

Many other infections can actually cause neuropsychiatric symptoms

The concept of infections as a cause of neurologic or psychiatric symptoms has been around for many years. The most well-known connection between infection and these types of symptoms occurs in rheumatic fever. Hippocrates described a condition with symptoms similar to those of rheumatic fever in 400 BC.[29]

Rheumatic fever is an autoimmune condition which occurs after an infection with group A *Strep*. Due to molecular mimicry, antibodies directed at the *Strep* bacteria may attack the heart, skin, joints, and brain. Symptoms of rheumatic fever can be delayed by several weeks to months after the *Strep* infection.[30] One particular sign of rheumatic fever is known as Sydenham chorea (SC), which is a disorder that causes continuous motor movements (chorea) of the arms, legs, and head and difficulty walking. In addition to the abnormal movements seen in SC, studies have shown that 82% of these patients experience OCD.[31,32] If chorea reoccurs, the incidence of OCD becomes 100%. ADHD-like symptoms, memory and mood issues, and even symptoms of psychosis can be seen with SC.[33–36] Interestingly, patients with Sydenham chorea, like those with PANS and PANDAS, have measurable anti-neuronal antibodies.[37–40] MRI, CT, and PET scans in patients with SC show abnormalities in a part of the brain called the basal ganglia. This is a similar pattern as that seen in studies of patients with PANS and PANDAS.[41–44]

Infection with *Mycoplasma* has been linked to Tourette syndrome.[45] OCD and vocal and motor tics have also been found with *Mycoplasma* infections.[46,47] Influenza infection has been linked to tics and abnormal neurologic symptoms as far back as 1931.[48]

> **Symptoms of rheumatic fever can be delayed by several weeks to months after the Strep infection.**

Epstein-Barr virus has been linked to various neurologic and psychiatric syndromes.[49,50] *Borrelia burgdorferi* can produce OCD and other psychiatric disorders and is greatly underdiagnosed[51–55] (Lyme disease and other tick-borne infections are discussed extensively in Chapters 9 and 16).

Toxoplasma and other viral infections can also produce PANS symptoms.[56–60] Several articles have outlined a relationship between COVID-19 infection and neuropsychiatric symptoms.[61,62]

Stress as a cause of OCD and tics

We all know that psychological stress and adversity can cause anxiety and depression. Researchers have also found that stress can cause OCD.[63–65] Stress has been shown to increase symptoms in children with tic disorders.[66]

ENVIRONMENTAL FACTORS AND NEUROPSYCHIATRIC SYMPTOMS

Nearly 100% of our patients with PANS and PANDAS have evidence of mold exposure. Mycotoxins are organic poisons released by molds. There is evidence in the literature that mycotoxins are neurotoxins[67] and exposure can cause neuropsychiatric symptoms.[68]

We have been the first to link mycotoxins to PANS and PANDAS as both a cause (in the case of PANS) and a contributor to altered immune response (in the case of both). Chapter 5 outlines the role of mold exposure in immune dysregulation and the contribution of mycotoxins to human sickness.

Electromagnetic frequency (EMF) exposure is a topic of recent interest. There has been no direct link noted in the literature between EMF exposure and PANS. There have been several theoretical and basic science articles expressing concern that low-level EMF exposure can lead to neuropsychiatric abnormalities and EMF sensitivity.[69–73]

Although no link between PANS and heavy metals has been clearly established in the medical literature, metals such as lead and mercury are known to cause neuropsychiatric symptoms, even at low levels.[74–77]

> Patients with Sydenham chorea, like those with PANS and PANDAS, have measurable anti-neuronal antibodies.

CHAPTER 2 REFERENCES

1. Younger DS, Mast PA, Bouboulis DA. PANDAS: Baseline immunoglobulin levels predict achievement of remission at one year following IVIG therapy. *J Neurol Neurosurg.* 2016;3(2):122–127

2. Behar SM, Porcelli S. Mechanisms of autoimmune disease induction. *Arthritis & Rheumatism: Official Journal of the American College of Rheumatology.* 1995;38(4):458–476

3. Oldstone MBA. Molecular mimicry as a mechanism for the cause and as a probe uncovering etiologic agent of autoimmune disease. *Curr Top Microbiol Immunol.* 1989;145:127–135

4. Porcelli S. Molecular mimicry and the generation of autoimmune diseases. *Rheumatol Rev.* 1993;2:41–50

5. Fourneau JM, Bach JM, van Endert PM, et al. The elusive case for a role of mimicry in autoimmune disorders. *Mol Immunol.* 2004;40(14–15):1095–1102

6. Damian RT. Molecular mimicry: antigen sharing by parasite and host and its consequences. *Am Naturalist.* 1964;98:129–149

7. Belkaid Y, Hand TW. Role of the microbiota in immunity and inflammation. *Cell.* 2014;157:121–141

8. Mathis D, Benoist C. Microbiota and autoimmune disease: the hosted self. *Cell Host Microbes*. 2011;10:297–301

9. Visser J, Rozing J, Sapone A, et al. Tight junctions, intestinal permeability, and autoimmunity: celiac disease and type 1 diabetes paradigms. *Ann N Y Acad Sci*. 2009;1165:195–205

10. Mu Q, Kirby J, Reilly CM, et al. Leaky gut as a danger signal for autoimmune diseases. *Front Immunol*. 2017;8:598

11. www.health.harvard.edu/blog/leaky-gut-what-is-it-and-what-does-it-mean-for-you-2017092212451, accessed 10/20/2021

12. Arrieta MC, Bistritz L, Meddings JB. Alterations in intestinal permeability. *Gut*. 2006;55(10):1512–1520

13. Swedo SE, Leonard HL, Kiessling LS. Speculations on antineuronal antibody-mediated neuropsychiatric disorders of childhood. *Pediatrics*. 1994;93(2):323–326

14. Swedo SE, Leonard H, Kiessling L. Neuroimmunologic variant of childhood psychiatric disorders? *AJDC*. 1993;147:480

15. Swedo SE, Kilpatrick K, Schapiro M, et al. Antineuronal antibodies in Sydenham's chorea and obsessive-compulsive disorder. *Pediat Res*. 1991;29(4 pt 2):369a

16. Kiessling LS, Marcotte AC, Culpepper L. Antineuronal antibodies in movement disorders. *Pediatrics*. 1993;92:39–43

17. Husby G, van de Rijn I, Zabriskie JB, et al. Antibodies reacting with cytoplasm of subthalamic and caudate nuclei neurons in chorea and acute rheumatic fever. *J Exp Med*. 1976;144:1094–1110

18. Swedo SE, Leonard HL, Mittleman BB, et al. Identification of children with pediatric autoimmune neuropsychiatric disorders associated with streptococcal infections by a marker associated with rheumatic fever. *American Journal of Psychiatry*. 1997;154(1):110–112

19. Swedo SE, Leonard HL, Garvey M, et al. Pediatric autoimmune neuropsychiatric disorders associated with streptococcal infections: clinical description of the first 50 cases. *American Journal of Psychiatry*. 1998;155:264–271

20. Murphy ML, Pichichero, ME. Prospective identification and treatment of children with pediatric autoimmune neuropsychiatric disorder associated with group A streptococcal infection (PANDAS). *Archives of Pediatrics & Adolescent Medicine*. 2002;156(4):356–361

21. Perlmutter SJ, Leitman SF, Garvey MA, et al. Therapeutic plasma exchange and intravenous immunoglobulin for obsessive-compulsive disorder and tic disorders in childhood. *Lancet*. 1999;354(9185):1153–1158

22. Giedd JN, Rapoport JL, Garvey MA, et al. MRI assessment of children with obsessive-compulsive disorder or tics associated with streptococcal infection. *American Journal of Psychiatry*. 2000;157(2):281–283

23. Frick LR, Rapanelli M, Jindachomthong K, et al. Differential binding of antibodies in PANDAS patients to cholinergic interneurons in the striatum. *Brain, Behavior, and Immunity*. 2018;69:304–311

24. Frankovich J, Thienemann M, Pearlstein J, et al. Multidisciplinary clinic dedicated to treating youth with pediatric acute-onset neuropsychiatric syndrome: presenting characteristics of the first 47 consecutive patients. *Journal of Child and Adolescent Psychopharmacology*. 2015;25(1):38–47

25. Guyatt GH. Evidence-based medicine. *ACP J Club*. 1991;114:A–16

26. Sackett DL, Rosenberg WMC, Muir Gray JA, et al. Evidence based medicine: what it is and what it isn't. *BMJ*. 1996;312(7023):71–72

27. Haynes RB, Devereaux PJ, and Guyatt GH. Clinical expertise in the era of evidence-based medicine and patient choice. *BMJ Evidence-Based Medicine*. 2002;7(2):36–38

28. Swedo SE, Leckman JF, Rose NR. From research subgroup to clinical syndrome: modifying the PANDAS criteria to describe PANS (pediatric acute-onset neuropsychiatric syndrome). *Pediatr Therapeut*. 2012;2(2):113

29. Quinn RW. Did scarlet fever and rheumatic fever exist in Hippocrates' time? *Rev Infect Dis*. 1991;13(6):1243–1244

30. Shulman ST, Bisno AL. Non-suppurative post-streptococcal sequelae: rheumatic fever and glomerulonephritis. In Bennett J, Dolin R, Blaser M, editors. *Mandell, Douglas, and Bennett's Principles and Practice of Infectious Diseases*. 8th ed. Philadelphia, PA. Elsevier. 2020;2:2300–9

31. Maia DP, Teixeira AL Jr, Quintão Cunningham MC, et al. Obsessive compulsive behavior, hyperactivity, and attention deficit disorder in Sydenham Chorea. *Neurology*. 2005;64(10):1799–1801

32. Swedo SE, Leonard HL, Casey BJ, et al. Sydenham's chorea: physical and psychological symptoms of St. Vitus dance. *Pediatrics*. 1993;91(4):706–713

33. Asbahr FR, Negrão AB, Gentil V, et al. Obsessive-compulsive and related symptoms in children and adolescents with rheumatic fever with and without chorea: a prospective 6-month study. *Am J Psychiatry*. 1998;155(8):1122–24

34. Ridel KR, Lipps TD, Gilbert DL. The prevalence of neuropsychiatric disorders in Sydenham's chorea. *Pediatr Neurol*. 2010;42(4):243–8

35. Harsányi E, Moreira J, Kummer A, et al. Language impairment in adolescents with Sydenham chorea. *Pediatr Neurol*. Epub 2015;53(5):412–6

36. Punukollu M, Mushet N, Linney M, et al. Neuropsychiatric manifestations of Sydenham's chorea: a systematic review. *Dev Med Child Neurol*. 2016;58(1):16–28

37. Kirvan CA, Swedo SE, Heuser JS, et al. Mimicry and autoantibody-mediated neuronal cell signaling in Sydenham chorea. *Nat Med*. 2003;9(7):914–920

38. Church AJ, Dale RC, Cardoso F, et al. CSF and serum immune parameters in Sydenham's chorea: evidence of an autoimmune syndrome? *J Neuroimmunol*. 2003;136(1–2):149–153

39. Church AJ, Cardoso F, Dale RC, et al. Anti-basal ganglia antibodies in acute and persistent Sydenham's chorea. *Neurology*. 2002;59(2):227–231

40. Kotby AA, El Badawy N, El Sokkary S, et al. Antineuronal antibodies in rheumatic chorea. *Clin Diagn Lab Immunol*. 1998;5(6):836–839

41. Giedd JN, Rapoport JL, Kruesi MJ, et al. Sydenham's chorea: magnetic resonance imaging of the basal ganglia. *Neurology*. 1995;45(12):2199–2202

42. Traill Z, Pike M, Byrne J. Sydenham's chorea: a case showing reversible striatal abnormalities on CT and MRI. *Dev Med Child Neurol*. 1995;37(3):270–273

43. Aron AM. Sydenham's chorea: positron emission tomographic (PET) scan studies. *J Child Neurol*. 2005;20(10):832–833

44. Goldman S, Amrom D, Szliwowski HB, et al. Reversible striatal hypermetabolism in a case of Sydenham's chorea. *Mov Disord*. 1993;8(3):355–358

45. Müller N, Riedel M, Blendinger C, et al. *Mycoplasma pneumoniae* infection and Tourette's syndrome. *Psychiatry Research*. 2004;129(2):119–125

46. Ercan TE, Ercan G, Severge B, et al. *Mycoplasma pneumoniae* infection and obsessive-compulsive disease: a case report. *Journal of Child Neurology* 2008;23(3):338–340

47. Muller N, Riedel M, Forderreuther S, et al. Tourette's syndrome and *Mycoplasma pneumoniae* infection [letter]. *American Journal of Psychiatry*. 2000;157,481–482

48. Von Economo C. *Encephalitis Lethargica: Its Sequelae and Treatment*. London: Oxford University Press, 1931

49. Fagundes CP, Jaremka LM, Glaser R, et al. Attachment anxiety is related to Epstein-Barr virus latency. *Brain Behav Immun*. 2014;41:232–238

50. Khandaker GM, Stochl J, Zammit S, et al. Childhood Epstein-Barr virus infection and subsequent risk of psychotic experiences in adolescence: a population-based prospective serological study. *Schizophr Res*. 2014;158(1–3):19–24

51. Fallon BA, Kochevar JM, Gaito A, et al. The underdiagnosis of neuropsychiatric Lyme disease in children and adults. *Psychiatric Clinics of North America*. 1998;21(3):693–703

52. Riedel M, Straube A, Schwarz MJ, et al. Lyme disease presenting as Tourette's syndrome [letter]. *Lancet*. 1998;351:418–419

53. Fallon BA, Nields JA. Lyme disease: a neuropsychiatric illness. *American Journal of Psychiatry*. 1994;151:1571–1583

54. Fallon BA, Nields JA, Parsons B, et al. Psychiatric manifestations of Lyme borreliosis. *Journal of Clinical Psychiatry*. 1993;54:263–268

55. Johnco C, Kugler BB, Murphy TK, et al. Obsessive-compulsive symptoms in adults with Lyme disease. *Gen Hosp Psychiatry*. 2018;51:85–89

56. Flegr J, Horáček J. Toxoplasma-infected subjects report an obsessive-compulsive disorder diagnosis more often and score higher in obsessive-compulsive inventory. *Eur Psychiatry*. 2017;40:82–87

57. Akaltun İ, Kara SS, Kara T. The relationship between toxoplasma gondii IgG antibodies and generalized anxiety disorder and obsessive-compulsive disorder in children and adolescents: a new approach. *Nord J Psychiatry*. 2018;72(1):57–62

58. Miman O, Mutlu EA, Ozcan O, et al. Is there any role of toxoplasma gondii in the etiology of obsessive-compulsive disorder? *Psychiatry Res*. 2010;177(1–2):263–5

59. Breitschwerdt EB, Greenberg R, Maggi RG, et al. Bartonella henselae bloodstream infection in a boy with pediatric acute-onset neuropsychiatric syndrome. *J Cent Nerv Syst Dis*. 2019;11:1–8

60. Khanna S, Ravi V, Shenoy PK, et al. Viral antibodies in blood in obsessive compulsive disorder. *Indian J Psychiatry*. 1997;39(3):190–5

61. Banerjee D, Viswanath B. Neuropsychiatric manifestations of COVID-19 and possible pathogenic mechanisms: Insights from other coronaviruses. *Asian J Psychiatr*. 2020;54:102350:1–19

62. Boldrini M, Canoll PD, Klein RS. How COVID-19 affects the brain. *JAMA Psychiatry*. 2021;78(6):682–683

63. Adams TG, Kelmendi B, Brake CA, et al. The role of stress in the pathogenesis and maintenance of obsessive-compulsive disorder. *Chronic Stress* (Thousand Oaks). 2018;2:1–11

64. Rosso G, Albert U, Asinari GF, et al. Stressful life events and obsessive-compulsive disorder: clinical features and symptom dimensions. *Psychiatry Research*. 2012;197(3):259–264

65. de Silva P, Marks M. The role of traumatic experiences in the genesis of obsessive-compulsive disorder. *Behaviour Research and Therapy*. 1999;37(10):941–951

66. Godar SC, Bortolato M. What makes you tic? Translational approaches to study the role of stress and contextual triggers in Tourette syndrome. *Neuroscience & Biobehavioral Reviews*. 2017;76(A):123–133

67. Bennett JW, Klich M. Mycotoxins. *Clin Microbiol Rev*. 2003;16(3):497–516

68. Ratnaseelan AM, Tsilioni I, Theoharides TC. Effects of mycotoxins on neuropsychiatric symptoms and immune processes. *Clin Ther*. 2018;40(6):903–917

69. Pall ML. Millimeter (MM) wave and microwave frequency radiation produce deeply penetrating effects: the biology and the physics. *Rev Environ Health*. 2021;1–12

70. Pall ML. Scientific evidence contradicts findings and assumptions of Canadian Safety Panel 6: micro-waves act through voltage-gated calcium channel activation to induce biological impacts at non-thermal levels, supporting a paradigm shift for microwave/lower frequency electromagnetic field action. *Rev Environ Health*. 2015;30(2):99–116

71. Pall ML. Wi-Fi is an important threat to human health. *Environ Res*. 2018;164:405–416

72. Salford LG, Nittby H, Brun A, et al. The mammalian brain in the electromagnetic fields designed by man with special reference to blood-brain barrier function, neuronal damage and possible physical mechanisms. *Progress of Theoretical Physics Supplement*. 2008;173:283–309

73. Terzi M, Ozberk B, Deniz OG, et al. The role of electromagnetic fields in neurological disorders. *Journal of Chemical Neuroanatomy*. 2016;75(B):77–84

74. Bouchard MF, Bellinger DC, Weuve J, et al. Blood lead levels and major depressive disorder, panic disorder, and generalized anxiety disorder in US young adults. *Arch Gen Psychiatry*. 2009;66(12):1313–1319

75. www.aacap.org/AACAP/Families_and_Youth/Facts_for_Families/FFF-Guide/Lead-Exposure-In-Children-Affects-Brain-And-Behavior-045.aspx, accessed 8/10/2021

76. Gump BB, Dykas MJ, MacKenzie JA, et al. Background lead and mercury exposures: psychological and behavioral problems in children. *Environ Res*. 2017;158:576–582

77. Brinkel J, Khan MH, Kraemer A. A systematic review of arsenic exposure and its social and mental health effects with special reference to Bangladesh. *Int J Environ Res Public Health*. 2009;6(5):1609–1619

THE PROBLEM: OVERLOAD, OVERWHELM, OVERFLOW

It's not stress that kills us, it's our reaction to it.
~ **HANS SELYE**

KEY POINTS

▸ The three steps involved in disease development or progression can be represented by the terms *overload*, *overwhelm*, and *overflow*

▸ The flowerpot analogy illustrates the mechanisms of disease development and helps identify therapeutic targets for healing

▸ About 25% of people don't efficiently process or remove toxins and toxicants from their body

In our model, the process that starts human illness (including PANS and PANDAS) consists of three steps. We call this the "illness triad." These steps are:

1. Overload
2. Overwhelm
3. Overflow

To best understand this process, I would like to introduce a visual representation called the flowerpot analogy (FPA) that was developed by Dr. Ellen Antoine. Understanding this picture and how it represents the human ecosystem in sickness and in health is vital to help you get the most out of this book.

I invite you to picture your patient as a flower in a flowerpot as in the diagram below.

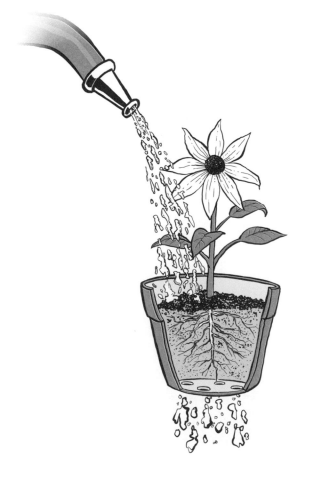

In a perfect world, a flower (reflecting health) would be strong and vibrant. Ideally, there would be a watering can full of clean water and nutrients to feed the flower and help it grow.

Unfortunately, in this picture you can see that there is a fire hose above the flower. The hose represents everything that your patient is exposed to every day. It represents the things

> **About 25% of people do not detoxify as well as others in the general population, possibly due to genetic factors.**

coming into the body that we have control over (what we eat and drink—including chemicals in the food supply—relationships, and the social media to which we are exposed) and some things we can't control or may not know we are exposed to (infectious diseases, environmental pollution, heavy metals, mold). Stress can be included in the fire hose and should also be thought of as a toxin.

The flowerpot itself represents the patient's physical body. Inside an actual flowerpot you would find soil and roots, but inside your patient's body there is a lot of complex biochemistry, including normal metabolic compounds, nutrients, the immune system, hormones, any toxins they could not biotransform and remove, and any active or dormant infections. The holes in the bottom of the flowerpot represent the patient's detoxification ability. The detox system must also deactivate some of our own chemical byproducts, which we make every day. Once compounds are made into a water-soluble form, they are excreted—some through sweating, some through urinating, and some through bowel movements.

About 25% of people do not detoxify as well as others in the general population, possibly due to genetic factors. This makes these people the "canaries in the coal mine." They are more susceptible to toxins (natural compounds in our environment) or toxicants (man-made chemicals) than the general population. Since the holes in the bottom of the flowerpot represent detoxification, imagine that these patients have rocks or mud obscuring and clogging them.

Health is the dynamic balance between what comes into your body and what you process and neutralize or get rid of. If the flow from the hose is too high, it causes an OVERLOAD on the system. High levels of toxins and toxicants in the body (the flowerpot) or chronic infections can also overload the system. If the volume in the flowerpot is too high and/or the person cannot detoxify well, the system becomes OVERWHELMED, and the flowerpot OVERFLOWS all over the floor.

The OVERFLOW on the floor (the puddle) represents symptoms your patient is experiencing or diagnoses they have been given. This puddle could include diagnoses like PANS or ADHD or generalized anxiety disorder. It could also include nonspecific symptoms like headache, nausea, or an urgent need to urinate, all of which are concerning symptoms but may not yet meet the criteria for a specific diagnosis.

Once symptoms are identified or a diagnosis is made, medical procedures, prescription medications, or supplements are used to mop up the puddle to remove the symptoms. This is not wrong in and of itself. In our practice we use prescription medications, supplements, and other adjunctive therapies when needed to help with symptoms or manage PANS. Many in the natural health community have labeled prescription medications as evil or unnecessary. This is unfortunate. Medications are very helpful in relieving suffering and managing various medical conditions.

The point is that your patient will not get better if you just mop up the floor. You must address the

> **Turning down the hose, treating what is in the flowerpot, mopping up the puddle, and optimizing detoxification are more vital parts of the process than establishing a diagnosis.**

right (flowerpot) side of the diagram to create long-lasting recovery for your patient and their family. More on this in the next chapter on our Fully Functional process (which is the solution).

One more note on the puddle. Even though many parents come to us to have us "make the diagnosis" of PANS or PANDAS, the diagnosis itself is not the crucial matter. Dr. Jeff Bland, a colleague of ours who was instrumental in the genesis of functional medicine thirty years ago, calls this focus on the diagnosis, rather than the root cause, the "disease delusion." What is more important is a systems approach. Turning down the hose, treating what is in the flowerpot, mopping up the puddle, and optimizing detoxification are more vital parts of the process than establishing a diagnosis.

In the next chapter we present the Fully Functional process, which we use to restore health to patients with PANS and PANDAS. Chapter 4 provides a broad overview of the process. Chapters 5 through 19 provide clear, clinically relevant illustrations of how we use the five pillars of the Fully Functional process to successfully treat patients with PANS and PANDAS.

We believe we have the most organized, systems-based approach to PANS and PANDAS. It considers the whole ecosystem of the patient (the flowerpot, the hose, the puddle, etc.) so that long-term recovery can occur. As we have seen in our practice and in our own child, PANS does not have to be an identity, and future flares are not inevitable for most patients.

If we only addressed one area of the system (the puddle) with a limited number of "mop-like" interventions (antibiotics, steroids, and IVIG), we would have a much lower success rate, and the patients would continue to have frequent flares after treatment. If system inputs (the hose), total toxic load, infections, immune system dysregulation, and detoxification are not addressed, long-term recovery is much less common. Over the last decade, we have found that our process gives our patients the best chance to achieve a long-term recovery.

CHAPTER 3 REFERENCES

1. Pizzorno L, Bland JS. The disease delusion: conquering the causes of chronic illness for a healthier, longer and happier life. *Integr Med (Encinitas)*. 2014;13(5):52–56

CHAPTER 4

THE SOLUTION:
THE FULLY FUNCTIONAL® PROCESS

If you can't describe what you are doing as a process,
you don't know what you're doing.
~ W. EDWARDS DEMING

KEY POINTS

▸ The Fully Functional process is an effective solution to address all diseases, including PANS and PANDAS

▸ The Fully Functional process has five essential steps: IDENTIFY, REDUCE, OPTIMIZE, SUPPORT, and PERSONALIZE

In the last chapter I defined the problem (the illness triad) that makes these children get sick (the OVERLOAD that OVERWHELMED their system and caused it to OVERFLOW with signs and symptoms of PANS and PANDAS). This illness triad is the reason that people develop illness at any age.

I will now outline the process that has allowed us to help hundreds of children (and their families) heal. It is known as the Fully Functional process and was originally created by Dr. Ellen Antoine. This unique approach is based upon her extensive clinical experience and it serves as the lens through which we approach every patient. In this chapter, I will discuss the "bones" of this process. In the chapters following, I will break down each of the five sections (or *pillars*, as we call them) of the process, and delve into the specifics, while illustrating practical ways we apply the principles to help our patients heal. Paying close attention to each of these pillars is a vital part of the true, lasting solution to PANS and PANDAS.

The Fully Functional process has five pillars:
1. Identify
2. Reduce
3. Optimize
4. Support
5. Personalize

In this chapter, we will reference the flowerpot analogy often. If you have not already done so, head to Chapter 3 to read all about the flowerpot analogy, which explains why people become ill in the first place. This information is necessary to fully understand the process of treatment and recovery going forward.

IDENTIFY

The first step in the process is the IDENTIFY pillar. Think back to the flowerpot analogy.

We need to clearly IDENTIFY three things: what is in the hose, what is in the flowerpot, and what is in the puddle.

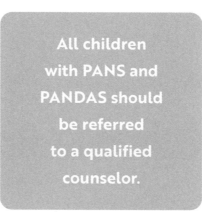

Identifying what is in the patient's puddle is usually where the process starts, because parents seek us out due to symptoms or diagnoses their children have. Perhaps the central "puddle" question we need to answer is: Does this child have PANS or PANDAS? The criteria for these diagnoses can be found in Chapter 1 of this book. But even if the child does not meet these classic criteria for PANS and PANDAS, the Fully Functional process can still help them recover from their symptoms.

Since illness can always be traced back to the illness triad of overload, overwhelm, and overflow, our process is not just for PANS and PANDAS. In addition to the symptoms included in the PANS criteria, our patients with these disorders also commonly complain of muscle and joint pain, headaches, and digestive issues.

All children with PANS and PANDAS should be referred to a qualified counselor.

Next, we need to identify what is in the hose. The hose includes three main inputs to the system (both good and bad). The first are foods the child eats both in and out of the house. The second input includes potential toxins (poisons produced in nature, like mycotoxins from mold) as well as toxicants (poisons or pollutants produced by man through manufacturing). The third major component in the hose is stress, and includes stressful family or peer relationships, the stress of illness (anxiety, OCD, emotional lability), and unsupportive school systems.

Finally, we must IDENTIFY what is in the flowerpot. This is really a deep dive into the structure and function of the body. It is basically split into two parts. The first is a good physical examination. This comprehensive, nutrition-oriented examination must be done in person by a trained PANS/PANDAS physician. We discuss vital parts of the physical examination in PANS and PANDAS in Chapter 6.

The second part of IDENTIFYING what is in the flowerpot typically involves laboratory and/or radiology testing. As mentioned in Chapter 2, testing of any type is not required to diagnose PANS and PANDAS, but can help support the diagnosis. More importantly, testing can provide an initial direction to begin treatment. The patient evaluation may include laboratory testing (blood, urine, stool, and environmental testing), radiology tests like MRI, and specialty consultations with other physicians or psychologists. In Chapters 7, 8, and 9, we explore specifics about these tests and their interpretation. In Appendix A, I have provided a summary of the laboratory and radiology tests we use in children with PANS and PANDAS.

REDUCE

Once we have IDENTIFIED what's in the hose, what's in the puddle, and what's in the flowerpot, healing starts when we REDUCE the things that are negatively impacting the child's health.

First, you must "turn down the hose." This involves removing inflammatory foods and foods to which the child may be reacting. This includes true food allergies, food sensitivities, and foods that may trigger other types of immune reactions. Reducing stress is also very important. All children with PANS and PANDAS should be referred to a qualified counselor. Reducing environmental toxins often involves remediation of mold and filtration of the air and water. Elimination of toxic (non-supportive) relationships, if possible, is important as well.

Next, we REDUCE what is in the puddle. Getting to the root cause of the patient's symptoms can take time. While we wait for lab results, treating the symptoms helps ease suffering for the patient. As you can learn in Chapter 10, there are many ways to reduce the symptoms in PANS and PANDAS. Some therapeutic modalities we discuss in this chapter include medications, supplements, herbals, counseling (such as psychotherapy and neurolinguistic programming [NLP], cognitive behavioral therapy [CBT], and mindfulness practices).

Finally, you must REDUCE the overwhelm in the flowerpot. This involves REDUCING infections with natural or prescription antimicrobials. This encompasses treating bacterial infections, viral infections, and yeast overgrowth. It also involves REDUCING the overwhelm caused by toxins and toxicants. This is reliably done through the next pillar, which is OPTIMIZING detoxification.

OPTIMIZE

When we speak of the OPTIMIZE pillar, we are really talking about optimizing the patient's detoxification processes. People process toxins and toxicants through their liver (a process called biotransformation) and then urinate, sweat, or have bowel movements to remove these substances once the liver has processed them. Lymphatic drainage is also a process that can support detoxification. Sleeping and dreaming can be thought of as a "mental detox."

There are several modalities we will discuss to help optimize detoxification in patients, including infrared sauna, binders, and supplements.

SUPPORT

The three main categories we speak about when discussing SUPPORT are:

1. Structural support (muscles, bones, cell membranes, mucous membranes, and any structural components of the body)
2. Biochemical support (the "roots and dirt" in the flowerpot). This includes the communication chemicals of your patient's body like hormones, nutrients, cytokines, etc. It also encompasses supporting each individual system in the body, like the nervous system, the gastrointestinal system, and the immune system, among others.
3. Personal support (relationships, spiritual health, personal support through the medical team). This is the stake in the ground that helps hold the plant up. The importance of self-care for the caregiver is discussed in appendix D.

PERSONALIZE

The final pillar of the Fully Functional process is PERSONALIZE. It has two aspects. The first is using the data gathered in the IDENTIFY stage to refine the therapeutic approach. Lab

> **People process toxins and toxicants through their liver (a process called biotransformation) and then urinate, sweat, or have bowel movements to remove these substances once the liver has processed them.**

results do matter and may alter the course of the patient's treatment. The second aspect of the PERSONALIZE pillar is that the patient (or parents) must PERSONALIZE this journey for themselves so that they can find what works best for them and their family. This will help them better navigate their child's health journey in the future.

CHAPTER 5

IDENTIFY: ENVIRONMENTAL TOXINS, TOXICANTS, STRESS, AND SYMPTOMS

Where there's a will, there's a detective story.
~ CAROLYN WELLS

KEY POINTS

▸ Curiosity, diligence, and listening to the patient are the keys to the best medical care
▸ Children with PANS and PANDAS are often initially diagnosed with other neuropsychiatric disorders
▸ Toxins are proteins made by or derived from living organisms which may adversely affect the human body, such as mycotoxins made by molds, or the venom of animals or insects
▸ Toxicants are substances not made by living organisms which may adversely affect the human body, such as heavy metals or industrial chemicals
▸ Food can act as a toxin itself or may contain toxicants
▸ Mycotoxins are among the worst toxins known to man, as they disrupt the immune system and are direct neurotoxins
▸ Proper home inspections and testing for molds are vital if a home has had known water damage or excess humidity
▸ Stress and adverse childhood experiences should be considered toxic exposures

The IDENTIFY pillar is all about gathering information. In the IDENTIFY chapters (5–9), we are going to discuss what we can find and how these things can negatively impact health. The REDUCE chapters that follow will provide information on how we can eliminate or REDUCE things that are negatively impacting our health.

Before we get into the specifics of identifying what is in the puddle (symptoms), what is in the hose (things coming into the body), and why this matters, we should discuss how we gather information. As "medical detectives" of sorts, we approach clinical problems by staying curious and asking lots of the right questions. This is essential to IDENTIFY what is in the hose, the puddle, and the flowerpot. It is often a case of "the devil is in the details." Patients and parents aren't always aware of what is significant.

In our medical practice, information gathering begins with an extensive patient intake

> **Excellent medical care is provided when the physician approaches the patient with an attitude of intense curiosity**

form with questions addressing all aspects of the patient's history. We not only ask about major life events, diagnoses, drug allergies, and current medications, but we also make a timeline of the patient's life. It is very helpful to look at exactly when the patient's symptoms started. Digging into the details about that time period may provide clues to the etiology of the illness or information that helps refine the treatment plan. Was there an illness or fever just prior to

the onset of symptoms? Was there a major life stressor or a move to a new home? Even the most minor of details may provide a vital clue to cracking the case.

In our residency in emergency medicine at Albert Einstein Medical Center in Philadelphia, we were told never to trust anyone with your patient's medical history. It is important to speak with the patient (and parents) before reviewing old records; many things (including errors) get written there. Sometimes conclusions in the medical record are based upon assumptions or opinions with little supporting data or experience.

Assumptions are dangerous and just plain bad medicine. They are not congruent with excellent patient care. Assumptions are different from a hypothesis or a differential diagnosis. Assumptions start off with a guess that is devoid of any acceptable evidence. They may come from a place of disbelief or a bias that says that if a patient's symptoms don't fit into a box, they must be "all in their head."

A very common assumption that we see with the children we treat is that their behavior is due to simple defiance or poor parenting. A second assumption which is just as disturbing is that these children are suffering from mental illness and just need medication to deal with symptoms when a correctable physical cause for the behaviors exists.

Excellent medical care is provided when the physician approaches the patient with an attitude of intense curiosity and provides the benefit of the doubt to the patient and family while independently verifying all aspects of their history, performing a comprehensive physical examination, and ordering testing as needed. The final step of providing excellent medical care involves

> **Children with sleep disturbance who are suspected of having sleep-disordered breathing should be referred to a specialist for a sleep study.**

continued monitoring of the outcomes of the treatment plan. This feedback is essential as it allows for course correction when a particular treatment is not helpful or results in increased symptoms.

The Value of Journaling Symptoms and Responses

In this chapter we will be taking a close look at what is in the patient's environment that could be contributing to their illness. Having the parents keep a journal of what's going on with their child's symptoms can be really helpful in tracking whether a specific food, location, activity, or medication could be making the behavior worse. It can also be helpful to know if the child responds better to one antibiotic or supplement than another. We tell parents that

this journaling does not have to be fancy or even have complete sentences or punctuation. A simple jotting down of stimulus and response is very helpful in personalizing care.

IDENTIFYING WHAT'S IN THE PUDDLE (SYMPTOMS AND DIAGNOSES)

There are many diagnoses that children with PANS and PANDAS symptoms are given before we see them. They often come to see us with diagnoses like OCD, avoidant restrictive food intake disorder (ARFID), generalized anxiety disorder, major depressive disorder, Tourette syndrome, oppositional defiant disorder, ADHD, and psychosis, to name a few. As noted at the end of Chapter 3, the diagnosis itself does not matter. Although it might seem like a zen sort of thing to say, we tell parents to IDENTIFY which symptoms or behaviors that they want to get rid of and we will start working there together.

While some practitioners use scales to follow specific symptoms like OCD or anxiety, we have not found these to be predictive of how a patient will progress. For this reason, we do not routinely follow these scales. It is very important, as noted in Chapter 1, to remember that PANS and PANDAS are neuropsychiatric disorders which, by definition, are not better explained by other neurologic conditions.

It can be helpful to see a psychologist or psychiatrist to obtain a specific diagnosis to help with obtaining an IEP for school, but this is not required to successfully treat PANS and PANDAS. Emergent referral to psychiatry (in the hospital setting) is recommended for children who are extremely violent or are a danger to self or others.

Children with sleep disturbance who are suspected of having sleep-disordered breathing should be referred to a specialist for a sleep study. Parents will usually report snoring and occasionally they will report witnessing periods of apnea during sleep.

IDENTIFYING WHAT'S IN THE HOSE (THINGS COMING INTO THE BODY)

Hippocrates famously said "all disease begins in the gut" nearly 2,500 years ago. We, too, will start the hose discussion by identifying which foods the patient is eating. We ask our parents to fill out a log of everything that their child is eating and drinking for at least three days before coming to see us.

Since this step is not about impressing us, we preface this by saying we want the parents to give the child what they typically would eat during that period. It is important to be as specific as possible when recording this information (amount, brand, and origin of food eaten). This step is especially important for children who have restrictive eating. In those cases, we also have parents track weight and compare height and weight to age-adjusted norms. We don't track weight at home if it adds undue stress to the child, as it can contribute to OCD.

Food choices

There are few, if any, neutral foods. Foods people consume either promote health or illness. Inflammation in the brain is one of the drivers of flares in PANS and PANDAS. Many of the treatment interventions employed by physicians treating these children focus on decreasing inflammation with medications like steroids and NSAIDS. We discuss the science behind inflammation in Chapter 12 and look at these medications specifically. But many of the fundamental treatment strategies in the Fully Functional process focus on naturally decreasing inflammation in these patients. We will begin this discussion by looking at foods that may cause inflammation and other harmful health effects.

Sugar

For many years, the regulatory bodies in the United States have recommended a food pyramid which was based upon faulty science. Fat (especially animal fat) has been declared unhealthy, and grains (which are converted into sugars in the body) have been celebrated as an important component of a healthy diet. Grains do have fiber, which does lower the

> There are few, if any, neutral foods. Foods people consume either promote health or illness.

blood sugar spike seen when refined sugars like candy are eaten. Still, in major studies,[1] the dietary intake of more than half of the children in the United States is classified as poor (due to excess processed sugars).

Numerous studies have shown that refined sugars such as table sugar and high-fructose corn syrup can lead to inflammation in the body.[2–5] High-fructose corn syrup recently underwent a clever name change to "corn sugar" as part of a PR campaign to make it seem more natural. When parents record what their child is eating, we emphasize that they should be specific about brands and check the "added sugar content" on the label.

One thing we emphasize numerous times in this textbook is that we never recommend restricting or changing the diet of children with food restrictive behaviors or weight loss. We also don't recommend eliminating all grains in most children as it may result in unintended weight loss.

Food additives

Many chemicals are added to food to make the color more appealing, to make the food taste better, or to increase its shelf life. There are at least 150 peer-reviewed articles in the medical literature which clearly document the harmful effects of food additives and preservatives. A great summary of these articles and the associated science is available in the American Academy of Pediatrics policy titled "Food Additives in Child Health."[6] This policy notes that exposure to food additives and preservatives may contribute to disruption of normal hormone pathways, neuro-developmental pathway disruption, obesity promotion, suppression of the immune system, cancer promotion, decreased birth weight, and cardiac toxicity. The article also notes that these additives cause oxidative stress, which can be harmful to the body.[7] For more information on testing for oxidative stress, see Chapter 7. For more information on the effects of oxidative stress on the body and strategies to correct it, see Chapter 12.

It is important to note that many food additives like monosodium glutamate (MSG) can be difficult to identify since they are allowed to be listed on food labels as *natural flavors*.

What about GMOs and pesticides?

Humans have been modifying plant characteristics for many, many years. The multitude of apple varieties at the grocery store is a product of mixing (crossing) different types of plants together.[8] This simple type of plant modification is called *crossing*. Genetic modification (also called genetic engineering) of plants is a different process.[9]

> **We never recommend restricting or changing the diet of children with food restrictive behaviors or weight loss.**

In genetic modification, plant DNA is extracted from plants that have a desirable characteristic (disease resistance or increased fruit production). This DNA is then inserted into cells of another plant. This can be done by inserting metal particles coated with the new DNA or by using a bacterium or virus to carry the DNA into the new cell.

The first genetically modified crops (soybeans) came to market in the mid-1990s. Soon after, a whole array of genetically modified crops was released. It is now estimated that more than 90% of the corn in the United States is genetically modified. An ongoing debate exists as to whether the actual process of genetic modification will cause long-term health effects. Although no short-term issues have been identified in high quality studies, the most well-known of these studies (which is often cited to promote the idea of GMO safety) was actually authored by an employee of Dupont (a major producer of genetically modified crops).[10]

The bigger question when considering the safety of GMO foods is not necessarily the actual genetic modification process but why the modification was performed. If it were to help a plant resist frost or drought, that would be one thing. However, most crops produced in the United States (corn, for example) are modified for the purpose of being resistant to herbicides (like glyphosate).[11] These crops are often marketed as "Roundup Ready."

> There is some good evidence that glyphosate and other pesticides directly impair the immune system.

Roundup is a trademarked herbicide used to stop weeds from growing. If plants are genetically modified to be resistant to this chemical, much higher doses can be used (and are used) to eliminate weeds and increase the yield of crops since they will not be choked out as often. It has been demonstrated that these grains contain high residues of glyphosate.

Currently, there is a controversy in the regulatory community as to whether glyphosate poses a cancer risk in humans. The US Environmental Protection Agency (EPA) says it does not, but the World Health Organization's International Agency for Research on Cancer (IARC) says it is likely a human carcinogen. An editorial article from the medical literature suggests that the IARC considered more peer-reviewed human studies than the EPA did and looked at studies using the actual products used in farming (not just pure glyphosate).[12]

In the last few years, the company that produces Roundup has been the target of several successful lawsuits alleging that this product causes cancer. As of this writing, the parent company is asking for an appeal to the US Supreme Court. Although the patients' legal victories have resulted in multi-million-dollar settlements, this does not necessarily prove that this chemical is harmful scientifically. But the chemical-resistant garb required for farm workers exposed to glyphosate in the fields certainly seems to contradict the assertion that this chemical is "nontoxic." Given that this chemical has only been used for the past three decades, we may see more long-term effects in the coming years.

Aside from cancer, there is some good evidence that glyphosate and other pesticides directly impair the immune system.[13,14] In addition, glyphosate-resistant weeds have emerged and will likely drive the need for higher doses of herbicides to keep these so-called super-weeds at bay.[15]

Gluten

In the past few years, you may have noticed quite a bit of talk about gluten. Gluten intake is one of the questions we ask our patients about since it can negatively affect health.

Gluten is a structural protein found in wheat products. It can be found as a contaminant in other grains, such as oats, and anything processed, prepared, or cooked in a location which also prepares gluten-containing foods. Gluten is also present in some foods that you might not think of, such as licorice, soy sauce, and many barbecue sauces. Gluten gives breads and other dough elastic properties and makes them chewy.

There are a few problems that gluten-containing foods can cause. The first is that some people have a true allergy to wheat. This is not very common, and most people know that if they have this, they should completely avoid gluten.

Second, we have celiac disease, which is an autoimmune condition. Patients with celiac disease have a genetic risk factor (HLA DQ2 or HLA DQ8) present >90% of the time. When these genetically susceptible people eat gluten, they may produce antibodies that trigger an autoimmune reaction that can cause gastrointestinal issues. They can also have neurologic symptoms, including gluten ataxia. Some patients with celiac only get a skin rash called dermatitis herpetiformis. Patients with celiac disease can go many years without having symptoms and may not know they have this disease, but they must strictly avoid gluten for life. As much gluten as one-eighth of a grain of rice can cause symptoms in these patients.

Another issue we see quite often is gluten sensitivity (also sometimes called "non-celiac gluten sensitivity"). Gluten sensitivity can cause patients to have any combination of headaches, joint pain, brain fog, concentration and memory issues, and digestive complaints.

There is still controversy in the medical community about the existence of gluten sensitivity. Some patients have erroneously been told that celiac disease or true allergies are the only documented issues related to gluten. Since about 2010, several articles confirming the phenomenon of gluten sensitivity causing symptoms in various bodily systems have appeared, including some in major peer-reviewed gastroenterology journals.[16] Numerous journal articles

have reported that gluten sensitivity is an underrecognized cause of neurologic and psychiatric illnesses.[17-22] We will explore the topics of testing for wheat allergy and celiac disease in Chapter 7.

Dairy

Dairy has been a staple in the American diet for many years. We have been told that dairy products like milk and yogurt are essential for children from a very young age. Many of the patients we see in the office have issues with dairy (whether they know it or not). Anecdotally, we have seen children with repeated bouts of ear infections avoid getting tympanostomy tubes and future infections by eliminating cow dairy. The professional medical literature only recognizes dairy

> **Numerous journal articles have reported that gluten sensitivity is an underrecognized cause of neurologic and psychiatric illnesses.**

issues due to true milk allergy (found with IgE blood or skin testing). However, in our practice we have seen childrens' respiratory, ear, and skin conditions improve with cow's dairy elimination even in the absence of true IgE allergy. Many of these children have IgG reactions on testing (not a true allergy, but an abnormal immune response nonetheless).

Non-allergy-related issues with dairy are often blamed on lactose intolerance, but this is not usually the case. In fact, some colorectal surgeons hold the position that some patients with inflammatory bowel disease have issues digesting dairy unrelated to lactose intolerance.[23]

There is a convincing body of literature to support the association of cow's milk consumption to autoimmune disease. One fascinating journal article[24] explains that the concept of molecular mimicry caused by infections, toxins, toxicants, and foods (including gluten and dairy) can be directly linked to autoimmunity. These links have been found or proposed in type 1 diabetes, autoimmune thyroid disease, autoimmune arthritis, and autoimmune encephalitis.

Trans fats, omega 6 fats, saturated fats

Trans fats (also called trans unsaturated fatty acids) occur in small amounts in dairy and meat, but the most common exposure to artificial trans fats occurs with purchased or prepared foods. Foods that contain trans fats commonly include commercial baked goods like cakes and cookies, shortening, microwave popcorn, refrigerated doughs (like biscuits), and margarine. The problem with trans fats is that they are very inflammatory. They have been strongly associated with cardiovascular disease.[25,26] Trans fats have been shown in mice to cause intestinal inflammation, which may affect the absorption of vital nutrients.[27]

Omega 6 fats are a type of polyunsaturated fat. They are essential for the formation of cellular membranes and other biochemical processes.

The relationship between omega 6 fats and inflammation is complex,[28–30] but we know that if the ratio of omega 6 fats to omega 3 fats (like those found in fish and nuts) is too high, it can cause inflammation.[31] Omega 6 levels are high in many processed foods.

> If the ratio of omega 6 fats to omega 3 fats (like those found in fish and nuts) is too high, it can cause inflammation.

Water

Fortunately, in the US most people have access to clean water in their home. Water-borne infectious diseases from parasites (like *Giardia*) or bacteria (like *Cholera*) are relatively rare.

Chemical exposures in the water supply, however, are much more common. The EPA has identified contamination with both farming chemicals (atrazine, glyphosate, trichloroethylene, and tetrachloroethylene) and disinfection byproducts (e.g., chloroform) in drinking water and has stated that elevated levels of these chemicals may be particularly harmful for children and the elderly.[32] Nitrates and nitrites from farming and livestock runoff have been associated with thyroid disease in children and pregnant women.[33–35] Maternal hypothyroidism is well-known to be a contributing factor to developmental issues in children.[36]

Heavy metal contamination of drinking water also occurs frequently in the US. Commonly seen heavy metals include cadmium, lead, arsenic, and mercury. There is extensive research[37–40] showing that heavy metals can cause neuropsychiatric disorders, even at levels within the "normal range" on blood testing. Heavy metals have also been shown to adversely affect the immune system.[41–45] Lead can often be found in the paint of older homes.

Many online sources[46–47] geared at both consumers and practicing physicians report that heavy metal poisoning is "rare" or "very rare," implying that heavy metals are not much of a concern. The problem with this statement is that you cannot properly apply statistics on the frequency of disease to the individual patient standing in front of you. After all, your patient at any point in time may represent one of those supposedly rare cases.

But is exposure to heavy metals actually rare? Several professional articles[48,49] have established the fact that there has been a logarithmic increase in heavy metal contamination in water and soil since the 1970s. This raises the question: Is heavy metal toxicity "rare" simply because we are not considering these toxins in cases of neuropsychiatric illness or developmental disorders? We need to consider organic causes in patients with neuropsychiatric illnesses, rather than assuming these diagnoses to be random events.

There are many companies that offer home water testing for heavy metals and contaminants. We usually recommend SimpleLab (formerly Simple Water). We direct patients to their website at www.simplewater.us. If a house was built before 1980, we recommend that patients hire a lead-based paint inspector to check the paint. Dust or chips from this type of paint can increase lead levels in the body.

Further discussion of testing patients for heavy metals can be found in Chapter 7.

Air pollution and other environmental chemicals

Air pollution is also known as "ambient particulates." Burning fossil fuels and vehicle exhaust are major causes. A quick search of the professional medical literature for the terms "air pollution" and "health" produces over five hundred references every year.

Exposure to high levels of air pollution has been shown to increase the risk of death, cardiac disease, and asthma.[50] Pollutants cause both oxidative stress and inflammation.[51,52] There is no standard index in most places in the US, so a patient's individual exposure to air pollution may be difficult to quantify unless you live in an area with known pollution that is regularly monitored, such as Los Angeles.

Patients may also be exposed to industrial chemicals through playing in fields which have been sprayed or playing near industrial sites. One of the herbicides commonly used in the United States is atrazine.[53] Even at low levels, atrazine causes reproductive abnormalities in amphibians. It has been banned in other countries due to links to cancer and the hypothesis that it is an endocrine disruptor. Endocrine disruptors bind to hormone receptor sites in the body. If these toxicants bind to these receptors, hormones cannot, and health effects can be seen. If our patients are considering renovating a home, we recommend a survey for hazardous chemicals and materials beforehand.

Environmental chemicals have been shown to suppress the immune system.[54] Since immune dysregulation is a prerequisite for the

> Endocrine disruptors bind to hormone receptor sites in the body.

development of PANS and PANDAS, careful attention to chemical exposures is important when trying to IDENTIFY what is in the hose.

Microplastics[55]

Microplastics are plastic particles that are between 1 micrometer and 5 millimeters in size.[56] They have been found in food, water, air, and soil. Sources of microplastics include larger plastics that degrade, microfibers from textiles,

> **Medical literature describes the capacity of EMFs to alter the normal function of the immune system by increasing allergic responses and inflammation.**

and microbeads used in cosmetics. Microplastic exposures have been linked to oxidative stress, DNA damage, damage to the immune system, and neurologic dysfunction.[57] Inflammation and increased cancer risk have been reported as well. Particular concern has been raised for children's exposures to microplastics.[58]

Electromagnetic fields (EMFs)

EMFs are present everywhere in the modern environment. EMFs are divided into two groups: extremely low frequencies (ELFs), which are in high-voltage towers and home wiring for electricity, and radio frequencies (RFs), which are those frequencies found in cell phones, Wi-Fi, and the like. From radio waves to cellular

telephones and Wi-Fi, we are continually bathed in RFs and ELFs.

Some children (and adults) have electromagnetic hypersensitivity (EHS) and develop symptoms when exposed to high levels of EMFs. In this case, health changes or worsened behavior/symptoms may be seen in an area with strong Wi-Fi. Beyond just those children and adults who are sensitive, there is a lot of information on the potential dangers of EMFs to both children and adults.

Initial concerns about EMFs were for risks of cancer. The US Department of Health and Human Services conducted a review and found evidence linking EMF exposure from cell phones to cancers in animals.[59] The same review noted that these frequencies caused damage in the brain, liver, and blood cells of mice.

Although controversial, there are some publications which have proposed a link between cell phone RF exposure and brain tumors based upon some early data.[60] Additional sources have proposed that cell phone exposures contribute to developmental disorders in children due to DNA damage to the brain.[61,62] Researchers in India found a link between the distance of cell phone towers and DNA damage and oxidative stress in white blood cells.[63]

One case-controlled, retrospective study looked at childhood cancer and the relation to distance from radio-frequency towers and found a 69% increased cancer risk in children in the UK who lived within 200 meters of a radio-frequency tower as compared to children who lived >600 meters away.[64] Although this was a retrospective study, no other known reasons for the difference in cancer rates were noted. The majority of studies on man-made EMFs have shown significant effects on animals, plants, and human cells. Additional medical literature describes the capacity of EMFs to alter the normal function of the immune system by increasing allergic responses and inflammation.[65]

Water damage and mold

People have been living in and around various types of molds for thousands of years. In fact, this passage from the Bible speaks directly about mold:

> The owner of the house must go and tell the priest, "I have seen something that looks like a defiling mold in my house." The priest is to order the house to be emptied before he goes in to examine the mold, so that nothing in the house will be pronounced unclean. (Leviticus 14:35–36, NIV)

Mold exposures aren't all bad. Mold is used to produce certain foods (blue cheese and Gorgonzola) as well as prescription medications like penicillin, lovastatin, mycophenolate mofetil, and cyclosporin. Other types of useful fungi include yeast and mushrooms.

Some types of mold exposures, however, can be harmful to people. We were able to directly connect mold exposure to PANS and PANDAS based upon our experience with our own daughter's illness and the hundreds of patients we have seen over the years. In this section, we will discuss the role that mold exposures play in the development of PANS and PANDAS.

Excluding the cheeses and medications listed above, we also encounter molds as environmental contaminants in foods, which can be harmful to our health. Grains such as corn, oats, wheat, and rice can all become contaminated with mold. This can happen while it is still in the field or after the grain is stored. The main issue with mold contamination of foods is that some of these molds produce poisons called *mycotoxins*, which have various effects on humans.

While it had previously been estimated that up to 25% of the grain supply is contaminated with mold,[66,67] recent studies[68] using different, more sensitive measurements have found that virtually 100% of grains are contaminated to some degree with mycotoxins. Coffee beans and peanuts can also become contaminated. One study showed that only 11% of coffee beans analyzed were mycotoxin free.[69] We have all seen visible mold on foods such as bread, cheese, and fruit that have been left for long periods of time.

Although we often think of mold in a home as occurring after a large water leak from faulty plumbing or due to a roof leak, any damp or humid area can harbor microbial growth. This can include any home with an indoor humidity

> **Virtually 100% of grains are contaminated to some degree with mycotoxins.**

level over 50%. Whole house humidification is not recommended for that reason. You can check humidity levels using a hygrometer that can be found online for around twenty dollars.

How mold affects the body

People with mold allergies can develop a stuffy nose, a cough, or itchy eyes when they are exposed to indoor molds. Mold is also a trigger for many people with asthma.[70] But the capacity of mold exposure to cause human illness extends far beyond allergies.

The principal mechanism by which molds adversely affect both animals and humans is through the release of mycotoxins, which are very small organic toxins. They are directly toxic to the nervous system and are linked to neuropsychiatric disorders and abnormalities in neurological testing.[71,72] Numerous articles have shown that mycotoxins impair immune response.[73–78]

This immune disruption can lead to longer, more severe bacterial and fungal infections. In addition to causing the immune system to be underactive (or deficient), mycotoxins have also been shown to cause elevations of antinuclear antibodies and anti-smooth muscle antibodies.[73] This suggests that mycotoxins trigger autoimmunity as well. So mycotoxins actually cause immune "dysregulation" where the immune system can be both underactive and overactive. This represents a loss of normal immune regulation.

Numerous articles have shown that mycotoxins impair immune response.

Immune dysregulation in PANS and PANDAS

Years ago, when we first started treating children with PANS and PANDAS, we learned (from researchers at the National Institute of Mental Health) that these disorders started when the immune system, rather than just attacking an infecting organism (like the *Strep* bacteria), attacked an area of the brain.[79]

This, then, would be a case of an autoimmune disorder caused by an infection. The autoimmune attack on the brain in PANS has been confirmed in several studies.[80] It has also been shown that approximately 40% of children with PANS and PANDAS will have an elevated ANA level when tested. But, reviewing both the published medical studies[81] and the patient data in our practice, we discovered that a significant number of patients with PANS and PANDAS also have some type of immune deficiency.

As many as 48% of these children have low levels of immunoglobulins.[82] In our practice, we have found that a significant number of these children have issues making antibodies when they are vaccinated (specific antibody deficiency). Children with PANS and PANDAS get sick more often than their siblings and get sicker than others in the family when they do catch something.

Testing your home for mold and mycotoxins

We will discuss how to test for mycotoxins in the body in Chapter 7. For now, we will discuss home testing, as mold may be a dangerous part of what is in the hose.

The US Environmental Protection Agency did a study and found that 85% of commercial buildings had evidence of water intrusion at some point and 43% had active water intrusion at the time of the study.[83] Based upon government census data from 2009, about 10% of homes had a water leakage from an external source and about 1% had leakage from an internal source.[84] According to population weighted averages from multiple studies, it is estimated that about 50% of homes have some degree of "dampness."[84]

The first step in evaluating your home for possible mold involves deciding what the risk is for mold in the home. It is important to remember that mold is not only present in older homes. Building materials like drywall and lumber are often exposed to humidity both before and during the building process. This can increase the chance of mold growth in a newly built home. We have seen plenty of cases in our practice where patients built a new home and discovered mold or water intrusion within the first few years.

A known water leak (from a leaky pipe, broken sump pump, overflowing bathtub, or roof leak) always increases the risk of mold and mycotoxins unless the affected area was immediately exposed and aggressively dried within twenty-four hours of the leak. Mycotoxins are odorless, but volatile organic compounds (VOCs) produced by molds can produce a musty odor in a home. So a musty odor indicates definite cause for concern, but the lack of an odor does not necessarily rule out mold. Any home that has had a significant leak (especially if not found for more than twenty-four hours), should be checked for mold and mycotoxins.

Humidity in the air and on surfaces can be tested with an inexpensive hygrometer, as previously discussed. There are hygrometers available that have prongs that can be inserted into drywall or wooden surfaces to indicate humidity.

If there is a risk of mold in the home or if a child is very ill and has mycotoxins in their system, a professional mold inspection is recommended. In many states there is no specific certification or qualification required for contractors to offer mold testing and remediation services or to call themselves "mold experts."

Dr. Ellen Antoine and I are two of the founding members of the International Society for Environmentally Acquired Illness (www.ISEAI.org). This worldwide, professional organization is dedicated to the treatment of chronic infections, environmental toxins like mycotoxins, and other environmental toxicants and their effects. ISEAI has a webpage dedicated to finding professional mold inspectors (called indoor environmental professionals or IEPs) who are well versed in the physical effects of mold on the human body. The web page is here: www.iseai.org/find-professional. This is always our first recommendation when looking for a professional to test or remediate a home. We have had patients get sicker after they tried to remediate on their own or hire someone who promises to do the whole job for a much lower price than the experts.

We recommend an in-person inspection as the very first step.

What should a mold inspection look like?

In our professional opinion, based upon years of experience speaking with certified mold inspectors and many encounters with patients who have become ill after a mold exposure, we recommend an in-person inspection as the very first step. The inspector should look first at the landscape outside the home and make sure it is not graded (slanted) toward the home, which can result in water intrusion into the basement.

They should inspect the roof and attic (by actually getting into the attic), the basement, and any crawl spaces present. The inspector should look for both signs of water intrusion (staining on the ceiling, for example) and for mold itself. Humidity should be checked with a high-quality, professional hygrometer. Professional inspectors should use a temperature gun to check for thermal cold spots on the walls of the home. Cold spots may indicate cracks or water intrusion behind a finished wall.

Next, the inspector may suggest spore trap testing for molds. This should be done both inside and outside the home. Spore counts inside the home should be at least 50% lower than outside the home. One issue with spore traps is that not all molds are airborne. Some harmful molds (like *Stachybotrys*) are more "sticky," tend to be settled, and may be underreported on spore trap testing. Spore trap testing alone does not constitute a proper home inspection.

There are some direct-to-consumer test plates that look like petri dishes. Unfortunately, these tests are not standardized in terms of results.

The environmental relative moldiness index (ERMI) test is available at www.envirobiomics.com or www.mycometrics.com/service.html. The ERMI was initially developed by the EPA to assess mold DNA in homes. Although this test was designed to be used primarily for research, it has some utility in testing water--damaged buildings.

ERMI information can be translated into a HERTSMI-2 score, which can be used to determine if a building is safe for occupation post-remediation. In our own practice we have unfortunately seen homes with significant mold issues and a "normal" ERMI and other homes with a high (abnormal) ERMI number in which extensive evaluations have failed to find mold. For this reason, if an ERMI test is used, it should

be interpreted with caution. A normal ERMI is considered less than (-2). A HERTSMI-2 score of less than 10 is considered to indicate a building is safe for reoccupation.

Tape testing

Tape testing is often performed by IEPs to determine whether residue in building materials is mold, and if so, what type.

Environmental mycotoxin testing

As noted previously, the major issue with mold exposures comes from the mycotoxins they produce. Realtime Labs (www.realtimelab.com) offers an environmental mycotoxin test. It measures four major families of mycotoxins. Samples are taken from the air handler filter in the home (or via swab) and tested for these mycotoxins.

> Studies have suggested that mold may be as common in schools as it is in US homes.

If a home has no evidence of visible mold, a positive environmental mycotoxin test may indicate hidden mold, past mold which is not active, or mycotoxins that have been transferred on belongings from another location. Since the samples are taken from the air handler filter, a positive result means that these mycotoxins can be blown into any room in the house via the vents. This test can also be matched up with tests from the patient. If similar mycotoxins are noted, the home may be the source.

Other exposures to mold

Unless homeschooled, children spend a significant amount of time in school every year. Leaks at schools are common. The US Government Accounting Office (GAO) found that about 30% of US schools tested had plumbing problems and 27% had roof problems.[85] Other studies have suggested that mold may be as common in schools as it is in US homes.[86]

It is very difficult (if not impossible) to get schools to test for mold or mycotoxins. Clues might be changes in a child's behavior during and after holiday or summer breaks. If the child deteriorates after starting school again, mold may be present in the school. Churches, homes of friends and relatives, and preschools may also harbor mold. Parents should document changes in their child when they stay in different places for any significant period of time. We have seen the onset of PANS and PANDAS occur following a trip for spring break. Many coastal locations have very high humidity at baseline and mold growth is extremely common in vacation homes. Red tides represent blooms of harmful algae in both freshwater and ocean water. These algae can also produce mycotoxins, which make people sick. Red tides occur nearly every year along Florida's gulf coast.

Actinomyces

It is not just mold (and its associated mycotoxins) that makes people sick in water-damaged buildings. We are now aware of specific bacteria that are common in water-damaged buildings. One specific bacterium that can make people sick is *Actinomyces* or Actinomycetes. This bacterium can cause human infections of the lungs, sinuses, and other areas.[87,88] *Actinomyces* was once thought to be a fungus and behaves in some ways like a fungus.

This bacterium can also produce endotoxins (similar to mycotoxins), which adversely affect human health. One report discusses the possible role of *Actinomyces* as a trigger for rheumatoid arthritis.[89] *Actinomyces* has been shown to stimulate inflammation and oxidative stress.[90] Testing for *Actinomyces* is available from a company called EnviroBiomics, Inc. (www.envirobiomics.com). Some people believe that this bacterium is a more important pathogen than mold in water-damaged buildings. Additional endotoxins from other bacteria are also thought to be in play. As with mold, some actinomycetes are used to produce drugs used by humans, such as some antibiotics and ivermectin.

STRESS AND ADVERSE CHILDHOOD EXPERIENCES

The last thing we will discuss IDENTIFYING in the hose is stress. Stress, of course, is part of the human condition. Of course, not all stress is bad. Exercise, for example, is a type of "good" stress to the cardiovascular system and muscles, and the result is improved health. This would be classified as "positive stress."

What we are specifically talking about is the effect of bad types of stress (termed "toxic stress").

For more than thirty years, medical literature[91,92] has affirmed the fact that stress impacts the immune system. Short-term stressors with a defined end point (public speaking or exercising) increase the immune response quickly. Increased numbers and improved function of immune cells are seen. In "brief naturalistic stressors" like facing a test in school, the number of immune cells does not change, but a different type of immune response (Th2) occurs. This response uses more antibodies and less natural killer cell activity. Natural killer cell activity is a stronger, more desirable type of immune activity.

Antibody production to previously dormant Epstein-Barr virus residing in the body may be seen due to decreased natural killer cell activity following a period of increased stress. Similar changes are seen in people with a significant stressful event such as the loss of a spouse. Chronic stress (caretaking, chronic illness) leads to even greater changes to immunity and decrease in both types (Th1 and Th2) of immu-

> **Chronic stress (caretaking, chronic illness) leads to even greater changes to immunity and decrease in both types (Th1 and Th2) of immunity.**

nity. In chronic stress, immune system changes are seen regardless of age. The immune changes associated with stress occur at least partly because sympathetic nerve fibers travel from the brain and connect to the bone marrow where immune cells are made.[93]

The studies above measured immune changes in the blood and some chemical levels. The greater question is, Can these changes affect how our patients heal? Several studies have shown that patients with significant fear or stress do not heal as well and spend longer in the hospital.[94] There is also interplay of the gut microbiome, the immune system, and stress, which can be affected by diet.[95]

One of the main things we try to manage and reduce in children with PANS and PANDAS is

inflammation. Stress causes increased inflammation in the body, which can then lead to disorders like heart disease, liver disease, diabetes, cancer, irritable bowel syndrome, neurodegenerative diseases, poor response to certain vaccines, and depression.[92–101]

A specific type of childhood stress is defined by the term adverse childhood experiences (ACEs). ACEs are things like abuse, neglect, and household challenges (like parental divorce or a parent with mental illness). Adversity in childhood has been shown to alter the molecular and genetic makeup in children and can change function and development of the neurologic and immune systems for years to come.[102] They have also been linked to poor health outcomes as adults.[103]

Although there are specific scales to measure ACEs and stress objectively, we do not use them in our practice; they constitute one more task for parents to complete and they don't really change management. The question about whether stress is currently impacting people is more of a yes/no question than a scale.

Non-supportive relationships

Non-supportive relationships can be their own toxin since they produce stress. Since we are trying to eliminate stress to decrease inflammation and shorten the time to complete recovery for the patient, we have to IDENTIFY these relationships as well.

These types of relationships could be with teachers in school to relatives and friends who don't understand PANS and PANDAS. Poor understanding of human suffering often brings out the worst in people. Parents may find that others are judgmental concerning their child or their parenting. Allowing these relationships in the life of the child or the family may increase stress and divert attention from the real enemy—PANS and PANDAS.

A simple way to discover these relationships is to have the parent ask the question: Is this person pushing my child (or me) toward healing or not?

School resources

Since behaviors of children with PANS and PANDAS often appear to others as willful defiance, schools may resort to punishment instead of working with the family to ease stress and attempt to preserve a positive view of school for the child.

Parental resources to address challenges with family, friends, and school are located in Appendix D.

CHAPTER 5 REFERENCES

1. Liu J, Micha R, Li Y, Mozaffarian D. Trends in food sources and diet quality among US children and adults, 2003–2018. *JAMA Network Open*. 2021;4(4):e21526

2. Aeberli I, Gerber PA, Hochuli M, et al. Low to moderate sugar-sweetened beverage consumption impairs glucose and lipid metabolism and promotes inflammation in healthy young men: a randomized controlled trial. *American Journal of Clinical Nutrition*. 2011; 94(2): 479–485

3. Schulze MB, Hoffmann K, Manson JE, et al. Dietary pattern, inflammation, and incidence of type 2 diabetes in women. *American Journal of Clinical Nutrition*. 2005; 82(3):675–684

4. Lopez-Garcia E, Schulze MB, Fung TT, et al. Major dietary patterns are related to plasma concentrations of markers of inflammation and endothelial dysfunction. *American Journal of Clinical Nutrition*. 2004;80(4):1029–1035

5. Giugliano D, Ceriello A, Esposito K. The effects of diet on inflammation: emphasis on the metabolic syndrome. *Journal of the American College of Cardiology*. 2006;48(4):677–685

6. Trasande L, Shaffer RM, Sathyanarayana S, et. al. Food additives and child health. *Pediatrics*. 2018;142 (2):e20181410

7. Cheignon C, Tomas M, Bonnefont-Rousselot D, et al. Oxidative stress and the amyloid beta peptide in Alzheimer's disease. *Redox Biol*. 2018;14:450–464

8. www.royalsociety.org/topics-policy/projects/gm-plants/how-does-gm-differ-from-conventional-plant--breeding, accessed 4/7/2022

9. www.royalsociety.org/topics-policy/projects/gm-plants/what-is-gm-and-how-is-it-done, accessed 4/7/2022

10. Delaney B, Goodman RE, Ladics GS. Food and feed safety of genetically engineered food crops. *Toxicological Sciences*. 2018;162(2):361–371

11. Seralini GE. Update on long-term toxicity of agricultural GMOs tolerant to roundup. *Environ Sci Eur*. 2020;32(18):1–7

12. Benbrook CM. How did the US EPA and IARC reach diametrically opposed conclusions on the genotoxicity of glyphosate-based herbicides? *Environ Sci Eur*. 2019;31(2):1–16

13. Mokarizadeh A, Faryabi MR, Rezvanfar MA, et al. A comprehensive review of pesticides and the immune dysregulation: mechanisms, evidence and consequences. *Toxicology Mechanisms and Methods*. 2015;25.4: 258–278

14. Peillex C, Pelletier M. The impact and toxicity of glyphosate and glyphosate-based herbicides on health and immunity. *Journal of Immunotoxicology*. 2020;17(1):163–174

15. Boerboom C, Owen M. *Facts about Glyphosate Resistant Weeds*. The Glyphosate, Weeds, and Crops Series. www.extension.purdue.edu/extmedia/gwc/gwc-1.pdf, accessed 4/6/2022

16. Fasano A, Sapone A, Zevallos V, Schuppan D. Nonceliac gluten sensitivity. *Gastroenterology*. 2015;148(6):1195–1204

17. Hadjivassiliou M, Sanders DS, Grünewald RA, et al,. Gluten sensitivity: from gut to brain. *Lancet Neurology*. 2010;9(3):318–330

18. Hadjivassiliou M, Gibson A, Davies-Jones GA, et al: Does cryptic gluten sensitivity play a part in neurological illness? *Lancet*. 1996;347(8998):369–371

19. Hadjivassiliou M, Grünewald RA, Davies-Jones GA. Gluten sensitivity as a neurological illness. *J Neurol Neurosurg Psychiatry*. 2002;72(5):560–563

20. Ford R, Kinvig P. The gluten syndrome: a neurological disease. *Medical Hypotheses*. 2009;73(3):438–440

21. Volta U, De Giorgio R. Gluten sensitivity: an emerging issue behind neurological impairment? *Lancet Neurology*. 2010;9(3):233–235

22. Jackson JR, Eaton WW, Cascella NG, Fasano A, Kelly DL. Neurologic and psychiatric manifestations of celiac disease and gluten sensitivity. *Psychiatr Q*. 2012;83(1):91–102

23. www.lacolon.com/blog/dairy-free-for-crohns-disease, accessed 4/8/2022

24. Vojdani A. A potential link between environmental triggers and autoimmunity. *Autoimmune Dis*. 2014;2014:1–18

25. Mozaffarian D. Trans fatty acids: effects on systemic inflammation and endothelial function. *Atheroscler Suppl*. 2006;7(2):29–32

26. Bendsen NT, Stender S, Szecsi PB, et al. Effect of industrially produced trans-fat on markers of systemic inflammation: evidence from a randomized trial in women. *Journal of Lipid Research*. 2011;52(10):1821–1828

27. Takuro O, Yoshitaka H, Saori M, et al. Trans fatty acid intake induces intestinal inflammation and impaired glucose tolerance. *Frontiers in Immunology*. 2021;12:1–14

28. Innes JK, Calder PC. Omega-6 fatty acids and inflammation. *Prostaglandins, Leukotrienes and Essential Fatty Acids*. 2108;132:41–48

29. Calder PC. n-3 polyunsaturated fatty acids, inflammation, and inflammatory diseases. *Am J Clin Nutr*. 2006;83(6 Suppl):1505S-1519S

30. Russo GL. Dietary n-6 and n-3 polyunsaturated fatty acids: from biochemistry to clinical implications in cardiovascular prevention. *Biochem Pharmacol*. 2009;77(6):937–946

31. Simopoulos AP. Evolutionary aspects of diet, the omega-6/omega-3 ratio and genetic variation: nutritional implications for chronic diseases. *Biomedicine & Pharmacotherapy*. 2006;60(9):502–507

32. www.epa.gov/sites/default/files/2015–10/documents/ace3_drinking_water.pdf, accessed 4/10/2022

33. http://www.epa.gov/safewater/pdfs/factsheets/ioc/nitrates.pdf, accessed 4/10/2022

34. Gatseva PD, Argirova MD. 2008. High-nitrate levels in drinking water may be a risk factor for thyroid dysfunction in children and pregnant women living in rural Bulgarian areas. *International Journal of Hygiene and Environmental Health*. 2008;211(5–6):555–9

35. Tajtakova M, Semanova Z, Tomkova Z, et al. 2006. Increased thyroid volume and frequency of thyroid disorders signs in schoolchildren from nitrate polluted area. *Chemosphere*. 2006;62 (4):559–64

36. Morreale de Escobar G, Obregon MJ, Escobar del Rey F. 2000. Is neuropsychological development related to maternal hypothyroidism or to maternal hypothyroxinemia? *Journal of Clinical Endocrinology and Metabolism*. 2000;85(11):3975–87

37. Bouchard MF, Bellinger DC, Weuve J, et al. Blood lead levels and major depressive disorder, panic disorder, and generalized anxiety disorder in US young adults. *Arch Gen Psychiatry*. 2009;66(12):1313–1319

38. www.aacap.org/AACAP/Families_and_Youth/Facts_for_Families/FFF- Guide/Lead-Exposure-In--Children-Affects-Brain-And-Behavior-045.aspx, accessed 4/10/2022

39. Gump BB, Dykas MJ, MacKenzie JA, et al. Background lead and mercury exposures: Psychological and behavioral problems in children. *Environ Res*. 2017;158:576–582

40. Brinkel J, Khan MH, Kraemer A. A systematic review of arsenic exposure and its social and mental health effects with special reference to Bangladesh. *Int J Environ Res Public Health*. 2009;6(5):1609–1619

41. Mishra KP: Lead exposure and its impact on immune system: a review. *Toxicol In Vitro*. 2009;23(6):969–72

42. Lutz PM, Wilson TJ, Ireland J, et al. Elevated immunoglobulin E (IgE) levels in children with exposure to environmental lead. *Toxicology*.1999;134:63–78

43. McCabe MJ, Lawrence DA. Lead, a major environmental pollutant, is immunomodulatory by its differential effects on CD4+ T cell subsets. *Toxicology and Applied Pharmacology*. 1991;111:13–23.

44. Sun L, Hu J, Zhao Z, Li L, Cheng H. Influence of exposure to environmental lead on serum immunoglobulin in preschool children. *Environmental Research*. 2003; 92:124– 128.

45. Lawrence DA, McCabe MJ. Immunomodulation by metals. *International Immunopharmacology*. 2002; 2:293–302

46. www.webmd.com/a-to-z-guides/what-is-heavy-metal-poisoning, accessed 11/19/2022

47. www.healthline.com/health/heavy-metal-poisoning, accessed 11/19/2022

48. www.emedicine.medscape.com/article/814960-overview, accessed 11/19/2022

49. Zhou Q, Yang N, Li Y, et al. Total concentrations and sources of heavy metal pollution in global river and lake water bodies from 1972 to 2017. *Global Ecology and Conservation*. 2020;22: e00925:1–11

50. Brunekreef B, Holgate ST. Air pollution and health. *Lancet*. 2002; 360: 1233–42

51. Bayram H, Sapsford RJ, Abdelaziz MM, et al. Effect of ozone and nitrogen dioxide on the release of proinflammatory mediators from bronchial epithelial cells of nonatopic nonasthmatic subjects and atopic asthmatic patients in vitro. *J Allergy Clin Immunol*. 2001;107:287–94

52. Blomberg A, Krishna MT, Bocchino V, et al. The inflammatory effects of 2 ppm NO2 on the airways of healthy subjects. *Am J Respir Crit Care Med*. 1997;156:418–24

53. www.epa.gov/national-aquatic-resource-surveys/indicators-atrazine, accessed 4/10/2022

54. Gleichmann E, Kimber I, Purchase IFH. Immunotoxicology: suppressive and stimulatory effects of drugs and environmental chemicals on the immune system. *Archives of Toxicology*. 1989;63(4):257–273

55. Jenner LC, Rotchell JM, Bennett RT, et al. Detection of microplastics in human lung tissue using µFTIR spectroscopy. *Science of the Total Environment*. 2022;831:1–10

56. Hartmann NB, Hüffer T, Thompson RB, et al. Are we speaking the same language? Recommendations for a definition and categorization framework for plastic debris. *Environ. Sci. Technol.* 2019;53:1039–1047

57. Prokić MD, Radovanović TB, Gavrić JP, et al. Ecotoxicological effects of microplastics: examination of biomarkers, current state and future perspectives. *Trends in Analytical Chemistry*. 2019;111:37–46

58. Street ME, Bernasconi S. Microplastics, environment and child health. *Italian Journal of Pediatrics*. 2021;47(75):1–3

59. www.ntp.niehs.nih.gov/whatwestudy/topics/cellphones/index.html, accessed 4/11/2022

60. Carlberg M, and Hardell L. Evaluation of mobile phone and cordless phone use and glioma risk using the Bradford Hill viewpoints from 1965 on association or causation. *BioMed Research International*. 2017;2017:1–17

61. Sage C, and Burgio E. Electromagnetic fields, pulsed radiofrequency radiation, and epigenetics: how wireless technologies may affect childhood development. *Child Development*. 2018;89(1):129–136

62. Divan H, Kheifets L, Obel C, et al. Prenatal and postnatal exposure to cell phone use and behavioral problems in children. *Epidemiology*. 2008;19:523–529.

63. Zothan S, Zosangzuali M, Lalramdinpuii M, et al. Impact of radiofrequency radiation on DNA damage and antioxidants in peripheral blood lymphocytes of humans residing in the vicinity of mobile phone base stations. *Electromagnetic Biology and Medicine*. 2017;36:295–305

64. Draper G, Vincent T, Kroll ME, Swanson J. Childhood cancer in relation to distance from high voltage power lines in England and Wales: a case-control study. *BMJ*. 2005;330:1290

65. Johansson O. Disturbance of the immune system by electromagnetic fields: a potentially underlying cause for cellular damage and tissue repair reduction which could lead to disease and impairment. *Pathophysiology*. 2009;16(2–3):157–177

66. Bryden WL. Mycotoxins in the food chain: human health implications. *Asia Pac J Clin Nutr*. 2007;16 Suppl 1:95–101

67. Thielecke F, Nugent AP. Contaminants in grain-a major risk for whole grain safety? *Nutrients*. 2018;10(9):1–23

68. De Saeger S, Audenaert K, Croubels S. Report from the 5th international symposium on mycotoxins and toxigenic moulds. *Toxins*. 2016;8(146):1–37

69. García-Moraleja A, Font G, Mañes J, et al. Analysis of mycotoxins in coffee and risk assessment in Spanish adolescents and adults. *Food Chem Toxicol*. 2015;86:225–33.

70. www.cdc.gov/niosh/topics/indoorenv/moldsymptoms.html#:~:text=Inhaling%20or%20 touching%20mold%20or,(non%2Dsensitized)%20people, accessed on 4/11/2022

71. Bennett JW, Klich M: Mycotoxins. *Clin Microbiol Rev*. 2003;16(3):497–516

72. Ratnaseelan AM, Tsilioni I, Theoharides TC. Effects of mycotoxins on neuropsychiatric symptoms and immune processes. *Clin Ther*. 2018;40(6):903–917

73. Gray MR, Thrasher JD, Crago R, et al. Mixed mold mycotoxicosis: immunological changes in humans following exposure in water-damaged buildings. *Arch Environ Health*. 2003;58(7):410–20

74. Shigesaka M, Ito T, Inaba M, et al: Mycophenolic acid, the active form of mycophenolate mofetil, interferes with IRF7 nuclear translocation and type I IFN production by plasmacytoid dendritic cells. *Arthritis Res Ther*. 2020;22:264

75. Al-anati L, and Petzinger E: Immunotoxic activity of ochratoxin A. *Journal of Veterinary Pharmacology and Therapeutics*. 2006;29:79–90

76. Assaf H, Azouri H, Pallardy. Ochratoxin A induces apoptosis in human lymphocytes through down regulation of Bcl-xL. *Toxicological Sciences*. 2004;79:2:335–344

77. Bulgaru CV, Marin DE, Pistol GC, Taranu I. Zearalenone and the immune response. *Toxins* (Basel). 2021;13(4):248

78. Wu Q, Wu W, Franca TCC, et al. Immune evasion, a potential mechanism of trichothecenes: new insights into negative immune regulations. *International Journal of Molecular Sciences*. 2018;19(11):3307

79. Chang K, Frankovich J, Cooperstock M, et al. Clinical evaluation of youth with pediatric acute-onset neuropsychiatric syndrome (PANS): recommendations from the 2013 PANS consensus conference. *Journal of Child and Adolescent Psychopharmacology*. 2015;25(1):3–13

80. Swedo SE, Leonard HL, Kiessling LS. Speculations on antineuronal antibody-mediated neuropsychiatric disorders of childhood. *Pediatrics*. 1994;93(2):323–326

81. Frankovich J, Thienemann M, Pearlstein J, et al. Multidisciplinary clinic dedicated to treating youth with pediatric acute-onset neuropsychiatric syndrome: presenting characteristics of the first 47 consecutive patients. *Journal of Child and Adolescent Psychopharmacology*. 2015;25(1): 38–47

82. Calaprice D, Tona J. Treatment of pediatric acute-onset neuropsychiatric disorder in a large survey population. *Journal of Child and Adolescent Psychopharmacology*. 2017 28(2):92–103

83. Burton LE, Baker B, Hanson D. Baseline information on 100 randomly selected office buildings in the united states (BASE): gross building characteristics. *Proceedings of Healthy Buildings*. 2000;1:151–156

84. www.iaqscience.lbl.gov/prevalence-building-dampness, accessed 4/11/2022

85. www.gao.gov/assets/hehs-95-61.pdf, accessed 4/11/2022

86. Mudarri D, Fisk WJ. Public health and economic impact of dampness and mold. *Indoor Air*. 2007;17:226–235

87. Park JH, Cox-Ganser JM, White SK, et al. Bacteria in a water-damaged building: associations of actinomycetes and non-tuberculous mycobacteria with respiratory health in occupants. *Indoor Air*. 2017;27(1):24–33

88. Gajdács M, Urbán E. The pathogenic role of Actinomyces spp. and related organisms in genitourinary infections: discoveries in the new, modern diagnostic era. *Antibiotics* (Basel). 2020;9(8):1–19

89. Lorenz W, Trautmann C, Kroppenstedt RM, et al. Actinomycetes in moist houses, the causative agent of rheumatoid symptoms? *Proceedings: Indoor Air*; 2002:58–63

90. Hirvonen MR, Ruotsolainen M, Savolainen K, Nevalainen A. Effect of viability of actinomycete spores on their ability to stimulate production of nitric oxide and reactive oxygen species in RAW 264.7 macrophages. *Toxicology*. 1997;124:105–114

91. Segerstrom SC, Miller GE. Psychological stress and the human immune system: a meta-analytic study of 30 years of inquiry. *Psychol Bull*. 2004;130(4):601–630

92. Ade R, Cohen N. Psychoneuroimmunology: interactions between the nervous system and the immune system. *Lancet*. 1995;345(8942):99–103

93. Felten SY, Felten D. Neural-immune interaction. *Progress in Brain Research*. 1994;100:157–162

94. Gouin JP, Kiecolt-Glaser JK. The impact of psychological stress on wound healing: methods and mechanisms. *Immunol Allergy Clin North Am*. 2011;31(1):81–93

95. Foster JA, Rinaman L, Cryan JF. Stress & the gut-brain axis: regulation by the microbiome. *Neurobiology of Stress*. 2017;7:124–136

96. Slavich GM, Irwin MR. From stress to inflammation and major depressive disorder: a social signal transduction theory of depression. *Psychological Bulletin*. 2014;140(3),774–815

97. Liu YZ, Wang YX, Jiang CL. Inflammation: The common pathway of stress-related diseases. *Front Hum Neurosci*. 2017;11:316

98. Maydych V. The interplay between stress, inflammation, and emotional attention: relevance for depression. *Front Neurosci*. 2019;13(384):1–8

99. www.bluezones.com/2019/05/how-stress-makes-us-sick-and-affects-immunity-inflammation--digestion, accessed 4/10/2022

100. Furman D, Campisi J, Verdin E, et al. Chronic inflammation in the etiology of disease across the life span. *Nat Med*. 2019;25:1822–1832

101. Fourati S, et al. Pre-vaccination inflammation and B-cell signaling predict age-related hyporesponse to hepatitis B vaccination. *Nat. Commun*. 2016;7(10369):1–12

102. Boullier M, Blair M. Adverse childhood experiences. *Paediatrics and Child Health*. 2018;28(3):132–137

103. Monnat SM, Chandler RF. Long-term physical health consequences of adverse childhood experiences. *Sociological Quarterly*. 2015;56(4):723–752

IDENTIFY: THE PHYSICAL EXAM IN PANS AND PANDAS

To study the phenomena of disease without books is to sail an uncharted sea, while to study books without patients is not to go to sea at all.
~ SIR WILLIAM OSLER

> ## KEY POINTS
>
> ▸ The in-person physical exam is an essential step in the evaluation of children with PANS and PANDAS
> ▸ Establishing rapport is vital to a successful clinical encounter
> ▸ Fever is not a disease but a marker of a healthy immune response

It's been said that the physical exam is a dying art. Some clinicians believe that it has been supplanted by laboratory and radiology testing. Sadly, patients are increasingly having telemedicine visits and may view these as a suitable replacement for in-person visits, which they most certainly are not.

Although telemedicine visits may be fine for some follow-up and may be necessary during a public health emergency, an in-person exam is absolutely a best practice for any new patient. The physical examination by an experienced physician is vital to excellent medical care. Without an in-person visit, it is impossible to do an adequate neurologic examination to rule out other possible diagnoses. In the more than thirty years I have practiced medicine, I have seen many cases where the wrong diagnosis or treatment was given simply because no one bothered to do a good physical examination.

This chapter will outline what we consider to be important parts of the physical examination and will also provide examples of findings which may support the diagnosis of PANS or PANDAS, or which may alert the physician to another possible diagnosis.

> The physical examination by an experienced physician is vital to excellent medical care.

ESTABLISHING RAPPORT

The first (and maybe most important) step in the patient encounter is establishing rapport. Establishing a good relationship with the patient and their family will make everything that follows easier.

Parents of children with PANS and PANDAS (and the children themselves) are under a great deal of stress. They both have quite a bit of anxiety. For these reasons, we have had to become skilled at establishing rapport in difficult situations to help extract information and convince patients and parents to do what we ask them to do.

If you have ever noticed two people in love (or on a very good first date) at a restaurant, you may notice that they mirror one another. They may use the same gestures, the same vocal tone, and the same facial expressions. When we are in rapport with people, these things tend to happen naturally. This feels good. We tend to want to spend time with people who are like us.

The good news is, through the knowledge of how to establish rapport (taken from the field of neurolinguistic programming, or NLP), we can speed this process up and achieve rapport more quickly and completely. Chapter 21 contains more information on the uses and history of NLP.

When speaking with a parent or child, the first NLP technique we use is called *mirroring*. That means matching vocal tone, facial expression, posture, and gestures. It should not be done as a 100% mimic of their behavior; that will be noticeable, and this may prevent rapport. We then try "pacing and leading." This is helpful with a patient or parent who is very anxious, closed off, or argumentative. We start by mirroring their tone, volume, and gestures without directly opposing them or being argumentative. After a minute or so, when we notice that we are in rapport, we begin to change the tone (for example, lower the volume or speed of the conversation). Typically, we are able to lead the patient (or the parent) to a calmer place.

Children with PANS and PANDAS often arrive at our office very anxious, as they may be getting blood drawn to help IDENTIFY what is in the flowerpot. We have found that going into the room with a starched, white jacket and a serious demeanor will prevent immediate rapport. In these cases, we usually remove our white jacket and use another NLP technique, which is known as a *pattern interrupt*.

Upon entering the exam room, we may drop something on purpose or ask the child if they are there to "deliver a refrigerator." This interrupts the normal pattern of what a physician might do or say. They often laugh and look at their parents. This gives us time to read the room. We also start the dialogue with parents about any pets that might be in the home. We can usually get the child to give us the name of the animal or we may suggest an outlandish name for their pet to get the child to laugh.

We then try to pace and lead them to help them become calmer. We say "great job" and "that's right" each time we have the child change position. We also use the phrase "almost done" or "most children your age don't do this as well as you do."

Often, we try to explain PANS in childlike terms so that they can understand that this is an illness and is not forever.

Before blood draws, we usually use some conversational hypnosis or a simple technique to help the child "turn off the power" to their arm so that the blood draw is much easier. This simple technique is described in Chapter 21 in the section on hypnosis.

THE PHYSICAL EXAMINATION IN PANS AND PANDAS STEP BY STEP

1. How does the patient look from the door?

When we took our oral exams for our emergency medicine boards, we were given cases to discuss with the exam proctors. We had to talk our way through how we might manage a patient with a particular emergency medical condition. During this examination we were encouraged to always ask the question, "How does the patient look from the door of the room they are in?" This can change your treatment approach. The first look can signal an emergency that requires quick action from one that can wait for tests and a more thorough exam.

A child in the midst of a flare with PANS or PANDAS typically looks scared or anxious. They may have a distant "deer in the headlights" look. They may be sullen or withdrawn. Sometimes children may look completely normal outside the home (in school or even in our office) and really melt down when they get home. This is an example of "holding it together" because they don't want to feel "abnormal" around strangers. Children with PANS and PANDAS may also appear pale and have dark circles under their eyes. If they are food restricting, they may be thin. We often ask parents to bring a photo of their child from when they were well. The difference can be striking. The physical exam should always be performed with the parent in the room.

2. Vital signs

One of the reasons that we always advocate for a physical examination for all PANS and PANDAS patients is that this helps obtain much needed information about health status. Individual components of this category along with age adjusted normals are listed below.

a. Weight (kg)

Getting an accurate weight in children is very important. A sudden decrease in weight in a child who is food restricting can prompt the need for admission for assisted feeding. Weight changes to measure fluid loss can be helpful. Normal weights by age and height can be plotted by age on a standard pediatric chart. These charts may be found at www.cdc.gov/growthcharts.

A useful automatic calculator from the CDC for BMI (for older children) based on age can be found here: www.cdc.gov/ healthyweight/ bmi/ calculator.html.

In our office, we have a bioimpedance machine, which measures weight and body composition in children over the age of twelve. This is more useful than BMI as it shows muscle and adipose composition of the body as well as BMI. This can be helpful to track the needs to gain muscle and fat in children with food restriction. We don't usually reveal these numbers to the child as it may worsen OCD. InBody (www.inbodyusa.com) is one company that makes a good bioimpedance machine.

> Getting an accurate weight in children is very important.

b. Temperature

Normal body temperature[1] actually ranges from 97.5° to 98.9°F (36.4° to 37.2°C). Multiple studies have shown that parental touch misses a fever when present about 11% of the time.[2] Although oral thermometers are considered the standard, there are many good digital probe thermometers, tympanic thermometers, and skin thermometers. Skin and ear thermometers typically use infrared technology. Mercury thermometers should not be used due to the risk of mercury exposure if they break. Other types of glass thermometers are acceptable but may also pose a risk of injury from broken glass. Digital stick thermometers from most major drug stores are typically reliable. The Exergen temporal scanner is well rated by consumer sites.

Fever is technically described as a temperature of at least 100.4°F (38°C). Although we track fever as a vital sign, in adults and in children older than three months fever itself is not concerning in the vast majority of cases. Since some bacteria and viruses cannot survive at higher temperatures, the body, in its infinite wisdom, increases its temperature. Some clinicians (and many parents) still believe that high fever can lead to neurologic injury or a seizure. With a few exceptions, that is just not the case.[3–5] Treatment of fever has not been shown to decrease the risk of febrile seizures.[6] Neurologic injury occurs only when fever is higher than 107°F.[7] This is really only seen from exposure to environmental heat, as in "forgotten baby syndrome," when someone leaves a child in a hot car.

Children should be seen by a physician urgently regardless of how high a fever is if they have concerning symptoms or signs such as delirium, lethargy, decreased level of consciousness, intractable vomiting, dehydration, severe headache, or meningeal signs. Children who are immunocompromised may need to be seen or referred for inpatient care. Fever produced by heat exposure (as mentioned previously) needs an evaluation in the ED.

We recommend treating a fever only if it makes the child significantly uncomfortable. This is usually above 102°F. When considering treating a fever, the only commercially approved medications in the United States are acetaminophen and ibuprofen.

In high doses, or in chronically ill children, acetaminophen may cause liver damage. In vitro studies have shown that acetaminophen in normal dose concentrations reduces glutathione (a vital antioxidant) in cells.[8,9] This effect has not been demonstrated in humans since those studies have not yet been done.

If a fever is to be treated, we typically recommend weight-based doses of ibuprofen (10 mg/kg per dose) every six hours with food. Tepid baths are not recommended since they are very unpleasant to the child and can cause shivering, which may actually increase the body temperature. The response or lack of response of a fever to medication does not tell you anything about the severity of the child's illness. Failure of the fever to come all the way down to normal also does not signal a serious illness. The goal of treating a fever with medication is to make the child feel comfortable. Some integrative practitioners advocate using acupressure to treat fever in children, but no studies have been done.

c. Heart rate

As we know, the normal heart rate (see table below) may increase with anxiety, pain, fever, dehydration, blood loss, or infection. Very high heart rates in children (>180/minute) can be due to cardiac issues. Heart rates may also increase with postural orthostatic tachycardia syndrome (POTS). Abnormally slow heart rates may be seen with abdominal pain, nausea, anxiety from blood draws, and cardiac issues. Some older children who are athletes may have resting heart rates in the 40s and 50s. The key to whether something is normal or not is guided by the patient history and whether it produces symptoms.

NORMAL HEART RATES BY AGE (TABLE 6.1)

Age	Normal range of heart rate (beats per minute)
2–6 years	75–120
6–12 years	75–110
12 years and up	60–100

d. Respiratory rate

The respiratory rate may increase with fever, acidosis, infection, pneumonia, or dehydration.

NORMAL RESPIRATORY RATES BY AGE (TABLE 6.2)

Age	Normal range of respiratory rates (breaths per minute)
Toddlers	24–40
Preschoolers	22–34
Elementary age	18–30
Adolescents	16–20
Adults	16–22

e. Blood pressure

Elevated blood pressure is uncommon in children unless they have kidney disease. Low blood pressures can be produced by blood loss, dehydration, or anxiety from blood draws. Having the right size cuff for the arm is very important. Arm cuffs are more accurate than wrist cuffs. Young, thin adolescents may have systolic blood pressures of 70–80 without symptoms.

NORMAL BLOOD PRESSURE BY AGE (TABLE 6.3)

Age	Normal blood pressure readings (systolic)	Normal blood pressure readings (diastolic)
Toddlers	95–105	53–66
Preschoolers	95–110	56–70
Elementary age	97–112	57–71
Adolescents	98–128	66–80
Adults	100–130	66–80

f. Oxygen level

Normal oxygen levels are above 95%. Values below 92% are considered abnormal. When measuring pulse ox, it is important that the probe looks like it is tracking with the pulse wave.

3. Hair and scalp

Dirty or greasy hair may be present if they have stopped bathing. Alopecia can be a sign of autoimmune disease. As we tell our patients, autoimmunity begets autoimmunity. Since PANS and PANDAS are autoimmune diseases, finding other autoimmune diseases should be expected.

4. Eyes

Children with PANS and PANDAS often have mydriasis. This is usually due to sympathetic overdrive due to anxiety. Slow reactivity to light can indicate very strong sympathetic activity. The child may complain of eye pain or headache when exposed to bright lights or sunlight. Children who are old enough should have a formal eye exam by an ophthalmologist. Significant visual changes, nystagmus, or ophthalmoplegia can be a warning sign of another neurologic issue. The presence of a Kayser-Fleischer ring, a brownish ring around the iris, can be a sign of Wilson's disease. Wilson's disease is a hereditary disease that causes copper to accumulate in the organs, including the brain. This can be a rare cause of abnormal behavior in children.

5. Ears

Other than checking for infection or effusion, there are no specific ear findings associated with PANS and PANDAS. As in autism, some children with PANS and PANDAS may develop severe sensitivity to sounds.

6. Nose

The nose should be checked for mucus (which could be from acute or chronic bacterial or fungal infections). The septum should be checked for deviation or for any inserted foreign bodies (like beads, food, or toys).

7. Lips and mouth

Dry lips can be a sign of dehydration. Open sores on the lips can be from herpes simplex 1 infection. Canker sores can be from viral infections, too, but are usually from food allergies or sensitivities. In our practice, we have discovered that carbonated sugary drinks like sodas are a common cause of canker sores.

8. Teeth

Dental decay is a common cause of flares. Flares may be seen after routine dental work and cleanings or with untreated dental decay. Metal fillings in teeth can be a source of heavy metals (mercury), which may affect the brain.

9. Throat

Strep infection may show up as any combination of swollen tonsils, red throat, white patches (pus) on the tonsils, or palatal petichiae. It is important to know that *Strep* infections and colonization may be present with no physical signs on exam and no throat symptoms.

10. Neck

The neck should be checked for swollen lymph nodes in the front and back. The thyroid should also be checked since autoimmune thyroid disease can sometimes cause thyromegaly.

11. Chest

The examination of the chest should start with looking at the ribs and spine (from the neck to the pelvis). Prominence of ribs may be seen during times of weight loss.

a. Auscultation

Many children have an innocent flow murmur. If there is any doubt about the murmur, an echocardiogram should be ordered to exclude congenital or rheumatic heart disease. The importance of heart auscultation is another reason an in-person physical exam is vital. This task cannot be performed remotely.

b. The lung exam

The lung exam is usually normal in PANS and PANDAS unless asthma or active infection is present.

12. The abdominal exam

The first step in the abdominal exam is a visual exam for abdominal swelling or distension. Auscultation for abnormal bowel sounds is next. Finally, the presence of hepatomegaly or splenomegaly or any tenderness in the abdomen should be noted. A visual genital with parents present exam may be undertaken after rapport is established with the child. A red ring around the outside of the rectum may signal a perianal *Strep* infection.

13. The extremity examination

The arms and legs should be examined to look for muscle mass and strength.

14. The neurologic examination
a. Mental status

PANS and PANDAS do not cause children to be sleepy or lethargic. Children with decreased mental status should be immediately referred to the ED for an urgent workup. Similarly, children who are becoming increasingly confused or violent also need to be seen urgently. Excluding structural or infectious causes of behavioral change in these children is vital.

b. Motor strength

New muscular weakness of any type is not a feature of PANS or PANDAS.

c. Romberg test

Children older than age eight should be able to cooperate with and should have a normal

Romberg exam. Piano-playing movements of the fingers may be seen in Sydenham chorea.

d. Gait examination

In most cases of PANS and PANDAS, the gait is normal. Abnormal or staggering gait may indicate a more serious neurologic problem and is also seen in Sydenham chorea.

e. Memory and concentration

These two components of the exam are best assessed by parent reports or changes in schoolwork.

15. The skin examination

There is no specific skin finding with PANS or PANDAS, although perianal *Strep* and other skin infections (like cellulitis or impetigo) can be triggers. Tenting of the skin can be a sign of dehydration. Dermatographia may be seen with allergies or mast cell activation.

16. Joint examination

Joint pain or swelling on examination can indicate an autoimmune disease like juvenile rheumatoid arthritis (JRA), although a nonspecific enthesitis is often seen in patients with PANS and PANDAS. Loose joints or increased flexibility can be from Ehlers-Danlos syndrome (EDS). This is a genetic disorder which results in abnormal collagen, which in turn leads to joint issues. Some variants of EDS predispose patients to vascular issues.[10]

CHAPTER 6 REFERENCES

1. www.hopkinsmedicine.org/health/conditions-and-diseases/fever, accessed on 4/17/2022.
2. Teng CL, Ng CJ, Nik-Sherina H, et al. The accuracy of mother's touch to detect fever in children: a systematic review. *Journal of Tropical Pediatrics*. 2008;54(1):70–73
3. Poirier MP, Collins EP, McGuire E. Fever phobia: a survey of caregivers of children seen in a pediatric emergency department. *Clin. Pediatr*. 2010;49:530–534
4. Richardson M, Purssell E. Who's afraid of fever? *Arch. Dis. Child*. 2015;100:818–820
5. Barbi E, Marzuillo P, Neri E, Naviglio S, Krauss BS. Fever in children: pearls and pitfalls. *Children* (Basel). 2017;4(9):1–19
6. Strengell T, Uhari M, Tarkka R, et al. Antipyretic agents for preventing recurrences of febrile seizures: randomized controlled trial. *Arch. Pediatr. Adolesc. Med*. 2009;163:799–804
7. www.seattlechildrens.org/conditions/a-z/fever-myths-versus-facts, accessed 4/17/2022
8. Dimova S, Hoet PH, Dinsdale D, et al. Acetaminophen decreases intracellular glutathione levels and modulates cytokine production in human alveolar macrophages and type II pneumocytes in vitro. *Int J Biochem Cell Biol*. 2005;37(8):1727–1737
9. Rousar T, Pařík P, Kucera O, et al. Glutathione reductase is inhibited by acetaminophen-glutathione conjugate in vitro. *Physiol Res*. 2010;59(2):225–232
10. www.ehlers-danlos.com/what-is-eds, accessed 4/24/2022

IDENTIFY: LABORATORY AND RADIOLOGY TESTING IN PANS AND PANDAS

A scientist in his laboratory is not a mere technician:
he is also a child confronting natural phenomena that
impress him as though they were fairy tales.
~ **MARIE CURIE**

KEY POINTS

▸ Lab and radiology testing is not required to establish the diagnosis of PANS or PANDAS but may help guide initial therapy and rule out other diagnoses
▸ Both conventional and high-quality specialty labs are needed for the most complete clinical picture
▸ Clinical training and experience are required to properly interpret labs and guide treatment
▸ Specialty consultation and radiology testing may be necessary in some cases
▸ Labs should be ordered only if they provide information which will change the treatment of the patient
▸ Conventional and specialty lab ordering information can be found in Appendix A

NOTE: *Before we draw labs in our office, we prescribe EMLA cream (a mixture of prilocaine and lidocaine). We send a diagram to show parents how to apply and cover with either 3M Tegaderm or plastic wrap. We have parents place this on both antecubital fossae about an hour before arriving at the office.*

As mentioned in Chapter 1, the diagnosis of PANS and PANDAS depends solely upon clinical criteria. Too often we have seen parents bring their children in who were told that their child does not have PANDAS because the *Strep* tests or ASO antibodies are negative during a flare. This is a basic misunderstanding of the pathophysiology of PANDAS. Most of the parents we see at our practice have already made the diagnosis of PANS or PANDAS based upon their own research.

So where does testing come in? Similar to the physical exam we discussed in Chapter 6, lab testing may help rule out other diseases which may look a bit like PANS and PANDAS but require very different treatments. Second testing provides valuable information to help guide us by giving a direction in which to pursue treatment—like a starting point. Testing can also help monitor changes in inflammation or total body burden of toxins or infections. Perhaps the most important principle is that we never delay treatment while waiting for lab results.

> **Never delay treatment while waiting for lab results.**

TWO IMPORTANT NOTES ON TESTING AND INTERPRETATION

First, there are thousands of laboratory tests available with more being developed every day. Some are considered "conventional" labs in that they are provided by large laboratory companies and hospitals. Others, called "specialty tests," may look for specific imbalances within the body or may be more sensitive than conventional tests. Specialty tests are typically supplied by private companies.

Direct-to-consumer specialty testing which does not require a physician's order should not be used alone, since some of these tests are not as accurate and may not provide useful information. Both conventional and high-quality specialty testing is required for the most complete picture when treating children with PANS and PANDAS.

Second, interpretation of laboratory test results (and correctly deciding what they actually mean) depends on both context and the experience of the ordering physician. For example, a very elevated white blood cell count could indicate a serious infection or leukemia, could be a laboratory error, or could simply be from stress or pain alone.

Figuring out what a test result means when applied to a specific patient should only be done by an experienced physician. Otherwise, the results could be misinterpreted as far more or far less serious than they actually are. For this reason, and because laboratory ranges differ with each lab and by country of origin, normal reference ranges will not be routinely discussed in this chapter.

Some coaching programs have sprung up which advertise that they will teach their students (with no prior medical training) how to interpret labs and provide treatment recommendations in a very short period of time. We caution our patients that these short training programs provide no context and a very simplified view of testing which can result in misinterpretation. Although Dr. Ellen Antoine and I have each been board certified, practicing physicians for over thirty years, we continue to refine our knowledge about the nuances of laboratory interpretation.

Simply put, a trained PANS and PANDAS physician is an absolute must for this portion of the Fully Functional process, to make sure lab testing is ordered and interpreted correctly.

The following tests are what we find most useful every day in our patients. Careful attention must be paid to the amount of blood drawn per patient. Due to the volume of tests, the blood tests needed may be split and patients may need to be brought back 1–2 weeks later to complete the draw. This is further discussed in Appendix A.

> **Blood tests needed may be split and patients may need to be brought back 1–2 weeks later to complete the draw.**

LABORATORY TESTING

NOTE: *This chapter discusses conventional and specialty testing, but not testing for infections, which is discussed in Chapters 8 and 9.*

1. Complete blood count (CBC)

Since an elevated white blood cell count *may or may not* indicate infection, and since the white blood cell count can remain low, even in the face of a significant infection, it is best to use this as a trend to follow rather than an absolute indicator of health or disease. Some infections which may act as triggers for PANS can lower the white blood cell count (like EBV). Low hemoglobin and/or hematocrit can be from bleeding, nutritional deficiencies, malnutrition, diseases which affect nutrient absorption like celiac disease, and some hereditary disorders. Platelets are typically normal in patients with PANS or PANDAS.

2. Comprehensive metabolic panel (CMP)

The CMP can help look for liver issues (sometimes seen in toxic exposures, fatty liver, or infections like Epstein-Barr virus), dehydration (elevated BUN or creatinine, low GFR, elevated sodium, elevated chloride, low bicarbonate), and elevated blood sugar. A low albumin level in the blood may indicate inadequate protein levels in the body from food restriction, a protein-poor diet, or malabsorption.

3. High sensitivity C-reactive protein (hs-CRP)

The hs-CRP is a measure of total body inflammation. The value should ideally be below 1, but many labs list a normal value as anything below 3. Elevated CRP is seen in about 20% of our patients with PANS and PANDAS. In adults, values above 3 have been associated with a risk for cardiovascular disease.[1] The erythrocyte sedimentation rate (ESR) is sometimes used to measure inflammation in humans, but we don't typically use this as it is not as specific as the hs-CRP. Since the CRP is nonspecific, does not change management, and is only positive in 20% of our patients, we don't routinely check hs-CRP to help reduce the amount of blood we collect.

4. HLA-DQ2 and HLA-DQ8 antibody testing

This is a blood test for genes that indicate increased risk for celiac disease. If one or both are abnormal, the risk of celiac disease is increased. Even if they are abnormal, however, it does not mean that a patient has active celiac disease. This requires additional testing as below.

> **Celiac disease is a common cause of iron deficiency.**

5. Celiac antibody panel

The celiac antibody blood panel tests several things. The most significant is the tissue transglutaminase IgA level. If a patient has an elevated tissue transglutaminase IgA (TTG-IgA) and abnormal HLA gene(s) along with symptoms suggestive of celiac disease, this is considered positive for celiac. The diagnosis can be definitively confirmed by small bowel biopsy, but patients who have positive genetics with elevated IgA antibodies and symptoms should be advised that celiac disease is very likely, and gluten should be avoided strictly. There are several other antibodies in the panel which, if elevated, don't indicate celiac. In our experience,

these other antibodies are commonly elevated in cases of significant gluten sensitivity. The panel also contains a total IgA level. If the IgA level is below the normal range and the TTG-IgA is normal, the test is considered nondiagnostic since the test relies on the IgA level to TTG.

6. Iron, TIBC, and ferritin

The iron and TIBC are blood tests used to look for iron deficiency. The ferritin is also low in iron deficiency and may drop before the serum iron does. Ferritin can also act as a measure of inflammation. It can be significantly elevated in chronic illness, acute inflammatory diseases like infections, and hemochromatosis. Iron levels can be low due to poor intake, blood loss, or in situations where there is poor intestinal absorption. Celiac disease is a common cause of iron deficiency.

7. 25-OH vitamin D levels

Vitamin D is actually a steroid hormone, not a vitamin. There are many receptors for this hormone in the body. Vitamin D helps control blood calcium levels and is vital to immune function.[2] Multiple studies have shown that significant proportions of adults are deficient in vitamin D (25-OH vitamin D level <20 ng/mL).[3,4] We have found that many children are deficient as well.

Vitamin D exists in several forms in the body, but 25-OH vitamin D is the most useful to measure as it accurately reflects tissue levels.[5] Even though the lower limit of normal lab values for 25-OH vitamin D are often listed as 20 ng/mL, the optimal level for the favorable extra-skeletal benefits of vitamin D is likely around 60 ng/mL.[6–8]

We generally recommend levels of 50–70 ng/mL in children with normal kidney function. Even though most complications from vitamin D toxicity occur at 25-OH vitamin D levels of >200 ng/ mL, most of the current literature defines the safe upper limit in the blood to be 100–120 ng/mL.[9]

Researchers have found an inverse relationship between vitamin D levels and depression and anxiety.[10,11] An inverse relationship between vitamin D levels and the incidence of ADHD has been seen as well.[12–14] One study showed an inverse relationship between serum vitamin D levels and OCD.[15] One Norwegian study[16] of children with PANDAS showed higher rates of vitamin D deficiency in children with PANDAS as compared to controls.

8. Thyroid hormone testing

In children without known thyroid disease, we measure blood levels of TSH, free T4, and thyroid antibodies (anti-thyroglobulin antibodies and thyroid peroxidase antibodies). The normal blood level of TSH is usually listed as between 0.5 and 5 mU/ L. In adults, optimal levels are around 1.5 mU/ L. TSH levels may be at the higher range of normal in children since they are growing and there is more of a demand on their body metabolically. Free T4 measures the actual unbound T4 thyroid hormone. Normal values vary. If outside the reference range, a free T3 and reverse T3 are measured as well.

Free T4 must be converted to free T3 (by removing one iodine) before it binds to body tissue receptors. Reverse T3 (rT3) is a stereo-isomer and an inactive form of T3. It can bind to receptors but does not work like the normal isomer of T3.[17] Reverse T3 levels can increase in conditions of stress, such as chronic inflammation, starvation, cancer, and critical illness.

Sometimes the TSH can be normal with low free T3 and normal T4. This is sometimes called the *euthyroid sick syndrome.* In these cases, the TSH is normal even though Free T3 is low because the rT3 is elevated.[18] Anti-thyroglobulin antibodies (ATG antibodies) and thyroid peroxidase antibodies (TPO antibodies), when elevated, indicate autoimmune thyroid disease (Hashimoto's thyroiditis).

There is a form of autoimmune thyroiditis which can cause neuropsychiatric changes. It is

> Researchers have found an inverse relationship between vitamin D levels and depression and anxiety.

called steroid-responsive encephalopathy associated with autoimmune thyroiditis (SREAT). Patients with SREAT can present with altered mental status, seizures, or psychosis. SREAT does not clinically resemble PANS or PANDAS, as significantly altered mental status is a hallmark of this disorder. It is correctable with high-dose IV steroid medication.[19]

If a low TSH and high T3 is noted, additional testing for hyperthyroidism should be considered. Hypothyroidism can cause confusion, depression, or a lack of focus, while hyperthyroidism can cause neuropsychiatric changes such as anxiety or mania.

9. Copper and ceruloplasmin levels

Wilson's disease[20,21] is a genetic disorder in which people do not eliminate copper from the body. The buildup of copper damages the liver and brain. It can also cause neuropsychiatric changes. Ceruloplasmin is a copper storage protein in the blood. If ceruloplasmin levels are significantly low, genetic testing and a twenty-four-hour urinary copper level can be performed. Copper levels may also be low in Wilson's disease. If liver damage has occurred, the serum copper may be elevated. Definitive diagnosis relies on liver biopsy.

10. Antinuclear antibody (ANA) testing

About 40% of children with PANS or PANDAS have an elevated ANA level. Significant elevation of the ANA titer with altered mental status suggests lupus cerebritis rather than PANS or PANDAS. Patients suspected of having lupus cerebritis need urgent evaluation and treatment in a hospital setting.

In children with significant joint pain, anti-CCP antibodies and rheumatoid factor are tested as well. In our practice, many patients with an ANA that was initially elevated have a negative value on retesting when their symptoms have improved. In this way, the ANA can serve as a measure of immune system dysregulation.

11. Quantitative total immunoglobulins (IgA, IgM, IgG) with IgG and IgA subclasses

Studies have shown that low levels of at least one of these immunoglobulins is seen in about 48% of patients with PANS and PANDAS.[22] When low levels of immunoglobulins are seen in patients with frequent illness (of the ears, nose, sinuses, or lungs), this supports the diagnosis of common variable immunodeficiency (CVID). This test is useful to obtain because CVID is a diagnosis which is approved as an indication for IVIG.

12. Pneumococcal antibody testing and diphtheria/tetanus IgG antibody testing

Fully vaccinated children should have measurable levels of antibodies to these immunizations. The pneumococcal vaccines typically contain proteins from multiple different strains of pneumococcal bacteria. One of the tests we commonly order (in addition to diphtheria and tetanus IgG antibody titers) is a "23 serotypes test." If any of these three tests show inadequate antibody production, it may indicate an immune deficient state known as "specific antibody deficiency."

IVIG is also approved to treat patients with specific antibody deficiency with frequent infections. If the initial 23 serotypes test shows a lack of antibodies, immunologists commonly request repeat immunization with pneumococcal vaccine and retesting of levels after a month. We don't usually advocate active immunization during an autoimmune PANS or PANDAS flare, so repeat testing is not usually an option at that time.

13. Autoimmune encephalitis antibody panel

These panels measure antibodies to neuronal structures. If titers are elevated, this indicates autoimmunity to structures in the central nervous system. We use a test from LabCorp for this purpose. It is called the autoimmune encephalopathy panel. It tests twenty-three different antibodies, including GAD-65 and NMDA-R antibodies. We mainly use it to try to exclude these other forms of encephalopathy which may require different treatments. They are not usually positive in PANS and PANDAS patients unless other disease entities exist.

There is another commercially available test called the Cunningham panel. It measures four anti-neuronal antibodies and calcium/calmodulin-dependent protein kinase 2 (CaMKII) activity. We rarely use this test, not because it is an inaccurate test, but because it does not change management at all. It is also expensive and not covered by insurance.

There is an erroneous belief among some parent groups (and possibly some clinicians) that the Cunningham panel is a required part of the workup for PANS and PANDAS, and that a positive Cunningham panel "proves" you have PANS or PANDAS. This is not the case. On the company's website, they state that the sensitivity of the test is 88% and the specificity is 83%, so the test may be falsely negative 12% of the time and falsely positive 17% of the time. The company lists the PANS and PANDAS diagnostic criteria on their website, which, as discussed in Chapter 1, are composed solely of signs and symptoms. PANS and PANDAS are clinical diagnoses.

> About 40% of children with PANS or PANDAS have an elevated ANA level.

The one time we may use the test is if we are working on getting IVIG approved. If we have had a denial, we may order the panel and, if positive, use it at the peer-to-peer consultation to try to get IVIG approved.

14. Transforming growth factor beta 1 (TGFβ-1)

Human TGFβ-1 is a marker of inflammation within the body. It inhibits activity of natural killer cells, which are a type of white blood cell that helps fight against infections.[23] It is also involved in suppression of the immune response.[24,25]

TGFβ-1 receptors are found on virtually every body tissue. Levels are increased in patients with Epstein-Barr virus and some cancers.[26] Blood levels of TGFβ-1 are also elevated in patients with neuroinflammatory diseases (like progressive multiple sclerosis).[27] There is also some connection between TGFβ-1 and neuroborreliosis (Lyme disease affecting the brain).[28]

Since TGFβ-1 is a natural anti-inflammatory compound in the body, it will be elevated in response to inflammation. Lack of elevation has been noted in patients who went on to develop symptoms of chronic Lyme disease. Clinically, we find that TGFβ-1 levels are elevated in patients with mold exposure, although the experimental evidence of this from peer-reviewed references has not yet been seen.

Since there are several infections (and likely mold exposure) that elevate the TGFβ-1 levels, it is not a marker which *proves* any single diagnosis. It is best used as a marker of progress or trends. For these reasons, TGFβ-1 is not a must-have lab study. In the past, we considered levels >2800 pg/mL abnormal. Some conventional labs recently increased the upper limits of normal on their assays. We are currently collecting data to see how this reference range change affects test interpretation and utility. Trends in serial measurements are typically more valuable than the absolute numbers.

15. Complement C4a

The complement system is part of the innate immune system.

Complement proteins are proteins that float around in the bloodstream. In the bloodstream they are actually "pro-proteins," which means they contain additional attached sections that must be cleaved off by enzymes before they are active. When an immune response is triggered, the complement proteins are cleaved or trimmed, and the proteins become active. There are many different complement proteins.

Complement pathways amplify the immune response and lead to the death of invading organ-

> C4a (like TGFβ-1) tends to go up when patients are ill with either infection or toxin exposure and go down when they recover.

isms. Complement C4a levels are much higher after exercise in patients with chronic fatigue syndrome (CFS) than they are in sedentary patients without CFS.[29] Blood levels of C4a are also increased in patients with Alzheimer's disease.[30]

Both complement C3a and C4a have been linked to Lyme disease in observational studies.[31] Clinically, we find that elevated C4a levels are seen in concert with mold exposures. As with TGFβ-1, the literature support is not strong, and the concept is based upon clinical experience. In our practice we have found that C4a (like TGFβ-1) tends to go up when patients are ill with either infection or toxin exposure and go down when they recover.

It is most useful to look at the trend of this lab rather than an absolute number. Because it can be elevated from several different causes, an elevated level does not lead to one specific diagnosis. For this reason, C4a is not a must-have lab study.

Some practitioners state that C4a must be shipped to a particular lab in the United States to be accurately processed. There is, however, no published data which describes the reasoning behind this or proves that this is necessary. In our practice, trends in C4a measurements from conventional labs like LabCorp tend to track well with patient symptoms and known mold exposures or infections. Many labs that are unfamiliar with this test will mistakenly run a complement C4 (which is not useful in this case) in error. Some labs may not have the reagents necessary; it is best to verify this before drawing the lab. We consider C4a levels less than 2800 ng/mL (through LabCorp) to be normal. We do not routinely measure C3a as we have not found it as useful, and eliminating it helps decrease the amount of blood taken and the subsequent patient expense.

Some conventional labs are currently in the process of changing reference ranges for complement C4a. It appears that the upper limits of normal for this test may soon be increased from 650 ng/ mL (currently) to as high as 22,000. This is reportedly due to changes in ELISA testing methodology. Whether this reference range change has to do with increased rates of inflammation among the population or whether it is due to differences in the assay is unknown. As with any similar change, the impact of these changes upon the accuracy and clinical application of these tests is not known at this time.

16. Heavy metals

As noted in Chapter 5, exposure to heavy metals is harmful to the human brain and many other tissues in the body. Conventional testing for heavy metals like lead, mercury, and arsenic involves measurement of blood levels through companies like LabCorp or Quest Diagnostics.

Although some sources[32] question the accuracy of hair testing for heavy metals, the US Environmental Protection Agency (EPA) reports that hair testing for heavy metals, if properly conducted, is an accurate method of measurement.[33] The EPA states:

> It appears to be that if hair and nail samples are collected, cleaned, and analyzed properly with the best analytical methods under controlled conditions by experienced personnel, the data are valid. Human hair and nails have been found to be meaningful and representative tissues for biological monitoring for most of these toxic metals.

Hair testing is available from Mosaic Diagnostics (formerly Great Plains lab) and Doctor's Data. Both are CLIA-certified laboratories. We don't use hair testing in our practice.

Urine testing for heavy metals is available from LabCorp and Quest Diagnostics. Both twenty-four-hour tests and spot testing are available. Urine tests are also available from Mosaic Diagnostics and Doctor's Data as well. In our practice, we use the Metabolomix urine test from Genova Diagnostics. It gives a spot test for multiple heavy metals. If any of the initial heavy metal testing is positive, confirmatory testing may be performed. We do not use provoked heavy metal testing in children.

17. Nonmetal toxins

Tests for "nonmetal toxins" such as glyphosate and solvent-based, industrial chemicals, are available from several specialty labs. We do not recommend these tests since there are no specific antidotes or chelating agents for these chemicals, so the testing does not change our management. General detoxification measures, as discussed in Chapter 17, are sufficient in these cases.

18. Nutrients

Nutrients can be divided into macronutrients (protein, fat, carbohydrates), B vitamins, antioxidants (vitamins A, E, K, C, glutathione, CoQ10,

> **Studies suggest a role for magnesium in the treatment of depression and anxiety.**

and alpha lipoic acid), minerals (magnesium and zinc), essential fatty acids, and essential amino acids. Adequate nutrients are vitally important for the body to perform the vital processes of life. They are especially important in the process of making and regulating neurotransmitters and the immune system. Vitamin D is not included here since it is tested mainly on LabCorp or Quest labs as noted previously. Nutrients can be measured through LabCorp and Quest where noted. For new patients, we use a specialty lab called Metabolomix by Genova Diagnostics, which measures levels of all the nutrients in this section. To follow up on these values, we may use LabCorp or Quest testing.

a. Magnesium[34]

Magnesium is a cofactor for more than three hundred biochemical (enzymatic) reactions in the body. It is essential for proper nerve conduction and reduces excitotoxicity in the central nervous system, which can cause apoptosis. An increase in excitatory neurotransmitters (excitotoxicity) has been implicated in OCD.[35]

Studies suggest a role for magnesium in the treatment of depression and anxiety.[34] Lower nutritional intake of magnesium is directly associated with increases in the incidence of depression.[36,37] Perspectives on the role of magnesium in mental health are well documented in a review article from French researchers.[38] A study in a mouse model has shown conclusively that lower magnesium levels are associated with anxiety and HPA axis dysfunction.[39] Magnesium deficiency has been associated with sleep disorders, including frequent waking.[40,41]

Magnesium can be measured in standard labs from LabCorp or Quest. Red blood cell magnesium (RBC magnesium) levels are generally considered more representative of total body magnesium status than plain serum magnesium levels since magnesium stores can be significantly depleted before the serum level drops.[42] Low RBC magnesium levels have been demonstrated in patients with chronic fatigue syndrome.[43] Optimal RBC magnesium is between 4.2–6.8 mg/dL.

b. Zinc

Like magnesium, zinc is a mineral that is a vital cofactor for hundreds of enzymatic functions in the body.[44] It is important for proper functioning of the immune system and controls cellular proliferation and division.[45] There is a role for zinc supplementation in patients with depression and psychosis, even if serum levels are normal as there may be genetic mutations which affect zinc transporter molecules.[46] Several prescription medications used for psychiatric disorders can impede zinc absorption.[47] Zinc exhibits an inhibitory effect in the limbic region of the brain by acting as an inhibitory modulator at the NMDA glutamate receptor.[47] Adding zinc to fluoxetine has been shown to significantly decrease OCD when compared with placebo plus fluoxetine.[48]

Patients with elevated serum copper to zinc ratios have higher levels of anxiety.[49] An optimal copper to zinc ratio is about 1:1. Increased copper to zinc ratio has been associated with decreased

> **Vitamin B6 supplementation can reduce anxiety and appears helpful in depression.**

educational development.[50]

Serum zinc levels are available at LabCorp and Quest. The optimal range of values for zinc is 80–115 μg/dL. Some sources advocate checking red blood cell zinc levels as they are thought to be more accurate. There is no evidence that this is true, although serum levels decrease in response to inflammation or illness and RBC values do not.[51] If we follow up on these levels after the initial visit, we measure serum levels through a conventional lab.

d. Vitamin B6[52]

Vitamin B6 (pyridoxine) is a water-soluble vitamin. It is also known as pyridoxal-5-phosphate ("P-5-P"). It is a cofactor for more than a hundred enzymatic reactions. B6 is involved in metabolic reactions and the biosynthesis of neurotransmitters. It also supports healthy sleep. Vitamin B6 supplementation can reduce anxiety and appears helpful in depression.[53] Deficiencies in vitamins B2, B6, and B9 have been associated with ADHD in adults, and B6 levels specifically are inversely associated with symptom severity.[54] Optimal vitamin B6 levels are 5.1–65 μg/ L. This nutrient is measured by LabCorp and Quest. Caution is warranted as doses of vitamin B6 greater than 500 mg daily, over time can result in toxicity, which can cause neuropathy and ataxia.[55,56]

> **B12 deficiency and high homocysteine has been associated with OCD.**

e. Vitamin B9 (folate)[57]

Folate is a water-soluble vitamin that is needed to make DNA and other genetic material. Folate deficiency can cause megaloblastic anemia, weakness, and depression. Individuals who have significant MTHFR SNP mutations (tested via LabCorp, Quest, or other specialty labs) have difficulty converting dietary folate or folic acid supplements to 5-methylenetetrahydrofolate, which is the active form. This SNP can result in lower red cell folate levels.[58]

Research has shown that homozygous mutations of the MTHFR gene (677) may be associated with depression.[59] Lower levels of folate have been noted in patients with OCD.[60] Optimal levels of folate in the blood are >7.1 ng/mL. Red cell folate measurements are available but do not correlate as well with homocysteine levels or as a measurement of the adequacy of supplementation.[61,62] It is also more costly and is difficult to standardize.

f. Vitamin B12 (cobalamin)

Vitamin B12 (cobalamin) is a water-soluble vitamin that has a role in the formation of red blood cells and genetic material and is vital to neurologic function.[63] Deficiency of B12 can be caused by a lack of stomach acid and/or intrinsic factor. The use of PPIs and H2 blockers have been associated with B12 deficiency.[64]

In addition to macrocytic anemia, B12 deficiency can cause neuropathy, fatigue, confusion, and dementia. The combination of B12 deficiency and high homocysteine has been associated with OCD.[65,66] Serum B12 levels are available, but high methylmalonic acid (MMA) levels combined with elevated homocysteine are more accurate in measuring B12 deficiency than serum B12 levels.[67–69] Elevation of both MMA and homocysteine is an earlier predictor of subclinical B12 deficiency. Both LabCorp and Quest offer serum B12 levels, MMA levels, and homocysteine levels.

g. Glutathione

Glutathione (also known as γ-glutamyl-cysteinyl-glycine or GSH) is the body's master antioxidant and detoxifier. It is manufactured from the amino acids glycine, cysteine, and glutamate. It actually recycles other antioxidants so that they can neutralize oxidants. Glutathione levels can be measured through LabCorp or Quest or with specialty labs.

We further discuss the role of glutathione in the management of oxidative stress in Chapter

12 and its role in the biotransformation (detoxification) of compounds in Chapter 17.

19. Oxidative stress

Our body generates reactive oxygen species (ROS) like hydrogen peroxide, superoxide, and peroxynitrite through normal metabolic reactions. These are also known as free radicals or oxidants. High levels of oxidants can also be a result of exposure to environmental pollutants or from cooking fats like vegetable oils at high heats. Charred foods and processed foods are high in oxidants as well. If the amount of oxidants in the body outweighs the levels of antioxidants, a condition known as oxidative stress occurs. Oxidative stress is damaging to many bodily tissues and has been implicated in a wide range of disorders, including psychiatric and neurodegenerative disorders.

Metabolomix testing from Genova Diagnostics can demonstrate oxidative stress if levels of 8-OHdG or lipid peroxides are elevated.

For complete discussion of the effects of oxidative stress and strategies with which to manage it, see Chapter 12.

20. Organic acid testing

Levels of organic acids (like lactic acid, succinic acid, oxalic acid, etc.) provide objective measurements of metabolic efficiency in the body. They can provide evidence of yeast overgrowth, intestinal malabsorption, and efficiency of mitochondrial function. These markers should be viewed as trends rather than true diagnostic markers that rule in or rule out disease.

Specific interpretation of trends for these markers is beyond the scope of this book, but guides for interpretation with scientific references can be obtained from Genova Diagnostics.

Genova Diagnostics and Mosaic Diagnostics both provide test panels to measure organic acids and measures of oxidative stress. We use the Metabolomix test from Genovato measure organic acids, oxidative stress, and nutrients.

21. Stool testing

In residency, we were taught to order stool testing to look for pathogenic bacteria and parasites when patients have obvious GI complaints like diarrhea. We were also taught to test stool for C. diff toxin and for the presence of occult blood.

More comprehensive stool testing is valuable for both diagnostic and therapeutic reasons in patients with PANS and PANDAS.

Even though investigation of the human intestinal microbiome (the microorganisms located in the human intestines) and its contribution to health and disease is ongoing, the current medical literature contains strong evidence for the vital role of the microbiome to the human body. Although we often think of intestinal bacteria when we speak of the microbiome, it also contains viruses, parasites, fungi, and archaea.[70]

It was once thought that the microbiome was just composed of commensal organisms living in

> One of the main jobs of the intestinal microbiome is to train the human immune system and move it toward maturity.

the gut and sharing the food supply of humans without interacting with us. In recent years it has become increasingly clear that the microbiome/human relationship is actually symbiotic, with rich connections between the microbiome and its human host.

The brain communicates with the microbiome via cortical input to the intestines. The organisms of the microbiome communicate with the brain through chemical diffusion via the vagus nerve afferent fibers.[71] This two-way communication is known as the microbiota-gut-brain axis.[72] The number of organisms in the gut microbiome outnumbers the number of cells in the human body by a factor of ten to one and the number of bacterial genes is one hundred times greater than the amount of human genes in the entire body.[73–75]

One of the main jobs of the intestinal microbiome is to train the human immune system and move it toward maturity.[73,76] The microbiome regulates T-cell differentiation and Th1/ Th2 balance and Th17/Treg balance.[74–75]

Th1 immune reactions in general are involved in cellmediated immunity, which uses natural killer cells and cytotoxic T-cells. This helps clear infections. Th2 immune responses are involved with B-cell antibody production and thus prevention of infections. Th1 and Th2 cells secrete different cytokines. Although they are involved in distinct types of immune reactions, each has the ability to modulate activities of the other arm of this system. There should be a balance of the Th1/Th2 responses. If there is imbalance,

predisposition toward specific immune disorders may occur.[77] A Th2 dominant system can result in increased allergic-type immune reactions. It is important to note that the effect of the microbiome on the immune system is not localized to the gut. It also has a regulatory effect on systemic immune function and maturation.[77]

In addition to its role in immune function and maturation, the microbiome is involved in "programming" the stress response and helps regulate the HPA (hypothalamic, pituitary, adrenal) axis.[72,73,78] There is strong evidence that the microbiome functions as a key regulator for our stress pathways.[73] The intestinal microbiome is responsible for the production and regulation of neurotransmitters, neurotransmitter precursors, and neuroactive chemicals, including tryptophan, serotonin, acetylcholine, melatonin, catecholamines, GABA, dopamine, and histamine.[71–73] Disruption of the microbiome can affect the dynamic balance of these chemicals, which may further affect the stress response. Conversely, stress of various types can impact the microbiome and gut function.

> The role of the microbiome in the pathogenesis of neurologic and psychiatric disorders has been well documented.

The role of the microbiome in the pathogenesis of neurologic and psychiatric disorders has been well documented.[71–73,78] This association has been established for anxiety,[72,78] depression,[71,73,78] schizophrenia,[71,73,78] autism,[78] memory loss,[78] and ADHD.[71] There is a hypothesis that disruption of the microbiome may play a role in the etiology of OCD in patients with PANS and PANDAS.[79]

Several studies have demonstrated that prebiotics and various strains of probiotics are effective at improving symptoms of psychiatric disorders and HPA axis functionality in both animal and human subjects.[72,73,78] SSRIs, antipsychotics, and benzodiazepines may improve symptoms in patients with neuropsychiatric disorders due to their known antimicrobial properties.[71,73] It is also likely that changes in the microbiome contribute to the development of Parkinson's disease in some patients.[84]

There is a mountain of evidence that shows that alterations in the intestinal microbiome are involved

> **Extensive evidence has confirmed the link between increased intestinal permeability and various childhood diseases**

in the development of autoimmunity.[71,74–77,81–83] This includes both extra-intestinal autoimmunity as well as autoimmune diseases involving the gut, such as Crohn's disease and ulcerative colitis. One mechanism by which this autoimmunity develops is molecular mimicry.[74,76,83–90]

As previously noted, molecular mimicry occurs when there are structural similarities in host and microbial proteins. The immune system then attacks host tissue rather than just microbes. This can occur with some commensal organisms and with pathologic organisms like *Streptococcus pyogenes*. In PANDAS, antibodies to *Streptococcal* bacteria cross the blood-brain barrier and attack the basal ganglia.[91,92] These antibodies are also known as anti-tubulin antibodies. For further discussion, see Chapter 2.

There is evidence that there are differences in composition of the microbiome in patients with neuropsychiatric disorders and healthy controls.[73] Increased amounts of *Akkermansia mucinophila* and Th17-inducing-inducing *Streptococcal* species and decreased levels of *Prevotella* and *Parabacteroides* have been found in patients with multiple sclerosis.[76,81–83] Treatment with immunomodulatory agents in these patients has been shown to return the quantity of these bacteria to more normal levels with lower amounts of *Akkermansia* and higher amounts of *Prevotella* species.[76]

Research from the 1960s has demonstrated that patients with rheumatoid arthritis have higher levels of *Clostridium perfringens*.[76,82] A decrease in the ratio of firmiculites/ bacteroidetes has been found in patients with both lupus and type 1 diabetes.[81–83]

Diet-induced microbial population differences have been noted in people from different parts of the world, which may account for differences in the rates of inflammation and obesity.[77] Increased rates of intestinal colonization with *Candida albicans* have been shown in patients with type 1 diabetes,[82] and colonization may be linked to the development of autism spectrum disorders.[78]

Another significant factor in the development of both intestinal and systemic autoimmune conditions is increased intestinal permeability.[75,76,82,83] When permeability changes occur, luminal antigens and bacterial products pass into the lamina propria.[76,82]

Increased intestinal permeability is known in common parlance as "leaky gut." The concept of increased intestinal permeability has been dismissed by some in the medical establishment even though the evidence for the association of various diseases with this phenomenon has been well described for more than thirty years. Extensive evidence has confirmed the link between increased intestinal permeability and various childhood diseases such as eczema,[93] Crohn's disease,[94] celiac disease,[94] food allergies,[95] environmental allergies,[96] irritable bowel syndrome,[97] juvenile arthritis,[98] autism,[99] asthma,[100] type 1 diabetes,[101] ADHD,[102] Hashimoto's thyroid-

> **Butyrate regulates the size and function of the T-cell immune network in the gut.**

itis,[103] childhood obesity,[104] and COVID-related multisystem inflammatory syndrome in children (MIS-C).[105,106]

Short-chain fatty acids (SCFAs) such as butyrate, acetate, and propionate are metabolites exclusively produced by the intestinal microbiome. They are important for brain health.[73] SCFAs are involved with the interaction of microbes with host cells to induce cytokine release and also the translocation of microbial products to interact with the brain directly.[71,76,80] Reductions in SCFAs have consistently been reported in patients with Parkinson's disease.[80]

Butyrate administration has been shown to enhance remyelination in mice with experimentally induced MS.[76] SCFAs are considered to be anti-inflammatory and are significantly increased in patients with healthier ("non-Western")

diets.[77] Lower fiber diets lead to deficiencies of SCFAs. SCFAs are a source of energy for intestinal epithelial cells and microbes, influence the permeability of tight junctions, and affect host immunity.[82,83] Butyrate, specifically, regulates the size and function of the T-cell immune network in the gut.[75]

Secretory immunoglobulin A (SIgA) is produced by the human gut. It is involved in a process of immune exclusion by which it helps protect the human host from pathogenic microorganisms.[75,107] Reductions in SIgA are a good indicator of the immune state; decreased levels can be used as a surrogate marker for increased intestinal permeability. Studies in germ-free mice have shown that supplementation with Saccharomyces can promote release of SIgA.[108]

Fecal calprotectin, lactoferrin, and lysozyme are inflammatory stool markers which are elevated in the presence of significant GI inflammation. Elevated levels are often seen with inflammatory bowel diseases such as Crohn's disease and ulcerative colitis.[109–111]

Stool testing through most conventional laboratories provides testing for a limited number of pathogens, as well as perhaps testing for ova and parasites. There is much more useful information that can be gained from more detailed stool testing from companies such as Doctor's Data. The comprehensive stool analysis test from Doctor's Data is a three-day test which reports relative amounts of bacterial species, including beneficial bacteria, pathologic bacteria, and commensals. It also tests for parasites, yeast overgrowth, lactoferrin, calprotectin, lysozyme, short-chain fatty acids, pH, and occult blood. If pathologic bacteria or yeast are found, the test will also include susceptibility testing for prescription antimicrobials and natural compounds. Stool testing should not be performed in the absence of GI symptoms in patients with contamination OCD as this may worsen symptoms. Antibiotics, antifungals, and probiotics must be held to perform the testing for at least a week to avoid adversely affecting the results.

22. Urine mycotoxin testing

We outlined the role of mycotoxins and mold exposure with neuropsychiatric disorders and immune dysregulation in Chapter 5. We use urine testing to look for mycotoxins in the body. We have found that levels correlate with both exposure and symptoms as well as immune dysregulation.

We give the patient glutathione orally every day for about a week before the test. On the day of the test, the patient takes an additional bolus of oral glutathione and then collects urine for six hours at home. Details of the dosage we use can be found in Appendix B. The test is then sent to the testing company.

The best urine mycotoxin testing we have found is offered by Mosaic Diagnostics and Real-time Labs. We most commonly use the urine mycotoxin test from Realtime Labs.

23. Mold antibody testing

Within the past few years, some companies have begun to offer IgG antibody testing for mold exposures. We have not found any good literature support for this testing. For this reason, we do not use this testing modality.

24. Hormone testing

Sex hormone testing is not needed unless there are signs of precocious puberty or significant menstrual irregularities, or in the case of older children with food restriction (fat restriction) who may have low sex hormones (hormone production requires adequate levels of fat and cholesterol). Standard labs have reference ranges by age and sex.

25. Food allergy and sensitivity testing

Just as some foods like gluten and refined sugars can add to the inflammatory burden and worsen symptoms, food allergies and sensitivities can also cause inflammation and symptoms of IBS.[112] Food allergy testing can be performed through conventional labs such as LabCorp or Quest.

> **Eliminating foods based upon IgG reactions improves symptoms in patients with IBS, Crohn's disease, ulcerative colitis, and migraine headache.**

In our practice we use testing from Alletess. This lab provides testing for IgE food reactions (true allergies) for multiple foods. Alletess also provides testing for IgG food reactions. These are not true allergies since they are not IgE mediated. Some people consider IgG reactions to be food sensitivities or intolerances.

IgG food testing is not widely accepted as IgG reactions are sometimes considered to be normal immune responses.[113] However, the current literature shows that eliminating foods based upon IgG reactions improves symptoms in patients with IBS,[114] Crohn's disease,[115] ulcerative colitis,[116] and migraine headache.[117,118] In addition to the medical literature noted above, we have found similar trends in our adult and pediatric population in our practice.

Multiple food reactions (IgE or IgG) also provide indirect evidence of increased intestinal permeability.[119] When patient testing reveals multiple food or environmental allergies, Th2 immune dominance is suggested, which is a form of immune dysregulation.

Food allergy and sensitivity testing should never be performed in the absence of anaphylaxis in patients with food restriction. Patients with severe OCD without food restriction may start restricting excessively if they become aware of food test results. If we do perform IgG testing, we may choose not to eliminate all reactive foods, as management of patients with PANS and PANDAS sometimes means picking your battles. Since IgG food reactions cannot lead to anaphylaxis, a more liberal approach here may go a long way to patient cooperation and parental peace.

26. Urine pyrroles

In 1958, Dr. Abram Hoffer proposed that elevated levels of chemicals called "pyrroles" in the body were linked to mental health disorders. He measured a substance in the urine of his patients with mental health disorders which was called the "mauve factor."[120] The substances he measured were also known as "kryptopyrroles" or simply "pyrroles." Some practitioners suggest measuring urinary pyrroles in patients with neuropsychiatric symptoms. This test is available from many conventional labs. Proponents of this concept state that high urine pyrroles (known as pyroluria) are indicative of low levels of zinc and vitamin B6, and that replacing these nutrients will resolve neuropsychiatric complaints. The issue is that Dr. Hoffer's findings have not been replicated when tested through the years.[121,122]

Even if this theory had merit, testing for something that will not change what you do clinically does not make sense. Most of the patients we see are at least given a multivitamin with more than adequate amounts of vitamin B6 and zinc. It appears that the concept of pyrroluria is an example of a theory often repeated without questioning by some clinicians. For these reasons, we do not use this test.

RADIOLOGY TESTING

Whenever we start a clinical encounter with a patient with neuropsychiatric complaints, the first clinical question we answer is whether these symptoms could stem from a structural issue, such as a tumor. If there is any doubt at all, or if a patient with PANS or PANDAS is not getting better despite treatment, we order an MRI of the brain. We do not routinely use contrast for this study.

Younger children may require sedation. Pediatric specialty hospitals often have a sedation service for younger children needing these types of studies. These services sedate the children and closely monitor them for safety during the procedure.

SPECIALIST CONSULTATION

We refer children with frank dysphagia (as opposed to just "feeling like they can't swallow") to pediatric gastroenterology for an evaluation to see if they need endoscopy.

Extremely agitated or aggressive patients who may benefit from a trial of psychiatric medications are referred to psychiatry. Psychology consultation can be entertained if formal neuropsychological testing is desired to help support the ability to obtain an IEP at school.

CHAPTER 7 REFERENCES

1. Lagrand WK, Visser CA, Hermens WT, et al. C-reactive protein as a cardiovascular risk factor: more than an epiphenomenon? *Circulation*. 1999;100(1):96–102

2. Norman AW. From vitamin D to hormone D: fundamentals of the vitamin D endocrine system essential for good health. *American Journal of Clinical Nutrition*. 2008;88(2):491S–499S

3. Tangpricha V, Pearce EN, Chen TC, et al. Vitamin D insufficiency among free-living healthy young adults. *Am J Med*. 2002;112(8):659–662

4. Siddiqui I, Jabbar A. Prevalence and significance of vitamin D deficiency and insufficiency among apparently healthy adults. *Clinical Biochemistry*. 2010;43(18):1431–1435

5. Holick MF. Vitamin D: importance in the prevention of cancers, type 1 diabetes, heart disease, and osteoporosis. *American Journal of Clinical Nutrition*. 2007;79(3):362–371

6. Grant WB, Al Anouti F, Moukayed M. Targeted 25-hydroxyvitamin D concentration measurements and vitamin D_3 supplementation can have important patient and public health benefits. *Eur J Clin Nutr*. 2020;74:366–376

7. Gröber U, Spitz J, Reichrath J, et al. Vitamin D: update 2013: from rickets prophylaxis to general preventive healthcare. *Dermatoendocrinol*. 2013;5(3):331–347

8. Wacker M, Holick MF. Vitamin D: effects on skeletal and extraskeletal health and the need for supplementation. *Nutrients*. 2013;5(1):111–148

9. Jones G. Pharmacokinetics of vitamin D toxicity. *Am J Clin Nutr*. 2008;88:582S–6S

10. Ju SY, Lee YJ, Jeong SN. Serum 25-hydroxyvitamin D levels and the risk of depression: a systematic review and meta-analysis. *Journal of Nutrition, Health & Aging*. 2013;17(5):447–55

11. Akpınar Ş, Karadağ MG. Is Vitamin D important in anxiety or depression? what is the truth? *Curr Nutr Rep*. 2022;11(4):675–681

12. Kotsi E, Kotsi E, Perrea DN. Vitamin D levels in children and adolescents with attention-deficit hyperactivity disorder (ADHD): a meta-analysis. *ADHD Atten Def Hyp Disord*. 2019;11:221–232

13. Khoshbakht Y, Bidaki R, Salehi-Abargouei A. Vitamin D status and attention deficit hyperactivity disorder: a systematic review and meta-analysis of observational studies. *Advances in Nutrition*. 2018;9(1):9–20

14. Fasihpour B, Moayeri H, Shariat M, et al. Vitamin D deficiency in school-age Iranian children with attention-deficit/hyperactivity disorder (ADHD) symptoms: a critical comparison with healthy controls. *Child Neuropsychology*. 2020;26(4):460–474

15. Soyak HM, Karakükcü Ç. Investigation of vitamin D levels in obsessive-compulsive disorder. *Indian J Psychiatry*. 2022;64(4):349–353

16. Çelik G, Taş D, Tahiroğlu A, et al. Vitamin D deficiency in obsessive-compulsive disorder patients with pediatric autoimmune neuropsychiatric disorders associated with streptococcal infections: a case control study. *Noro Psikiyatr Ars*. 2016;53(1):33–37

17. Gomes-Lima C, Wartofsky L, Burman K. Can reverse T3 assay be employed to guide T4 vs. T4/T3 therapy in hypothyroidism? *Front Endocrinol* (Lausanne). 2019;10:1–5

18. Dentice M, Salvatore D. Deiodinases: the balance of thyroid hormone: local impact of thyroid hormone inactivation. *J Endocrinol*. 2011;209:273–82

19. Endres D, Perlov E, Stich O, et al. Steroid responsive encephalopathy associated with autoimmune thyroiditis (SREAT) presenting as major depression. *BMC Psychiatry*. 2016;16:184

20. Chaudhry HS, Anilkumar AC. Wilson Disease. [Updated 2021 Aug 11]. In: StatPearls [Internet]. Treasure Island (FL): StatPearls Publishing; 2022 Jan. www.ncbi.nlm.nih.gov/books/NBK441990, accessed 4/24/2022

21. www.my.clevelandclinic.org/health/diseases/5957-wilson-disease, accessed 4/24/2022

22. Frankovich J, Thienemann M, Pearlstein J, et al. Multidisciplinary clinic dedicated to treating youth with pediatric acute-onset neuropsychiatric syndrome: presenting characteristics of the first 47 consecutive patients. *Journal of Child and Adolescent Psychopharmacology*. 2015;25(1):38–47

23. Kriegel MA, Ming LO, Sanjabi S, et al. Transforming growth factor-beta: recent advances on its role in immune tolerance. *Current Rheumatology Reports*. 2006;8:138–144

24. Gilbert KM, Thoman M, Bauche K, et al. Transforming growth factor-beta 1 induces antigen-specific unresponsiveness in naive T cells. *Immunol. Invest*. 1997;26(4):459–72

25. Letterio JJ, Roberts AB. Regulation of immune responses by TGF-β. *Annual Review of Immunology*. 1998;16(1):137–161

26. Xu J, Ahmad A, Jones JF, et al. Elevated serum transforming growth factor β1 levels in Epstein-Barr virus-associated diseases and their correlation with virus-specific immunoglobulin A (IgA) and IgM. *Journal of Virology*. 2000;74(5):2443–2446

27. Nicoletti F, Di Marco R, Patti F, et al. Blood levels of transforming growth factor-beta 1 (TGF-beta1) are elevated in both relapsing remitting and chronic progressive multiple sclerosis (MS) patients and are further augmented by treatment with interferon-beta 1b (IFN-beta1b). *Clinical and Experimental Immunology*. 1998;113(1):96–99

28. Widhe M, Grusell M, Ekerfelt C, et al. Cytokines in Lyme borreliosis: lack of early tumour necrosis factor-alpha and transforming growth factor-beta1 responses are associated with chronic neuroborreliosis. *Immunology*. 2002;107(1):46–55

29. Nijs J, Nees A, Paul L, et al. Altered immune response to exercise in patients with chronic fatigue syndrome/myalgic encephalomyelitis: a systematic literature review. *Exerc Immunol Rev*. 2014;20:94–116

30. Bennett S, Grant M, Creese AJ, et al. Plasma levels of complement 4a protein are increased in Alzheimer's disease. *Alzheimer Dis Assoc Disord*. 2012;26(4):329–334

31. Stricker RB, Savely VR, Motanya NC, Giclas PC. Complement split products c3a and c4a in chronic lyme disease. *Scand J Immunol*. 2009;69(1):64–69

32. Frisch M, Schwartz BS. The pitfalls of hair analysis for toxicants in clinical practice: three case reports. *Environ Health Perspect*. 2002;110(4):433–6

33. www.cfpub.epa.gov/si/si_public_record_Report.cfm?Lab=ORD&dirEntryID=45357 accessed 11/19/2022

34. Kirkland AE, Sarlo GL, Holton KF. The role of magnesium in neurological disorders. *Nutrients*. 2018;10(6):730:1–23

35. Kuygun Karcı C, Gül Celik G. Nutritional and herbal supplements in the treatment of obsessive-compulsive disorder. *Gen Psychiatr*. 2020;33(2):e100159:1–6

36. Forsyth AK, Williams PG, Deane FP. Nutrition status of primary care patients with depression and anxiety. *Australian Journal of Primary Health*. 2012;18:172–176

37. Jacka FN, Overland S, Stewart R, et al. Association between magnesium intake and depression and anxiety in community-dwelling adults: the Hordaland Health Study. *Australian & New Zealand Journal of Psychiatry*. 2009;43(1):45–52

38. Noah L, Dye L, Bois De Fer B, et al. Effect of magnesium and vitamin B6 supplementation on mental health and quality of life in stressed healthy adults: post-hoc analysis of a randomised controlled trial. *Stress Health*. 2021;37(5):1000–1009

39. Sartori SB, Whittle N, Hetzenauer A, et al. Magnesium deficiency induces anxiety and HPA axis dysregulation: Modulation by therapeutic drug treatment. *Neuropharmacology*. 2012;62(1):304–312

40. Nielsen FH. Chapter 31: Relation between magnesium deficiency and sleep disorders and associated pathological changes. In Ronald Ross Watson, editor, *Modulation of Sleep by Obesity, Diabetes, Age, and Diet*. London, UK. Academic Press. 2015:291–296

41. Abbasi B, Kimiagar M, Sadeghniiat K, et al. The effect of magnesium supplementation on primary insomnia in elderly: A double-blind placebo-controlled clinical trial. *J Res Med Sci*. 2012;17(12):1161–9

42. Razzaque MS. Magnesium: are we consuming enough? *Nutrients*. 2018;10(12):1863:1–8

43. Cox IM, Campbell MJ, Dowson D. Red blood cell magnesium and chronic fatigue syndrome. *Lancet*. 1991;337(8744):757–760

44. www.ods.od.nih.gov/factsheets/Zinc-HealthProfessional, accessed 11/20/2022

45. MacDonald RS. The role of zinc in growth and cell proliferation. *J Nutr*. 2000;130(5S Suppl):1500S–8S

46. Petrilli MA, Kranz TM, Kleinhaus K, et al. The emerging role for zinc in depression and psychosis. *Front Pharmacol*. 2017;8:414:1–12

47. Frederickson CJ, Suh SW, Silva D, et al. Importance of zinc in the central nervous system: the zinc-containing neuron. *J Nutr*. 2000;130(5S Suppl):1471S–83S

48. Sayyah M, Olapour A, Saeedabad YS. Evaluation of oral zinc sulfate effect on obsessive-compulsive disorder: a randomized placebo-controlled clinical trial. *Nutrition*. 2012;28(9):892–5

49. Russo AJ. Decreased zinc and increased copper in individuals with anxiety. *Nutrition and Metabolic Insights*. 2011;4:1–5

50. Böckerman P, Bryson A, Viinikainen J, et al. The serum copper/zinc ratio in childhood and educational attainment: a population-based study. *Journal of Public Health*. 2016;38(4):696–703

51. Rodic S, McCudden C, van Walraven C. Relationship between plasma zinc and red blood cell zinc levels in hospitalized patients. *The Journal of Applied Laboratory Medicine*. 2022;7(6):1412–1423

52. www.ods.od.nih.gov/factsheets/VitaminB6-HealthProfessional, accessed 11/20/2022

53. Field DT, Cracknell RO, Eastwood JR, et al. High-dose Vitamin B6 supplementation reduces anxiety and strengthens visual surround suppression. *Hum Psychopharmacol*. 2022;37(6):e2852

54. Landaas ET, Aarsland TI, Ulvik A, et al. Vitamin levels in adults with ADHD. *BJPsych Open*. 2016;2(6):377–384

55. Moudgal R, Hosseini S, Colapietro P, et al. Vitamin B6 toxicity revisited: a case of reversible pyridoxine-associated neuropathy and disequilibrium. *Neurology*. 2018;90 (15 Supplement):P4.021

56. www.merckmanuals.com/professional/nutritional-disorders/vitamin-deficiency,-dependency,-and--toxicity/vitamin-b6-toxicity, accessed 11/20/2022

57. www.ods.od.nih.gov/factsheets/Folate-Consumer/#:~:text=Folate%20is%20a%20B%2Dvitamin,-foods%20and%20most%20dietary%20supplements, accessed 11/20/2022

58. www.lpi.oregonstate.edu/mic/vitamins/folate, accessed 11/20/2022

59. Lewis SJ, Lawlor DA, Davey Smith G, et al. The thermolabile variant of MTHFR is associated with depression in the British Women's Heart and Health Study and a meta-analysis. *Mol Psychiatry*. 2006;11(4):352–60

60. Atmaca M, Tezcan E, Kuloglu M, et al. Serum folate and homocysteine levels in patients with obsessive-compulsive disorder. *Psychiatry Clin Neurosci*. 2005;59(5):616–20

61. Farrell CL, Kirsch SH, Herrmann M. Red cell or serum folate: what to do in clinical practice? *Clinical Chemistry and Laboratory Medicine*. 2013;51(3):555–569

62. Galloway M, Rushworth L. Red cell or serum folate? results from the National Pathology Alliance benchmarking review. *J Clin Pathol*. 2003;56(12):924–6

63. www.ods.od.nih.gov/factsheets/VitaminB12-HealthProfessional, accessed 12/1/2022

64. Lam JR, Schneider JL, Zhao W, et al. Proton pump inhibitor and histamine 2 receptor antagonist use and vitamin B_{12} deficiency. *JAMA*. 2013;310(22):2435–2442

65. Yan S, Liu H, Yu Y, et al. Changes of serum homocysteine and vitamin B12, but not folate are correlated with obsessive-compulsive disorder: a systematic review and meta-analysis of case-control studies. *Front Psychiatry*. 2022;13:754165:1–13

66. Esnafoğlu E, Yaman E. Vitamin B12, folic acid, homocysteine and vitamin D levels in children and adolescents with obsessive compulsive disorder. *Psychiatry Research*. 2017;254:232–237

67. Vashi P, Edwin P, Popiel B, et al. Methylmalonic acid and homocysteine as indicators of vitamin B-12 deficiency in cancer. *PLoS One*. 2016 Jan 25;11(1):e0147843:1–13

68. Lindenbaum J, Savage DG, Stabler SP, et al. Diagnosis of cobalamin deficiency: II. relative sensitivities of serum cobalamin, methylmalonic acid, and total homocysteine concentrations. *Am J Hematol*. 1990;34:99–107

69. Sumner AE, Chin MM, Abrahm JL, et al. Elevated methylmalonic acid and total homocysteine levels show high prevalence of vitamin B12 deficiency after gastric surgery. *Ann Intern Med*. 1996;124:469–76

70. Williams SC. The other microbiome. *Proc Natl Acad Sci USA*. 2013;110(8):2682–4

71. Shoubridge AP, Choo JM, Martin AM, et al. The gut microbiome and mental health: advances in research and emerging priorities. *Mol Psychiatry*. 2022;27(4):1908–1919

72. Malan-Muller S, Valles-Colomer M, Raes J, et al. The gut microbiome and mental health: implications for anxiety- and trauma-related disorders. *OMICS*. 2018;22(2):90–107

73. Butler MI, Mörkl S, Sandhu KV, et al. The gut microbiome and mental health: what should we tell our patients?: Le microbiote Intestinal et la Santé Mentale : que Devrions-Nous dire à nos Patients? *Can J Psychiatry*. 2019;64(11):747–760

74. Mathis D, Benoist C. Microbiota and autoimmune disease: the hosted self. *Cell Host Microbe*. 2011;10(4):297–301

75. Belkaid Y, Hand TW. Role of the microbiota in immunity and inflammation. *Cell*. 2014;157(1):121–41

76. Miyauchi E, Shimokawa C, Steimle A, et al. The impact of the gut microbiome on extra-intestinal autoimmune diseases. *Nat Rev Immunol*. 2022 May 9:1–15

77. Wu HJ, Wu E. The role of gut microbiota in immune homeostasis and autoimmunity. *Gut Microbes*. 2012;3(1):4–14

78. Clapp M, Aurora N, Herrera L, et al. Gut microbiota's effect on mental health: the gut-brain axis. *Clin Pract*. 2017;7(4):987

79. Rees JC. Obsessive-compulsive disorder and gut microbiota dysregulation. *Med Hypotheses*. 2014;82(2):163–6

80. Tan AH, Lim SY, Lang AE. The microbiome-gut-brain axis in Parkinson disease: from basic research to the clinic. *Nat Rev Neurol*. 2022;18(8):476–495

81. Xu Q, Ni JJ, Han BX, et al. Causal relationship between gut microbiota and autoimmune diseases: a two-sample Mendelian randomization study. *Front Immunol*. 2022;12:746998:1–10

82. Gianchecchi E, Fierabracci A. Recent advances on microbiota involvement in the pathogenesis of autoimmunity. *Int J Mol Sci*. 2019;20(2):283:1–28

83. Chen B, Sun L, Zhang X. Integration of microbiome and epigenome to decipher the pathogenesis of autoimmune diseases. *J Autoimmun*. 2017;83:31–42

84. Behar SM, Porcelli S. Mechanisms of autoimmune disease induction. *Arthritis & Rheumatism: Official Journal of the American College of Rheumatology*. 1995;38(4):458–476

85. Oldstone MBA. Molecular mimicry as a mechanism for the cause and as a probe uncovering etiologic agent of autoimmune disease. *Curr Top Microbiol Immunol*. 1989;145:127–135

86. Porcelli S. Molecular mimicry and the generation of autoimmune diseases. *Rheumatol Rev*. 1993;2:41–50

87. Church AJ, Cardoso F, Dale RC, et al. Anti-basal ganglia antibodies in acute and persistent Sydenham's chorea. *Neurology*. 2002;59(2):227–231

88. Kotby AA, El Badawy N, El Sokkary S, et al. Antineuronal antibodies in rheumatic chorea. *Clin Diagn Lab Immunol*. 1998;5(6):836–839

89. Kirvan CA, Cox CJ, Swedo SE, et al. Tubulin is a neuronal target of autoantibodies in Sydenham's chorea. *J Immunol*. 2007;178(11):7412

90. Husby G, van de Rijn I, Zabriskie JB, et al. Antibodies reacting with cytoplasm of subthalamic and caudate nuclei neurons in chorea and acute rheumatic fever. *J Exp Med*. 1976;144(4):1094–1110

91. Swedo SE, Leonard HL, Kiessling LS. Speculations on antineuronal antibody-mediated neuropsychiatric disorders of childhood. *Pediatrics*. 1994;93(2):323–326

92. Swedo SE, Leonard HL, Mittleman BB, et al. Identification of children with pediatric autoimmune neuropsychiatric disorders associated with streptococcal infections by a marker associated with rheumatic fever. *American Journal of Psychiatry*. 1997;154(1):110–112

93. Jackson PG, Lessof MH, Baker RW, et al. Intestinal permeability in patients with eczema and food allergy. *Lancet*. 1981;1(8233):1285–6

94. Pearson AD, Eastham EJ, Laker MF, et al. Intestinal permeability in children with Crohn's disease and coeliac disease. *Br Med J* (Clin Res Ed). 1982;285(6334):20–1

95. Du Mont GC, Beach RC, Menzies IS. Gastrointestinal permeability in food-allergic eczematous children. *Clin Allergy*. 1984;14(1):55–9

96. Möller C, Magnusson KE, Sundqvist T, et al. Intestinal permeability as assessed with polyethyleneglycols in birch pollen allergic children undergoing oral immunotherapy. *Allergy*. 1986;41(4):280–5

97. Barau E, Dupont C. Modifications of intestinal permeability during food provocation procedures in pediatric irritable bowel syndrome. *J Pediatr Gastroenterol Nutr*. 1990;11(1):72–7

98. Picco P, Gattorno M, Marchese N, et al. Increased gut permeability in juvenile chronic arthritides. A multivariate analysis of the diagnostic parameters. *Clin Exp Rheumatol*. 2000;18(6):773–8

99. White JF. Intestinal pathophysiology in autism. *Exp Biol Med* (Maywood). 2003;228(6):639–49

100. Hijazi Z, Molla AM, Al-Habashi H, et al. Intestinal permeability is increased in bronchial asthma. *Arch Dis Child*. 2004;89(3):227–9

101. Liu Z, Li N, Neu J. Tight junctions, leaky intestines, and pediatric diseases. *Acta Paediatr*. 2005;94(4):386–93 (type 1 DM, autism, asthma, allergies, SIRS, IBD)

102. Özyurt G, Öztürk Y, Appak YÇ, et al. Increased zonulin is associated with hyperactivity and social dysfunctions in children with attention deficit hyperactivity disorder. *Compr Psychiatry*. 2018;87:138–142

103. Küçükemre Aydın B, Yıldız M, Akgün A, et al. Children with Hashimoto's thyroiditis have increased intestinal permeability: results of a pilot study. *J Clin Res Pediatr Endocrinol*. 2020;12(3):303–307

104. Küme T, Acar S, Tuhan H, et al. The relationship between serum zonulin level and clinical and laboratory parameters of childhood obesity. *J Clin Res Pediatr Endocrinol*. 2017;9(1):31–38

105. Hensley-McBain T, Manuzak JA. Zonulin as a biomarker and potential therapeutic target in multisystem inflammatory syndrome in children. *J Clin Invest*. 2021;131(14):e151467:1–3

106. Yonker LM, Gilboa T, Ogata AF, et al. Multisystem inflammatory syndrome in children is driven by zonulin-dependent loss of gut mucosal barrier. *J Clin Invest*. 2021;131(14):e149633:1–12

107. Mantis NJ, Rol N, Corthésy B. Secretory IgA's complex roles in immunity and mucosal homeostasis in the gut. *Mucosal Immunol*. 2011;4(6):603–11

108. Stier H, Bischoff SC. Influence of *Saccharomyces boulardii* CNCM I-745 on the gut-associated immune system. *Clin Exp Gastroenterol*. 2016;9:269–279

109. Bjarnason I. The use of fecal calprotectin in inflammatory bowel disease. *Gastroenterol Hepatol* (NY). 2017;13(1):53–56

110. Abraham BP. Fecal lactoferrin testing. *Gastroenterol Hepatol* (NY). 2018;14(12):713–716

111. van der Sluys Veer A, Brouwer J, Biemond I, et al. Fecal lysozyme in assessment of disease activity in inflammatory bowel disease. *Dig Dis Sci*. 1998;43(3):590–5

112. Barau E, Dupont C. Modifications of intestinal permeability during food provocation procedures in pediatric irritable bowel syndrome. *J Pediatr Gastroenterol Nutr*. 1990;11(1):72–7

113. www.aaaai.org/tools-for-the-public/conditions-library/allergies/igg-food-test, accessed 12/31/2022

114. Atkinson W, Sheldon TA, Shaath N, et al. Food elimination based on IgG antibodies in irritable bowel syndrome: a randomised controlled trial. *Gut*. 2004;53(10):1459–64

115. Bentz S, Hausmann M, Piberger H, et al. Clinical relevance of IgG antibodies against food antigens in Crohn's disease: a double-blind cross-over diet intervention study. *Digestion*. 2010;81(4):252–64

116. Jian L, Anqi H, Gang L, et al. Food exclusion based on IgG antibodies alleviates symptoms in ulcerative colitis: a prospective study. *Inflamm Bowel Dis*. 2018;24(9):1918–1925

117. Geiselman JF. The clinical use of IgG food sensitivity testing with migraine headache patients: a literature review. *Curr Pain Headache Rep*. 2019;23:79

118. Alpay K, Ertas M, Orhan EK, et al. Diet restriction in migraine, based on IgG against foods: a clinical double-blind, randomised, cross-over trial. *Cephalalgia*. 2010;30(7):829–37

119. Samadi N, Klems M, Untersmayr E. The role of gastrointestinal permeability in food allergy. *Ann Allergy Asthma Immunol.* 2018;121(2):168–173

120. Warren B, Sarris J, Mulder RT, et al. Pyroluria: fact or fiction? *J Altern Complement Med.* 2021;27(5):407–415

121. Gendler PL, Duhan HA, Rapoport H. Hemopyrrole and kryptopyrrole are absent from the urine of schizophrenics and normal persons. *Clin Chem.* 1978;24(2):230–3

122. Gorchein A. Urine concentration of 3-ethyl-5-hydroxy-4,5-dimethyl-delta 3-pyrrolin-2-one ("mauve factor") is not causally related to schizophrenia or to acute intermittent porphyria. *Clin Sci* (Lond). 1980;58(6):469–76

CHAPTER 8

IDENTIFY: INFECTIONS *(STREP, MYCOPLASMA,* AND OTHER BACTERIAL, PARASITIC, AND VIRAL INFECTIONS)

To array a man's will against his sickness is the supreme art of medicine.
~ **HENRY WARD BEECHER**

KEY POINTS

▸ PANDAS is associated with *Strep* pyogenes

▸ PANS may be associated with *Mycoplasma pneumoniae,* Influenza, COVID-19, *Toxoplasma gondii, Chlamydia pneumoniae,* and other organisms

▸ Various types of conventional and specialty testing may be needed to evaluate for these organisms

▸ Positive IFN-γ and IL-2 levels for organisms indicate that an active immune response is present, which implies that an infection is current, as opposed to a past infection

In this chapter we discuss laboratory testing for infections such as *Strep* and *Mycoplasma*. We also discuss other bacterial infections, parasitic infections, and viral infections. We discuss tick-borne infections in Chapter 9.

Testing for infections such as *Strep and Mycoplasma* can be challenging since these organisms can live in a biofilm that helps the infections evade the host immune system and may affect the sensitivity of laboratory testing. Biofilms are discussed in detail in Chapter 14.

GROUP A β-HEMOLYTIC *STREPTOCOCCUS*

As noted in Chapter 2, group A β-hemolytic *Streptococcus* (*Streptococcus pyogenes*) is the organism associated with PANDAS, and conclusive evidence has shown the association between this organism and autoimmune encephalitis.

Testing for *Strep*
1. *Strep* Culture

This test requires cooperation on the part of the child. It is not particularly comfortable, as the swab must contact both tonsils to be accurate and

> **Tests may be helpful if a rise and fall of titers is seen, even if the results never rise out of the normal range.**

can therefore cause a gag reflex. *Strep* cultures (if done correctly with a cooperative child) are very sensitive. *Strep* culture typically takes 24–72 hours to come back. The perianal area may be swabbed for *Strep* and sent for culture as well.

2. *Strep* antigen testing

This test measures for a specific antigen produced by *Strep* bacteria. Results typically take fifteen minutes to an hour.

3. PCR testing

PCR (polymerase chain reaction) testing is expensive and rarely performed.

4. ASO and anti-DNase titers[1]

ASO stands for anti-streptolysin (antibody); DNase is "deoxyribonuclease." These antibodies rise with active *Strep* infection and fall some period of time afterward. ASO titers and anti-DNase titers rise 1–3 weeks after the infection and peak at 3–5 weeks. They may be positive for up to twelve months. One issue with the ASO test is that it will be positive in some cases of group G and group C *Strep* and not just group A *Strep*. The sensitivity of an ASO titer is about 80–85%. If an anti-DNase titer is added to ASO titer, the sensitivity approaches 95%.[2] To give the most information, titers should be repeated after several weeks. We don't repeat this often, as blood draws can be traumatic for children. The tests may be helpful if a rise and fall of titers is seen, even if the results never rise out of the normal range.[3]

MYCOPLASMA PNEUMONIAE

Studies have demonstrated a link between *Mycoplasma pneumoniae* and tics, OCD, and Tourette syndrome.[4–6] In our practice, we have found a clinical correlation between food restriction and avoidance behaviors and *Mycoplasma* infection.

The adhesin molecules and glycolipids of the *Mycoplasma* cell membrane share homology with mammalian tissues and trigger autoimmunity in multiple organ systems through the process of molecular mimicry.[7] Central nervous system complications, including encephalitis, diplopia, mental confusion, and acute psychosis are the most common extrapulmonary manifestations of *Mycoplasma*. Anti-neuronal antibodies have been identified in 100% of patients with CNS involvement.[8]

Testing for *Mycoplasma*

We measure serum IgG and IgM antibody levels to *Mycoplasma pneumoniae* through conventional laboratories. Clinicians tend to think IgM antibodies are an indication of active infection, whereas IgG antibodies typically indicate past infection. In the case of *Mycoplasma*, however, patients who have been infected repeatedly over several years may fail to manifest an IgM response during an acute infection and may progress directly to IgG.[8,9] In addition, IgM antibodies may be persistent for several years, thus limiting the usefulness of serology in ruling in or ruling out acute infection.[8] Persistent infections with *Mycoplasma* are seen in patients with hypogammaglobulinemia.[10] Many patients with PANS and PANDAS have hypogammaglobulinemia.

In the case of *Mycoplasma*, high or increasing IgG antibodies alone may warrant a trial of antimicrobials, especially if food restrictive behavior is present. There is some evidence that *Mycoplasma pneumoniae* may be capable of an intracellular existence, which could establish a latent state to avoid the host immune system.[8]

We also use Infectolab testing for *Mycoplasma*. This test measures IFN-γ and Interleukin 2 (IL-2) levels to the organism. Elevated levels suggest that the immune system is dealing with an active infection. This test is useful in practice since it typically becomes negative when patients improve clinically, suggesting resolution of the active infection.

EPSTEIN-BARR VIRUS (EBV)

Epstein-Barr virus is a lymphotropic virus from the herpesvirus family. It is also known as human herpesvirus 4. It commonly causes a minor self-limited illness in young children. In teens and adults, it can cause acute mononucleosis.

> Epstein-Barr virus has been linked to anxiety and psychosis,

Mononucleosis usually presents with fever, sore throat, swollen lymph nodes, and fatigue, which can sometimes last for weeks after the infection.

During an episode of acute mononucleosis, patients may develop hepatomegaly and splenomegaly. Physical activity should be limited to avoid the risk of splenic rupture. The Epstein-Barr virus stays in the body inside B-lymphocytes and remains dormant (like varicella-zoster virus) for life. It can reactivate and cause a resurgence of symptoms months or years later.[11] Over 90% of adults have been exposed to EBV in their lifetime.[12]

In addition to some cancers, The Epstein-Barr virus has been linked to anxiety[13] and psychosis,[14] and this presentation does not typically include sore throat, fever, or lymphadenopathy. Some patients with PANS were shown to have had recent EBV infections in one Italian study.[15] Severe, acute presentations of EBV infection can be associated with encephalitis.[16] Articles have linked EBV reactivation to long-haul COVID-19 symptoms[17] and have shown that EBV can be a trigger for multiple sclerosis (MS).[18–22] The MS trigger is thought to occur due to molecular mimicry.

Testing for EBV

If EBV presents with acute mononucleosis, a heterophile antibody (IgM) test is typically performed. One common brand of this test is called the *Monopsot* test. The heterophile antibody test is 90–95% specific (there are very few false positives). Sensitivity in acute infection is only 70–90% (less in the first week of infection and in young children, in whom it may be 50% sensitive).[23] If a heterophile test is positive during acute illness, the diagnosis is confirmed. If negative and the suspicion is high, it could still be EBV or could be mononucleosis from cytomegalovirus (CMV) infection. If confirmation of the diagnosis is essential, EBV antibodies may be tested. Heterophile antibody tests have no role in the evaluation of past infection or reactivated EBV.

EBV antibody testing looks at four specific antibodies: VCA-IgM antibodies, VCA-IgG antibodies, EA-IgG antibodies, and NA-IgG antibodies. VCA stands for "viral capsid antigen."

The VCA-IgM antibody is virtually diagnostic of acute EBV infection.[24] In 90% of cases, the IgM is negative by four months. It has high sensitivity

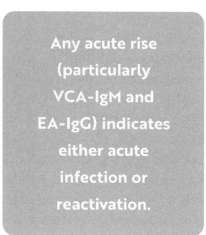

Any acute rise (particularly VCA-IgM and EA-IgG) indicates either acute infection or reactivation.

and specificity. The VCA-IgG antibody is usually positive early on and remains positive for life. EA stands for "early antigen." The EA-IgG antibodies rise later in the course of acute infection and typically disappear after recovery. They may remain positive in protracted cases. VCA-IgM and EA antibodies are active in the lytic phase of infection and indicate viral activity[25] (initial infection or reactivation). NA stands for "nuclear antigen." It typically occurs later in infection and may remain positive for life.

Antibody science can be confusing. The best advice for interpreting EBV antibodies is that any acute rise (particularly VCA-IgM and EA-IgG) indicates either acute infection or reactivation. Culture of EBV is not done outside of research settings. EBV viral load tests may be done in some settings (immunosuppressed organ transplant patients) but have considerable variability from lab to lab and are not helpful in diagnosing acute infection or reactivation.[24]

We also use Infectolab testing for EBV. This test measures IFN-γ and Interleukin 2 (IL-2) levels to the organism. Elevated levels suggest that the immune system is dealing with an acute infection or reactivated infection. This test is useful in practice since it typically becomes negative when patients improve clinically, suggesting resolution of the active infection.

CYTOMEGALOVIRUS

Cytomegalovirus (CMV) is also known as human herpesvirus 5.[26] Like EBV, this virus can cause acute mononucleosis. Congenital infections, which cause neurodevelopmental delays, can occur. Patients with solid organ transplants and hematopoietic stem cell transplants who are immunocompromised may develop severe complications and experience organ rejection. A possible link has been found between CMV infection and inflammatory bowel disorders.[27,28] Although some clinicians who treat children with PANS order IgG and IgM CMV titers for these patients, no link has been established between this organism and PANS. Over 95% of people test positive for CMV exposure by adulthood. Since there is no specific literature outlining treatment for CMV (except in transplant patients, HIV patients, and congenital infections) and no link has been established, we do not routinely test for this organism.

HUMAN HERPESVIRUS 6 (HHV-6)[29]

HHV-6 is another common virus that most people have been exposed to by the time they are adults. In children, it is the cause of a common, self-limited pediatric condition called exanthem subitum (also known as roseola infantum or sixth disease). Like CMV and EBV, HHV-6 can cause acute mononucleosis.

In some cases, HHV-6 can cause acute encephalitis or meningitis in children, which can present with altered mental status, seizures, and psychosis. Neurologic defects can persist after encephalitis. The presentation of encephalitis is impressive and would not be confused with PANS. There is an association between HHV-6 (and EBV) and chronic fatigue syndrome. The association with HHV-6 with chronic fatigue is stronger than that with EBV.[30] Although some clinicians who treat children with PANS order IgG and IgM HHV-6 titers for these patients, no

link has been established in the medical literature between this organism and PANS. We do not routinely test for or treat this organism in children with PANS.

COXSACKIEVIRUS A AND B[31]

Coxsackieviruses are members of the enterovirus family. They are common causes of routine viral exanthems (hand-foot-and-mouth disease) and enanthems (herpangina) in childhood. Neurologic complications can include aseptic meningitis, encephalitis, and acute flaccid paralysis. Acute respiratory diseases, myositis, and myopericarditis can also be seen with Coxsackievirus infections. Although some clinicians who treat children with PANS order IgG and IgM Coxsackievirus titers for these patients, no link has been established in the medical literature between this organism and PANS. We do not routinely test for or treat this organism in children with PANS.

INFLUENZA

The influenza viruses are ubiquitous pathogens that cause quite a bit of human suffering. We, as clinicians and humans, are familiar with common presentations of the influenza viruses, such as cough, pharyngitis, nasal congestion, headache, fever, and GI complaints. There are some more serious neurologic complications of influenza, including encephalitis, which, although rare, can be fatal. Other rare but reported complications include Guillain-Barré syndrome, transverse myelitis, and, historically, some movement disorders resembling Parkinson's disease.[32]

In 1917, Dr. Constantin von Economo described a new clinical syndrome associated with influenza that he called encephalitis lethargica (EL).[33] He described sleep disturbance, ocular motility issues (ophthalmoplegic palsies), and ptosis. Autopsies showed inflammation in the midbrain. In the winter of 1920, cases with chorea and hemichorea were noted. Months to years later, some of these patients developed Parkinsonian symptoms.[34] Howard and Lees published a report[35] of four patients in 1987 with EL and described clinical diagnostic criteria that included basal ganglia involvement, ophthalmoplegia, obsessive-compulsive behavior, akinetic mutism, and somnolence or sleep inversion.

Similar symptoms are commonly seen in

Similar descriptions from other articles from the medical literature at the time included *defiance, emotional instability, crying spells, tantrums,* and *irregular sleep habits*.[37] Most of the children with behavioral changes were between the ages of seven and eighteen. Researchers at the time commented that the behavioral changes were similar to those seen in traumatic brain injury.[38]

In the 1920s and 1930s, many of these children were admitted to state institutions or penal institutions. Unfortunately, some were treated

> Several articles have been published which detail the effects of COVID on the brain and describe neuropsychiatric symptoms related to the response of the body to infection.

patients with PANS. In fact, a subtype of encephalitis lethargica exists that is known as "pseudo-psychopathic encephalitis lethargica." In an article from 1929 (translated to English in 1931),[36] von Economo described children with EL thus:

[these children] "annoy strangers on the street, pluck their clothing, make faces at them or abuse them; they tramp, beg, lie, steal, write on the walls, squander all the money they can lay hands on in sweets, cannot be controlled at school, run away from home and spend their time at the cinema and in the streets, indulge in sexual misbehavior of every kind and make other dangerous acts." Children with encephalitis lethargica presented a wide variety of behaviors that were regarded as aberrant, delinquent, or in extreme cases, even psychopathic.

with frontal lobotomy.[38] It was hypothesized that damage to the basal ganglia was responsible for the behavioral changes in these children.[39] Viral fragments have not been found in the preserved brains of these patients, which may suggest a post-viral autoimmune attack.[38] The lack of viral infiltration in these histological sections has resulted in the very existence of this condition becoming controversial (much like PANS itself).[40]

Neurologic complications of influenza have continued into the twenty-first century. They were reported with the H1N1 outbreak in 2009.[32,41] Influenza is not known to be persistent in the body after the acute episode of illness subsides. Although there are rapid antigen tests that are used during the episode of acute illness, these tests have no value if delayed. In addition, there is no known antiviral treatment for post-influenza behavioral changes. Of all types of PANS, the initial onset after influenza or just before flares are not commonly reported by parents. Except in acute illness, we do not test for influenza.

SARS-COV-2 VIRUS (COVID)

The COVID pandemic likely began in late 2019. While some patients experienced little more than cold symptoms, a significant portion of patients developed severe respiratory distress. At the time of this writing, the world death toll from COVID is approximately 6.4 million.[42]

While disease in children was generally mild and self-limited, pediatric deaths in the United States total 1,538 at the time of this writing.[43] As of October 2021, 140,000 children lost a primary or secondary caregiver.[44]

Multisystem Inflammatory Syndrome of Children (MIS-C) is an inflammatory condition associated with COVID infection.[45] The exact pathophysiology is unknown, but it can be serious and even deadly. The diagnostic criteria for MIS-C include fever plus at least two of the following: diarrhea, conjunctival redness, abdominal pain, vomiting, and dizziness/ hypotension. Symptoms typically start two to six weeks after COVID infection and are most-commonly seen in children ages 8–9. MIS-C shares some findings in common with Kawasaki disease, such as coronary artery aneurysms, but unlike Kawasaki disease MIS-C patients may demonstrate coagulopathy (elevated D-dimer, PT, aPTT), shock, and gastrointestinal symptoms.[46] Subsequent analysis has identified a unique inflammatory cytokine signature, and treatment with interleukin (IL) blocking agents and IVIG has shown benefit. MIS-C tends to occur in the convalescent stage of COVID, weeks after exposure.

This delay in the onset of symptoms is similar to the delay seen in PANS and PANDAS.

Several articles[47,48] have been published which detail the effects of COVID on the brain and describe neuropsychiatric symptoms related to the response of the body to infection. It seems to be an interplay between infection and increased coagulability. The inflammatory cyto kines IL-6, IL-1, IL-10, and TNF-α levels are increased during infection. Blood-brain barrier (BBB) permeability is increased from cytokine induced damage. A retrospective study of over 1.2 million patients published in the *Lancet Psychiatry* in 2022 showed that patients who had had COVID had a persistently increased risk of psychosis, dementia, cognitive deficits, and epilepsy over a two-year follow-up period.[49]

Although children with PANS and PANDAS can develop a disease flare with any illness, we have not seen an increase in flares or the onset of PANS related to COVID infection in our practice. One case study[50] from Italy described two children who developed symptoms of PANS following COVID infection.

TOXOPLASMA GONDII

Toxoplasma gondii is an exclusively intracellular parasite which causes an infection in humans called toxoplasmosis.[51] As many as forty million people in the United States may be infected with *Toxoplasma gondii*, although most are asymptomatic. Infection may occur via contaminated foods (shellfish or meats), from ingesting contaminated water, or from coming into contact with contaminated soil or cat feces. Acute infection can cause swollen lymph nodes or flu-like symptoms, which may persist for a month or more. Ocular toxoplasmosis can produce blurred or impaired vision.

As in EBV, some patients with *Toxoplasma gondii* may have reactivation of the disease. Immunocompromised patients (including immunosuppression from medications) may develop more severe disease. Patients with AIDS can develop CNS infection, which may present as space-occupying lesions.

Toxoplasmosis has been associated with a 2.5x increased incidence of obsessive-compulsive disorder and a 2.7x increased risk of learning disorders.[52–54] Additional studies have supported a link between prior infection with *Toxoplasma gondii* and other mental illnesses.[55–60]

IgM and IgG testing is performed at most commercial labs. IgM antibodies typically decline after a short period, though they may be present up to a year after initial infection and are sometimes seen in chronic disease.[61] There are complexities to testing for *Toxoplasma gondii*; a single positive IgG or IgM titer may or may not represent active infection.[62] Testing for *Toxoplasma* antibodies is available through LabCorp or Quest Diagnostics.

CHLAMYDIA PNEUMONIAE

Studies have shown that serologic evidence of *Chlamydophila* infections (both *Chlamydia psittaci* and *Chlamydia pneumoniae*) is associated with increased odds ratios for schizophrenia.[63] These associations are amplified for people with certain HLA haplotypes. The association of these *Chlamydia* species with schizophrenia was shown to be highly significant, with an odds ratio of 9.43. *Chlamydia pneumoniae* has been shown to use monocyte migration to breach the blood-brain barrier in endothelial tissue samples taken from patients with Alzheimer's disease.[64] There is also some evidence that *C. pneumoniae* is involved in coronary artery disease and it

may be linked to multiple sclerosis.[65] *Chlamydia trachomatis*, which is a sexually transmitted disease, has not been linked to any neuropsychiatric conditions. No specific link between *Chlamydia* infections and PANS has been established.

Testing for these infections is performed using serologic tests (IgG and IgM) from LabCorp and Quest Diagnostics. We routinely test for antibodies to this organism in children with PANS.

> **Toxoplasmosis has been associated with a 2.5x increased incidence of obsessive-compulsive disorder and a 2.7x increased risk of learning disorders.**

We also use Infectolab testing for *Chlamydia*. This test measures IFN-γ and Interleukin 2 (IL-2) levels to the organism. Elevated levels suggest that the immune system is dealing with an active infection. This test is useful in practice since it typically becomes negative when patients improve clinically, suggesting resolution of the active infection.

NASAL SWABS

Multiple antibiotic-resistant coagulase-negative *Staph aureus* (MARCONS or MARCoNS) is defined as a strain of *Staph aureus* which resides in the nasopharynx and is resistant to at least two antibiotics upon testing.

The concept of MARCONS (and its connection to mold exposure) was first proposed in the

1990s. The hypothesis is that colonization with this particular strain of *Staph aureus* is associated with low melanocyte stimulating hormone (MSH) due to mold exposure.

Proponents of this theory advocate for testing for this bacterium using a nasal swab from a company called Microbiology Dx. If positive, some physicians recommend treatment of the colonization with a compounded nasal spray called "BEG spray," which contains Bactroban (mupirocin), EDTA (to break-up biofilms), and gentamicin.

As physicians, we know from our training and clinical experience that resistance to more than one antibiotic is common among *Staphylococcus aureus* bacteria, such as in the case of the ubiquitous MRSA. From that standpoint, MARCONS *as a concept* exists. The problem is that a PubMed search (as well as a simple Google search) fails to produce any peer-reviewed literature which uses the term *MARCONS*, demonstrates a relationship between *Staph* and low MSH, or connects these two concepts to mold exposure.

Google searches for MARCONS do return many blog posts from health and wellness practitioners (mostly non-physicians) which echo statements from the original proponents of the concept related to the existence, diagnosis, and treatment of MARCONS. None of these sources contain any peer-reviewed data to substantiate these statements.

The concept of MARCONS has been discussed extensively among our colleagues in the International Society for Environmentally Acquired Illness (www.iseai.org) and we have not collectively been able to find an evidence base for the MARCONS concept. One of our organizational cofounders collected patient data and found that treatment with BEG spray resulted in increased rates of resistance upon repeat testing (personal communication, ISEAI conference, 2018).

As noted in Chapter 14, *Staph* commonly produces biofilms, and the disruption of these

> Serologic evidence of *Chlamydophila* infections (both *Chlamydia psittaci* and *Chlamydia pneumoniae*) is associated with increased odds ratios for schizophrenia.

biofilms is essential to eradicating this potentially harmful bacteria. The Microbiology Dx nasal swab does quantify biofilms and identifies other bacteria and fungi present in the nose. If any bacterial growth or fungi are found on a Microbiology Dx swab, treatment to eradicate the organism and break down the biofilm is warranted.

Since we commonly treat empirically for nasal biofilms in our practice, we don't routinely run a nasal swab. If we do run the test, we are looking for fungal growth, other bacteria, and biofilms rather than *Staphylococcus aureus* alone.

CHAPTER 8 REFERENCES

1. www.emedicine.medscape.com/article/2113540-overview#a4, accessed 4/24/2022

2. Blyth CC, Robertson PW. Anti-streptococcal antibodies in the diagnosis of acute and post-streptococcal disease: streptokinase versus streptolysin O and deoxyribonuclease B. *Pathology*. 2006;38(2):152–156

3. Johnson DR, Kurlan R, Leckman J, et al. The human immune response to streptococcal extracellular antigens: clinical, diagnostic, and potential pathogenetic implications. *Clinical Infectious Diseases*. 2010;50(4):481–490

4. Müller N, Riedel M, Forderreuther S, Blendinger C, Abele-Horn M. Tourette's syndrome and *Mycoplasma pneumoniae* infection [letter]. *American Journal of Psychiatry*. 2000;157:481–482

5. Müller N, Riedel M, Blendinger C, et al. *Mycoplasma pneumoniae* infection and Tourette's syndrome. *Psychiatry Research*. 2004;129(2):119–125

6. Ercan TE, Ercan G, Severge B, et al. *Mycoplasma pneumoniae* infection and obsessive-compulsive disease: a case report. *Journal of Child Neurology*. 2008;23(3):338–340

7. Barile MF. *Mycoplasma*-tissue cell interactions. In Tully JG, Whitcomb RF, editors. *Mycoplasmas II. Human and Animal Mycoplasmas*. Volume 2. New York, NY. Academic Press. 1979;425–474

8. Waites KB, Talkington DF. *Mycoplasma pneumoniae* and its role as a human pathogen. *Clinical Microbiology Reviews*. 2004;17(4):697–728

9. Hammerschlag MR. *Mycoplasma pneumoniae* infections. *Current Opinion in Infectious Diseases*. 2001;14(2):181–6

10. Taylor-Robinson D, Gumpel JM, Hill A, et al. Isolation of *Mycoplasma pneumoniae* from the synovial fluid of a hypogrammaglobulinaemic patient in a survey of patients with inflammatory polyarthritis. *Ann Rheum Dis*. 1978;37(2):180–2

11. www.cdc.gov/epstein-barr/about-mono.html, accessed 5/23/2022

12. Tzellos S, Farrell PJ. Epstein-Barr virus sequence variation-biology and disease. *Pathogens*. 2012;1(2):156–174

13. Fagundes CP, Jaremka LM, Glaser R, et al. Attachment anxiety is related to Epstein-Barr virus latency. *Brain Behav Immun*. 2014;41:232–238

14. Khandaker GM, Stochl J, Zammit S, Lewis G, Jones PB. Childhood Epstein-Barr virus infection and subsequent risk of psychotic experiences in adolescence: a population-based prospective serological study. *Schizophr Res*.158(1–3):19–24, 2014

15. Falcini F, Lepri G, Bertini F, et al. From PANDAS to PANS: a nosographic entity in evolution throughout a descriptive analysis of a cohort of 103 Italian children and adolescents. *Pediatr Rheumatol*. 2014;1(suppl 1):1–2

16. Martelius T, Lappalainen M, Palomäki M. et al. Clinical characteristics of patients with Epstein-Barr virus in cerebrospinal fluid. *BMC Infect Dis*. 2011;11(281):1–6

17. Gold JE, Okyay RA, Licht WE, et al. Investigation of long COVID prevalence and its relationship to Epstein-Barr virus reactivation. *Pathogens*. 2021;10(6):1–15

18. Salvetti M; Giovannoni G, Francescac A. Epstein-Barr virus and multiple sclerosis. *Current Opinion in Neurology*. 2009;22(3):201–206

19. Bar-Or A, Pender MP, Khanna R, et al. Epstein-Barr virus in multiple sclerosis: theory and emerging immunotherapies. *Trends in Molecular Medicine*. 2020;26(3):296–310

20. Farrell RA, Antony D, Wall GR, et al. Humoral immune response to EBV in multiple sclerosis is associated with disease activity on MRI. *Neurology*. 2009;73(1):32–38

21. Sollid LM. Epstein-Barr virus as a driver of multiple sclerosis. *Science Immunology*. 2022;7(70):264–265

22. Wandinger KP, Jabs W, Siekhaus A, et al. Association between clinical disease activity and Epstein-Barr virus reactivation in MS. *Neurology*. 2000;55(2);178–184

23. Linderholm M, Boman J, Juto P, Linde A. Comparative evaluation of nine kits for rapid diagnosis of infectious mononucleosis and Epstein-Barr virus-specific serology. *J Clin Microbiol*. 1994;32(1):259–261

24. Johannsen EC, Kaye KM. Epstein-Barr virus (infectious mononucleosis, Epstein-Barr virus associated malignant diseases, and other diseases). In Bennett J, Dolin R, Blaser M, editors. *Mandell, Douglas, and Bennett's Principles and Practice of Infectious Diseases*. 9th ed. Philadelphia, PA. Elsevier. 2020;2:1872–1896

25. Wood RA, Guthridge L, Thurmond E, et al. Serologic markers of Epstein-Barr virus reactivation are associated with increased disease activity, inflammation, and interferon pathway activation in patients with systemic lupus erythematosus. *Journal of Translational Autoimmunity*. 2021;4:1–6

26. Britt WJ. Cytomegalovirus. In Bennett J, Dolin R, Blaser M, editors. *Mandell, Douglas, and Bennett's Principles and Practice of Infectious Diseases*. 9th ed. Philadelphia, PA. Elsevier. 2020;2:1857–1871

27. Thörn M, Rorsman F, Rönnblom A, et al. Active cytomegalovirus infection diagnosed by real-time PCR in patients with inflammatory bowel disease: a prospective, controlled observational study. *Scand J Gastroenterol*. 2016;51(9):1075–1080

28. Kandiel A, Lashner B. Cytomegalovirus colitis complicating inflammatory bowel disease. *Am J Gastroenterol*. 2006;101(12):2857–2865

29. Cohen JI. Human herpesvirus types 6 and 7 (exanthem subitum). In Bennett J, Dolin R, Blaser M, editors. *Mandell, Douglas, and Bennett's Principles and Practice of Infectious Diseases*. 9th ed. Philadelphia, PA. Elsevier. 2020;2:1891–1896

30. Ablashi DV. Summary: viral studies of chronic fatigue syndrome. *Clinical Infectious Diseases*. 1994;18:S130–33

31. Romero JR. Coxsackieviruses, echoviruses, and numbered enteroviruses (EV-A71, EVD-68, EVD-70). In Bennett J, Dolin R, Blaser M, editors. *Mandell, Douglas, and Bennett's Principles and Practice of Infectious Diseases*. 9th ed. Philadelphia, PA. Elsevier. 2020;2:2227–2237

32. Tsai JP, Baker AJ. Influenza-associated neurological complications. *Neurocrit Care*. 2013;18:118–130

33. Dickman MS. von Economo encephalitis. *Arch Neurol*. 2001;58(10):1696–1698

34. Ravenholt RT, Foege WH. 1918 influenza, encephalitis, parkinsonism. *Lancet* 1982;2:860–864

35. Howard RS, Lees AJ. Encephalitis lethargica: a report of four recent cases. *Brain: A Journal of Neurology*. 1987;110(1),19–33

36. von Economo C. 1931. *Encephalitis Lethargica, Sequelae and Treatment*. (K.O. Newman, trans.) Oxford University Press.

37. Jenkins RL, Ackerson L. The behavior of encephalitic children. *Am J Orthopsychiatry*. 1934;4:499–507

38. Vilensky JA, Foley P, Gilman S. Children and encephalitis lethargica: a historical review. *Pediatric Neurology*. 2007;37(2):79–84

39. Bond ED, Partridge GE. Post-encephalitic behavior disorders in boys and their management in hospital. *Am J Psychiatry*. 1926;6:25–103

40. Maurizi CP. Influenza caused epidemic encephalitis (encephalitis lethargica): The circumstantial evidence and a challenge to the nonbelievers. *Medical Hypotheses*. 2010;74(5):798–801

41. Surana P, Tang S, McDougall M, et al. Neurological complications of pandemic influenza A H1N1 2009 infection: European case series and review. *Eur J Pediatr*. 2011;170:1007–1015

42. www.worldometers.info/coronavirus, accessed 7/22/2022

43. www.covid.cdc.gov/covid-data-tracker/#demographics, accessed 6/10/2022

44. www.nih.gov/news-events/news-releases/more-140000-us-children-lost-primary-or-secondary--caregiver-due-covid-19-pandemic, accessed 6/10/2022

45. www.cdc.gov/mis/mis-c.html, accessed 6/12/2022

46. Gruber CN, Patel RS, Trachtman R, et al. Mapping systemic inflammation and antibody responses in multisystem inflammatory syndrome in children (MIS-C). *Cell*. 2020;183(4):982–995

47. Banerjee D, Viswanath B. Neuropsychiatric manifestations of COVID-19 and possible pathogenic mechanisms: insights from other coronaviruses. *Asian J Psychiatr*. 2020;54(102350):1–7

48. Boldrini M, Canoll PD, Klein RS. How COVID-19 affects the brain. *JAMA Psychiatry*. 2021;78(6):682–683

49. Taquet M, Sillett R, Zhu L, et al. Neurological and psychiatric risk trajectories after SARS-CoV-2 infection: an analysis of 2-year retrospective cohort studies including 1,284,437 patients. *Lancet Psychiatry*. 2022;9(10):815–827

50. Pavone P, Ceccarelli M, Marino S, et al. SARS-CoV-2 related paediatric acute-onset neuropsychiatric syndrome. *Lancet Child Adolesc Health*. 2021;5(6):e19-e21

51. www.cdc.gov/parasites/toxoplasmosis/index.html, accessed 6/13/2022

52. Flegr J, Horáček J. Toxoplasma-infected subjects report an obsessive-compulsive disorder diagnosis more often and score higher in obsessive-compulsive inventory. *Eur Psychiatry*. 2016;40:82–87

53. Akaltun İ, Kara SS, Kara T. The relationship between toxoplasma gondii IgG antibodies and generalized anxiety disorder and obsessive-compulsive disorder in children and adolescents: a new approach. *Nord J Psychiatry*. 2018;72(1):57–62

54. Miman O, Mutlu EA, Ozcan O, Atambay M, Karlidag R, Unal S. Is there any role of toxoplasma gondii in the etiology of obsessive-compulsive disorder? *Psychiatry Res*. 2010;177(1–2):263–265

55. Sutterland AL, Fond G, Kuin A, et al. Beyond the association: toxoplasma gondii in schizophrenia, bipolar disorder, and addiction: systematic review and meta-analysis. *Acta Psychiatr Scand*. 2015;132(3):161–179

56. Brown AS. Further evidence of infectious insults in the pathogenesis and pathophysiology of schizophrenia. *Am J Psychiatry*. 2011;168(8):764–766

57. Pedersen MG, Stevens H, Pedersen CB, et al. Toxoplasma infection and later development of schizophrenia in mothers. *Am J Psychiatry*. 2011;168:814–821

58. Niebuhr DW, Millikan AM, Cowan DN, et al. Selected infectious agents and risk of schizophrenia among US military personnel. *Am J Psychiatry*. 2008;165(1):99–106

59. Brown AS, Schaefer CA, Quesenberry CP Jr, et al. Maternal exposure to toxoplasmosis and risk of schizophrenia in adult offspring. *Am J Psychiatry*. 2005;162(4):767–773

60. Torrey EF, Bartko JJ, Yolken RH. Toxoplasma gondii and other risk factors for schizophrenia: an update. *Schizophr Bull*. 2012;38(3):642–647

61. Dhakal R, Gajurel K, Pomares C, et al. Significance of a positive toxoplasma immunoglobulin M test result in the United States. *J Clin Microbiol*. 2015;53(11):3601–3605

62. Montoya JG, Boothroyd JC, Kovacs JA. Toxoplasma gondii. In Bennett J, Dolin R, Blaser M, editors. *Mandell, Douglas, and Bennett's Principles and Practice of Infectious Diseases*. 9th ed. Philadelphia, PA. Elsevier. 2020;2:3355–3387

63. Fellerhoff B, Laumbacher B, Mueller N, et al. Associations between Chlamydophila infections, schizophrenia and risk of HLA-A10. *Mol Psychiatry*. 2007;12:264–272

64. MacIntyre A, Abramov R, Hammond CJ, et al. Chlamydia pneumoniae infection promotes the transmigration of monocytes through human brain endothelial cells. *J Neurosci Res*. 2003;71(5):740–750

65. Hammerschlag MR, Kohlhoff SA, Gaydos CA. Chlamydia pneumoniae. In Bennett J, Dolin R, Blaser M, editors. *Mandell, Douglas, and Bennett's Principles and Practice of Infectious Diseases*. 9th ed. Philadelphia, PA. Elsevier. 2020;2:2323–2331

IDENTIFY: TICK-BORNE INFECTIONS

I am a great admirer of mystery and magic.
Look at this life—all mystery and magic.
~ HARRY HOUDINI

KEY POINTS

▸ Lyme disease is not rare
▸ The concept of a "Lyme-endemic area" is becoming less predictive of the risk of infection
▸ Coinfections with organisms such as *Bartonella henselae*, *Babesia species*, and *Borrelia miyamotoi* are becoming more prevalent throughout the United States and worldwide
▸ Tick-borne infections can cause various neuropsychiatric symptoms and signs consistent with PANS
▸ Conventional two-tier testing for Lyme disease lacks appropriate sensitivity
▸ Specialty lab testing is usually required to properly diagnose tick-borne illnesses
▸ Positive IFN-γ and IL-2 levels for organisms indicate that an active immune response is present, which implies that an infection is current
▸ A significant number of adult patients with Lyme disease experience chronic symptoms, even after completion of recommended treatment regimens

INTRODUCTION

The diagnosis and treatment of Lyme disease has become a controversial subject in both the medical community and in popular culture. The role of tick-borne illnesses in PANS is also controversial. As is the case with many controversial topics, two very vocal groups at the extremes of opinion have arisen.

There are many medical practitioners who are of the opinion that Lyme disease is no big deal and can be handled definitively by two weeks of a macrolide such as azithromycin or a tetracycline antibiotic such as doxycycline or minocycline. There are other practitioners, however, who seem to tie every vague symptom a patient

> **Staying curious is the key to professional development as a physician.**

experiences to Lyme disease and then treat it aggressively, even in the absence of a positive test result.

As with many controversies in medicine, the truth often lies somewhere in the middle. One thing that does not allow for medical progress is when civil discourse is not allowed. We must strive to know more and be better. Staying curious is the key to professional development as a physician.

If a group of patients with a certain diagnosis or constellation of symptoms feels dismissed or not well cared for, we should listen. If they come to a physician and report that they were treated

for Lyme disease (or chronic fatigue or fibromyalgia) and have found recovery they did not think was possible, it's time to pull up a chair and really take notice.

In this chapter we resolve many of the controversies concerning the diagnosis and clinical presentations of tick-borne illnesses by using the published medical literature, a measure of common sense, and the curiosity with which we approached the topic at the launch of our own practice.

As physicians, we have dedicated our lives to understanding and improving the human condition. We have done this by studying core concepts like physiology, pathology, and pharmacology, and by developing good medical judgment. Healthy clinical curiosity does not require you to suspend clinical judgment; it allows you to further develop it to help more patients.

To resolve these controversies and better define a testing and treatment approach to tick-borne illnesses, we must be crystal clear when answering these fundamental clinical questions:

1. Does Lyme disease cause neuropsychiatric symptoms?
2. If so, are those symptoms similar to symptoms seen in children with PANS?
3. Can we tell whether Lyme disease is likely based upon where the patient lives?
4. How can we diagnose Lyme disease most accurately?
5. What about other tick-borne illnesses (sometimes called "co-infections" or "coinfections") like *Bartonella*, *Babesia*, *Borrelia miyamotoi*, and *Ehrlichia*?
6. Is there evidence for "chronic Lyme disease" or "post-treatment Lyme disease"?
7. How should Lyme disease be treated?
8. How should coinfections be treated?

The first six questions are answered in this chapter. Questions seven and eight are answered in Chapter 16 on the treatment of Lyme disease and coinfections.

BACKGROUND

A phenomenon initially called "Lyme arthritis" was first identified in Lyme, Connecticut, in 1975 after a cluster of cases of what was thought to be juvenile rheumatoid arthritis was reported.[1-3] It was subsequently noted that additional symptoms were often present in patients with this disorder, including a characteristic rash, neurologic signs and symptoms, and other constitutional symptoms such as fever, headache, fatigue, and myalgias.

For this reason, the disorder eventually became known as Lyme disease. A few years later, investigators discovered that the cause of Lyme disease was infection with the spirochete *Borrelia burgdorferi*, and improvement was seen in patients with antibiotic treatment.[4,5]

Lyme disease ("borreliosis") was not a new phenomenon, however. Tick-borne disease has been well described in the world medical literature since the early part of the 1900s. In 2011, *National Geographic* published an article detailing findings of the autopsy of the 5,300-year-old mummy Ötzi.[6] The article notes that *Borrelia burgdorferi* DNA was found in the mummy's tissues.

Approximately 35,000 cases of Lyme disease are reported in the United States each year.[7] This is felt to be a low estimate of true cases due to underreporting to state health departments (especially in endemic areas). Review of recent insurance data (2010–2018) shows that about 476,000 people in the United States are diagnosed and treated for Lyme disease each year.[8]

Since this data only reflects cases which were diagnosed and treated, it is logical to infer that the true number of people infected may be much higher. Lyme disease has also been reported in Europe and Asia.

Lyme disease is transmitted by the bite of an *Ixodes* tick. There are approximately fourteen species of *Ixodes* ticks.

There are three stages of Lyme disease which have been described in the medical literature. Due to the small size of the nymph form of the *Ixodes* tick, most people do not remember the initial tick bite.[9-11] Patients may initially present

> Tick-borne disease has been well described in the world medical literature since the early part of the 1900s.

for treatment with symptoms from any of the stages and do not typically manifest all three.

Stage one (early localized infection) typically occurs within several days of a tick bite from which *Borrelia* is transmitted and can last for weeks to months afterward. A skin rash may occur. It is called erythema migrans (formerly erythema chronicum migrans). The rash occurs at the site of the bite and *usually* starts as a homogenous red patch. There may be central clearing after a few days (it is often called a "bull's-eye rash"); the rash usually gets larger at a rate of 1 cm per day. At the middle of the rash, a necrotic center or vesicle may develop. The patch is typically painful or itchy.

Although many clinicians believe that erythema migrans (EM) must have a bull's-eye appearance for diagnosis, there are many serologic confirmed cases of Lyme with an atypical appearance. In fact, two-thirds of patients do not have central clearing in the lesion.[12] The best repository for these images will be found with a simple internet image search for erythema migrans. Although erythema migrans is often said to be pathognomonic for Lyme disease, it is not seen in approximately 20% of cases.[13] Reliance on patients remembering a "tick bite with a rash" will result in many missed diagnoses.

Stage two (early disseminated infection) begins several days to weeks after the tick bite. In this stage, patients may develop multiple annular skin lesions. These lesions are not as migratory as EM. They may coalesce or fade over time. During this period, patients may report headache, fever and chills, malaise, myalgia, and lymphadenopathy. Fatigue and lethargy (which may be constant throughout this period) may occur as well. Migratory pain or waxing and waning symptoms are common. During this stage, a significant proportion of patients (possibly 15%) develop neurologic symptoms such as meningitis, encephalitis, unilateral or bilateral facial palsy, and motor or sensory neuropathic symptoms.[9,14] Within the first few weeks of this stage of disseminated infection, about 5% of patients develop cardiac abnormalities such as heart block or myocarditis.[15,16]

Stage three (late disseminated infection) presents months after the initial infection. It is characterized by arthritis in large joints such as the knees. Monoarticular or polyarticular involvement may be seen. Some cases of antibiotic refractory arthritis have been seen, presumably due to a different strain of *Borrelia* in the northeastern US.[17]

Some patients also develop chronic neurologic manifestations (known as neuroborreliosis) at this time. These neurologic manifestations may include polyneuropathy and radicular pain.[18] EMG testing frequently demonstrates abnormalities in these patients.[19] In early studies, 89% of the patients with neuroborreliosis had mild encephalopathy, and abnormalities with memory were noted on neuropsychological testing.[18] Additional abnormalities with word finding and irritability were noted as well.

Question 1: Does Lyme disease cause neuropsychiatric signs and symptoms?

Since the initial reports describing Lyme disease, many articles have been published which describe neuroborreliosis and its neurologic and psychiatric consequences. In 1987, an article

> **Reliance on patients remembering a "tick bite with a rash" will result in many missed diagnoses.**

was published which described five patients with neuroborreliosis.[20] Presentations included cranial neuritis, encephalitis, and myelitis. Two of the patients experienced cerebral infarction. None of the patients had recalled a history of tick bite or EM rash. The delay in diagnosis in these patients was between three months and five years. All patients improved with high dose IV penicillin. Neurologic deficits disappeared, except in one of the patients with a multi-infarct presentation. Although this patient continued to have neurologic deficits, she improved to the point that she regained the ability to walk.

Another case report documents a patient who presented with a central facial droop and hemiparesis with normal neuroimaging, carotid studies, and echocardiogram.[21] The diagnosis of

> Due to the wide array of neurologic presentations, neuroborreliosis has been rightly called the "great imitator."

neuroborreliosis was established with serology, and resolution of symptoms occurred after a four-week course of IV antibiotics. Additional case reports have described "MS-like" lesions and vascular involvement on neuroimaging in patients with chronic meningoencephalomyelitis from neuroborreliosis.[22] In a larger systematic review of eighty-eight patients with confirmed cerebrovascular complications of neuroborreliosis, ischemic stroke was the most common finding in 89%.[23] Response to antibiotics in these cases was good (75% responded), but there was a mortality of 4.7%.

There is one case report of Lyme neuroborreliosis presenting as an intracranial mass lesion in a ten-year-old girl.[24] Lyme neuroborreliosis can also present initially with persistent headache as the sole finding in both children and adults.[25-27] Bilateral reversible sensorineural hearing loss[28] and demyelinating encephalopathy[29] have also been reported. One case report describes a patient with chronic polyneuropathy

who improved with IV antibiotics.[30] Subsequent sural nerve testing showed *Borrelia* DNA on PCR. There is also a case report of neuroborreliosis which mimicked ALS.[31] Symptoms and neurologic deficits resolved with doxycycline therapy.

Due to the wide array of neurologic presentations, neuroborreliosis has been rightly called the "great imitator."[32] A great review of neuroborreliosis was published in the *Journal of Neurology* in 1998.[33]

In addition to hard neurologic findings, neuroborreliosis has also been shown to affect cognition and memory. Deficits may persist for years after acute infection. These long-term measurable deficits may include issues with verbal memory, mental flexibility, verbal associative functions, and articulation.[34,35] Cognitive and attentional issues are also well established in case reports and controlled studies in children.[36-38]

In addition to the neurologic symptoms (memory loss, cranial neuropathy, polyneuropathy, meningitis, encephalopathy), neuroborreliosis is also responsible for various psychiatric presentations.[39-41] A comprehensive review was published in the *Psychiatric Clinics of North America* in 1998.[41] This review lists a variety of psychiatric impairments found in patients with Lyme disease, including personality changes, hallucinations (auditory, visual, and olfactory), depersonalization, mania, paranoia, obsessive-compulsive disorder, violent outbursts, and panic attacks.

In addition to these reviews, there are case reports of specific neuropsychiatric presentations associated with Lyme disease, including psychosis,[42,43] OCD,[44] Tourette syndrome in a child (Note: *reading the case, this was likely PANS*),[45] hallucinations,[46,47] and depression with suicidal ideation.[48]

These facts clearly demonstrate that infection with *Borrelia* causes neuropsychiatric signs and symptoms.

Question 2: Are the neuropsychiatric symptoms and signs of neuroborreliosis similar to symptoms seen in children with PANS and PANDAS?

An interesting review which outlines the similarity of neuropsychiatric symptoms seen in children with PANDAS and neuroborreliosis was published in 2012.[49]

In addition to symptoms and signs that neuroborreliosis and PANS have in common, several studies have shown that the mechanisms behind neuroborreliosis and PANS or PANDAS are identical. An in vitro study has shown that antibodies made to *Borrelia* OspA epitopes cross-react with human neural tissue from the brain, spinal cord, and dorsal root ganglia.[50] Another study documented anti-neuronal antibodies in patients with persistent symptoms of Lyme disease after treatment.[51]

As noted in Chapter 2, anti-neuronal antibodies have been found in patients with PANS and PANDAS. Inflammation and autoimmunity are prominent parts of PANS and PANDAS pathophysiology. Central nervous system inflammation,[52–55] inflammation-induced glial activation,[56] and autoimmunity[57,58] have been found in patients with neuroborreliosis as well. Early invasion of the central nervous system by Lyme spirochetes has been demonstrated.[59] Glial cell invasion allows *Borrelia* to be intracellular and avoid host defenses.[60] Disruption of the blood-brain barrier (demonstrated in in vitro studies) is part of the CNS invasion process.[61]

As we also noted in Chapter 2, CT, MRI, and PET scans in Sydenham chorea[62–65] and MRI scans in patients with PANDAS[66] show abnormalities which improve with treatment. Similarly, in neuroborreliosis, SPECT scans show abnormalities which improve with treatment.[67,68] Brain abnormalities on MRI are also seen with neuroborreliosis.[69,70]

These facts, as well as our extensive clinical experience treating these children, clearly demonstrate that symptoms of patients with neuroborreliosis are completely consistent with those seen in PANS.

> A common error in medicine is to assume that if a disease or disorder is "rare," then we need not look as closely for it.

Question 3: Can we tell whether Lyme disease is likely based upon where the patient lives?

Most people think of Lyme disease as being a disease which exists solely in the northeastern United States. After all, the original cases were first identified there. Often when physicians discuss patient cases, if someone mentions Lyme, the next question will be, "Is the patient coming from a 'Lyme endemic area'?" When we first started seeing patients with signs and symptoms of chronic infections, we asked the same question. Are patients in Indiana at risk for Lyme disease? What about patients in Oregon, or Illinois, or Kansas? Let's explore this further.

According to the latest CDC data, Lyme disease has been reported in every US state except Hawaii.[71] It has also been reported in fifty countries.[72]

The next question to ask, though, is whether the organism is in ticks in those areas or whether some of these reported cases represent patients who may have traveled elsewhere and contracted the disease. The immediate answer is that it just does not matter. If patients in states not considered endemic for Lyme are showing up with Lyme, it has to remain in the differential diagnosis in these states as well. A common error in medicine is to assume that if a disease or disorder is "rare," then we need not look as closely for it. The problem with this is that you cannot apply population statistics to an individual person. Any patient in front of you may be a patient with a rare disease. That said, as noted previously, Lyme disease is not rare.

When assessing the risk of Lyme in a specific area, it can be helpful to look for information on Lyme testing of ticks in a particular state. This is available online for many states by searching for Department of Natural Resources data on tick testing for a state.

In a well-done study performed in 2017, researchers compiled *canine* serological data for *Borrelia* antibodies from the forty-eight contiguous United States and used this data along with information on forestation and topography to compose a Bayesian model to help provide a *risk forecast* for pet owners, which would predict the risk of Lyme disease transmission to pets based upon current location.[73] As expected, the risk is greatest in the northeastern United States and in Michigan, but the maps show southern and western spread in contiguous areas with some isolated high-prevalence areas noted in the western United States. As with human testing, it is difficult to tell whether current numbers reflect true epidemiological differences in prevalence versus biases due to underreporting or under-testing.

Question 4: What is the best way to test for Lyme disease?

As previously shown, the seriousness and prevalence of Lyme disease are significantly underestimated. Similarly, the subject of testing for *Borrelia* species is also a complex discussion.

If a patient presents with *Streptococcal* pharyngitis or a urinary tract infection, microscopic examination of a sample or culture often reveals the offending organism. *Borrelia* species are very difficult to isolate or culture from blood samples. Culturing *Borrelia* requires a special BSK medium and takes several weeks at low temperature to grow. For this reason, detection of infection due to *Borrelia* commonly relies on the demonstration of antibodies to *Borrelia* species or, in some cases, PCR testing. PCR testing is not as sensitive or specific as antibody testing, especially in neuroborreliosis, where the sensitivity is only about 19%.[74]

The universal questions we must answer with all medical tests are, What are the sensitivity, specificity, and reproducibility of a given test? Next, we need to know whether follow-up testing is available and reliable—i.e., is there a "test of cure"?

The first thing to remember is that Lyme disease is a clinical diagnosis which is supported by laboratory testing.[33,75] In fact, the CDC states, "Lyme disease is diagnosed based on symptoms, physical findings (e.g., rash), and the possibility of exposure to infected ticks."[76] Since IgM and IgG serologic antibodies take several weeks to develop, the current recommendations[77–79] are to treat patients with an erythema migrans rash, even in the absence of other symptoms, if they have been in a "Lyme endemic area."

In the 2020 Infectious Disease Society of America (IDSA) guidelines,[79] the authors base the "incidence" of Lyme disease in each state on reported cases. This underestimates the true incidence as noted in the canine study previously reported.[73] The data from the canine study indicates that the areas of the United States that harbor Lyme disease are now quite wide and continue to expand. In addition, 20–30% of patients do not develop an erythema migrans rash and, if present, the rash may not have a classic bull's-eye appearance. Few patients recall a bite since the deer tick (especially the nymph form) is smaller than other common ticks, such as the dog tick.

If we see a patient beyond the initial bite period, laboratory testing is required. Various tests are used. The two most common tests are an enzyme immunoassay (EIA) and a Western blot test (WB), which reports IgG and IgM antibodies to *Borrelia burgdorferi*.

The current recommendations for Lyme disease testing from the CDC and the IDSA recommend "two-tier" testing.[79,80] First, an EIA test is performed, which reportedly has high sensitivity and low specificity. If positive or equivocal, it is typically followed by a WB test to confirm positivity, as the WB reportedly has a higher specificity. In 2019, the CDC approved a "modified two-tier test (MTTT)" protocol which uses a second EIA test to confirm positivity.[81] If an EIA test is negative, no follow-up is recommended

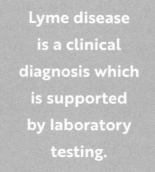

Lyme disease is a clinical diagnosis which is supported by laboratory testing.

since the sensitivity is reported to be very high; therefore, the negative predictive value would statistically be high as well.

However, studies have shown the sensitivity and specificity of EIA testing may vary depending on how the test is done and also by manufacturer of the test kits. Sensitivity in one study that compared test kits from several different manufacturers using patients with confirmed clinical Lyme disease manifestations (such as erythema migrans, neuroborreliosis, and Lyme arthritis) was between 35–70% for IgM (ELISA) and 60–78% for IgG (ELISA).[82] Concordance of test results in this study was shown to be between 56–67%. Some tests in this study were plagued by indeterminate or borderline results which could not be properly interpreted. The study also pointed out that some manufacturers may remove these indeterminate results when analyzing data, which could cause the sensitivity to appear much higher. Similarly, in a European study,[83] the authors note that:

Sensitivity was highly heterogeneous, with summary estimates: erythema migrans 50% (95% CI 40% to 61%); neuroborreliosis 77% (95% CI 67% to 85%); acrodermatitis chronica atrophicans 97% (95 % CI 94% to 99%); unspecified Lyme borreliosis 73% (95% CI 53% to 87%). Specificity was around 95% in studies with healthy controls, but around 80% in cross-sectional studies. Two-tiered algorithms or antibody indices did not outperform single test approaches.

In a meta-analysis of North American research, EIA testing was found to have similar issues with variable sensitivity.[84] The lower-than--optimal sensitivity appeared to be related to the manufacturer and type of test used.

The second stage of the two-tier test is a Western blot test. This test measures specific bands of IgM and IgG to *Borrelia*. The positivity of the test depends upon how many positive bands are seen of either IgM or IgG. A Western blot test is considered positive if at least two of three IgM bands are positive, or if at least five of ten IgG bands are positive.

As previously mentioned, the Western blot is currently recommended only if the ELISA is positive or equivocal. One potential issue is that most Western blot testing requires the lab technician to read the bands by visual inspection. They have a similar appearance to commercially available urine pregnancy tests. Because of this, there may be some variability between technicians reading the same study. There is not as much literature on the sensitivity or specificity of the Western blot alone since it is typically run as part of the two-tier test.

A C-6 ELISA test is now being used, often as a standalone test, due to a reported sensitivity greater than 90% and due to the fact that subjective interpretation by a laboratory technician is not required.

A very well-done study from New York compared C-6 ELISA testing to two-tier testing in patients with culture-proven Lyme disease.[85] It showed that the sensitivity of C-6 peptide was only 69.5% and the sensitivity of the two-tier test was 38.9%. The sensitivity in this study was also variably related to *Borrelia* with different RST genotypes which occur in the wild. In early infection, the two-tier test is even less sensitive. IgM antibodies should go down within thirty days of infection, followed by a rise in IgG antibodies. IgM antibodies and IgG antibodies may remain elevated for years after infection (even in patients who have had treatment).[86] It seems odd that these IgM antibodies are called "false positives" by some sources.[87]

Since we have documented persistence of IgM and IgG antibodies years after infection, the only way we would know that something was a "false positive" is if we had a reliable gold standard with which to compare it. Since we do not have this gold standard, a positive test in a patient with unexplained neuropsychiatric symptoms should not necessarily be counted as a false positive.

A new strain of *Borrelia* called *B. mayonii* has recently been detected in the Midwest. It is not well detected on Western blot testing.[88] *B. mayonii* has been identified in several rodents in the Midwest.[89] The prevalence of *B. mayonii* is still quite low.

It should be noted , though, that the CDC (on their website) lists two-tier testing or modified two-tier testing as part of the *case definition* for Lyme disease. The website also currently states:

> A surveillance case definition is a set of uniform criteria used to define a disease for public health surveillance. Surveillance case

The areas of the United States that harbor Lyme disease continue to expand.

definitions enable public health officials to classify and count cases consistently across reporting jurisdictions. Surveillance case definitions are not intended to be used by healthcare providers for making a clinical diagnosis or determining how to meet an individual patient's health needs. [90]

In our practice we often order tests through a company called IGeneX. IGeneX has developed an immunoblot IgG and IgM test which has a much higher sensitivity than traditional Western blots (reported to be 90%)[91] and a better specificity for many species of *Borrelia,* including *B. burgdorferi* B31, *B. burgdorferi* 297, *B. californiensis, B. mayonii, B. afzelii, B. garinii, B. spiel-*

> **Since the specificity of the Western blot test is so high, a positive result should be regarded as a true positive in a symptomatic patient.**

manii, and *B. valaisiana.*

Since IGeneX testing is not commonly used in hospitals and traditional lab settings, it is dismissed by some physicians. One common criticism is that it is not accurate since the testing is not "FDA approved." Interestingly, the US Department of Health and Human Services states that low- or no-risk lab tests developed in laboratories (LDTs) do not have to be FDA approved.[92] These tests are regulated under the Clinical Laboratory Improvement Amendments (CLIA)

and its accreditation bodies.[93] IGeneX is CLIA certified.[94] Many specialty lab tests used every day by conventional physicians (such as many send-out tests) are performed at CLIA-certified but not FDA-approved labs. One drawback to IGeneX is that the lab is not always covered by insurance and can be expensive.

We use Medical Diagnostic Laboratories (MDL) for Lyme disease Western blot testing as well. This lab is billed to insurance and, even if not covered, they tend to be much less expensive than IGeneX. This lab is CLIA certified. The sensitivity and specificity are not known but are likely comparable to traditional laboratories. The benefit of this lab is that antibody testing for Lyme and other coinfections is available in a panel that is very affordable, even without insurance.

LabCorp and Quest labs perform ELISA and Western blot testing. Sensitivity and specificity of the two-tier tests are likely comparable to most labs. LabCorp offered a C-6 peptide test at one point but it is currently unavailable. Since the specificity of the Western blot test is so high, a positive result should be regarded as a true positive in a symptomatic patient. A negative result (especially to the ELISA test) may be a false negative.

You have to know what you are ordering when ordering Lyme testing. Many commonly used labs report a quantitative total antibody (likely an ELISA test), which only reflexes to the Western blot if this test is positive. If the initial test has a low sensitivity, true positive cases of borreliosis could be missed.

We also use Infectolab testing for *Borrelia burgdorferi.* This test measures IFN-γ and Interleukin 2 (IL-2) levels to the organism. Elevated levels suggest that the immune system is dealing with an active infection. This test is useful in practice since it typically becomes negative when patients improve clinically, suggesting resolution of the active infection. Infectolab is also CLIA certified.

Some practitioners order a CD-57 lymphocyte count in patients suspected of having Lyme disease. One case report and one small study have reported decreased levels of CD-57 cells in patients with chronic Lyme disease and have suggested counts improve with successful antibiotic treatment.[95,96] Another similarly small study demonstrated no differences in patients with post-treatment Lyme disease (PTLD) and controls.[97] Due to a lack of clear supporting evidence, we do not routinely use this test in children with PANS.

In our experience, Lyme disease is underreported and underdiagnosed. Screening tests, to be valuable, should have a sensitivity much higher than current testing at all stages of infection.

Question 5: What about other tick-borne illnesses (sometimes called "coinfections")?

In this section, we discuss other tick-borne infections such as *Bartonella* species, *Babesia* species, *Borrelia miyamotoi*, *Ehrlichia*, and *Anaplasma*. They can occur both with Lyme disease (as a "coinfection") and as isolated infections in patients in whom Lyme disease is not seen.

The rate of coinfections (*Borrelia* plus another agent) can be as high as 39%, with *Borrelia* and *Babesia* coinfection being the most common pattern seen in greater than 80% of cases.[98] In one report from France, 45% of ticks were noted to contain coinfections, with some ticks carrying up to five pathogens at once.[99]

Human studies have reported multiple coinfections.[100–103] There is one case report of a patient with an eating disorder (anorexia) who was diagnosed with a polymicrobial tick-borne infection.[104] Coinfections may lead to more severe disease through alteration of host immune defenses.[103] Tick-borne coinfections are often missed, as the clinical picture can be complicated, leading to a delay in treatment and worsening of the patient's condition.[102,105]

> **Lyme disease is underreported and underdiagnosed.**

BARTONELLA SPECIES

Bartonella species are gram negative bacilli. The two main species we see outside the Andes Mountains are *Bartonella henselae* and *Bartonella quintana*.[106,107]

Bartonella quintana is typically spread by the common body louse and is the causative agent of trench fever (a self-limited, febrile illness), although it can also cause culture-negative endocarditis. This infection typically occurs in homeless populations. No animal vector has been found for *B. quintana*.[107]

B. henselae is most commonly associated with cat scratch disease, which comes from cat scratches that have been inoculated with feces from infected fleas. In immunocompetent patients, cat scratch disease usually causes a self-limited lymphadenopathy. Atypical cases can cause ophthalmic complications and fever of unknown origin in children.

In severe cases or in immunodeficient patients, *Bartonella henselae* infection can cause endocarditis or necrotizing, granulomatous inflammation. Immunocompromised patients may also develop bacillary angiomatosis, which produces multiple round vascular lesions on the skin.

In some cases, however, *Bartonella henselae* can cause significant neurologic manifestations, even in immunocompetent patients. Encephalopathy requiring ICU admission has been reported.[108] In addition, cranial nerve abnormalities, seizures, combative behavior, neuroretinitis, transverse myelitis, peripheral nerve abnormalities, and lethargy without coma have been seen.[108,109] These neurological complications are most commonly seen in children. Although *Bartonella* encephalopathy is usually reversible, there is one case report of a patient with encephalitis who had persistent severe dementia over a 2.5-year period.[110] MRI of the patient demonstrated diffuse white matter lesions in the brain. Persistent infection (bacteremia) with central nervous system involvement has been documented in both humans and other animal hosts.[111,112]

Most of the current literature states that tick-to-human transmission of *Bartonella* species has not been established.[107,113,114] One reference listed on the CDC website as evidence that transmission of *Bartonella* species via ticks does not occur is a review of some of the present literature.[114] Careful reading of this reference, however, shows that it discounts much of the evidence found in other papers and that it was written in an attempt to debunk the concept of *Bartonella* testing and treatment. It is interesting that while the authors do concede that *Bartonella* species have been identified in ticks (including *Ixodes scapularis* ticks), they subsequently proceed to deny the validity of any study which suggests that tick-to-human transmission can occur. Anyone who reads this article will notice that the strong bias toward disproving the concept of tick transmission of *Bartonella* species leads to several contradictions and ignores good evidence of probable links. This bias is evident from the first paragraph of the article.

The specter of human disease caused by *Bartonella* species is yet to be fully seen or appreciated by the medical establishment. Since 1993, over forty-five species of *Bartonella* have been isolated. Several of which (besides *B. henselae*

> *Bartonella henselae* can cause significant neurologic manifestations, even in immunocompetent patients.

and *B. quintana*) can cause human infections.[115]

Bartonella species have been isolated from *Ixodes* ticks[116–122] and Lone Star ticks.[123] In one article, coinfection of *Bartonella* with *Borrelia* and *Anaplasma* was noted in *Ixodes pacificus* ticks.[119] The chief argument against tick-borne transmission of *Bartonella* species is that there are no studies showing direct transmission from ticks to humans. In any case, the argument is largely academic because serious human infections with *Bartonella* species have been demonstrated. Proving the actual vector is only useful if prophylaxis is being considered.

Tick-borne pathogens (*Borrelia*, *Babesia*, *Rickettsia*, and *Ehrlichia* species) have been demonstrated to persist in blood donor samples.

Transmission of *Rickettsia* and *Babesia* via blood transfusion has been demonstrated.[124] Needle stick transmission of *Bartonella* species has been reported in veterinarians.[125,126]

> **Bartonella species have been identified in ticks (including *Ixodes scapularis* ticks).**

Detection of another *Bartonella* species (*Bartonella vinsonii* subsp. *berkhoffi*) with *Bartonella henselae* has been reported in two patients with neurologic symptoms.[127] Another article describes concurrent CNS infection of *Bartonella* and *Borrelia burgdorferi* and refers to this as a "novel tick-borne disease complex."[128] One report describes a mother and son with multiple symptoms who had serologic and skin biopsy evidence of *Bartonella* species (including *B. henselae*) after tick exposures.[129] Neither of the patients had contact with cats.

Bartonella skin lesions

Many patients report skin lesions associated with *Bartonella* infection. They are sometimes referred to as "violaceous striae," "bartonella tracks," or "*Bartonella*-Associated Cutaneous Lesions" (BACL). These lesions have a red or violet appearance and slightly resemble stretch marks seen with weight gain or growth in stature, which are referred to as *striae distensae*.

As with many other aspects of PANS, as well as tick-borne illness, there is some controversy around these skin lesions. One online editorial piece from the American Academy of Dermatology states that "there is not enough data to completely rule out the theory that rare cases of striae may be caused by Bartonella infection."[130] Nevertheless, the author is doubtful that these lesions are from infection, as noted in the title of the editorial. Instead, the author assumes the striae in these cases are from weight loss.

The biggest issue with this assumption is that the patients we see in our practice who have these lesions almost universally have no history of weight loss or sudden growth. The lesions also disappear or lighten after the patient receives treatment for *Bartonella*.

One of the articles quoted in the American Academy of Dermatology editorial (and in other places) to disprove the association of these lesions with *Bartonella* is a very small, retrospective study of teenage boys.[131] This article, from the journal *Pediatric Dermatology*, describes twelve boys (ages 11–17) who presented to an academic dermatology clinic with lesions resembling stretch marks. All were above the fiftieth percentile for height. Eight of the twelve had had a growth spurt before the onset of the skin changes. Eleven of twelve had a first degree relative with similar lesions. Four of the patients had itching near the lesions and no other symptoms were reported in these patients or the rest of the study group. The authors state that none had used steroids and "none had a prior infection with *Bartonella henselae* or *Borrelia burgdorferi*."

This information was obtained by telephone conversations with parents. There were no serologic tests of any type to establish or refute *Bartonella* as a cause of the lesions. In addition, the demographics of the group obviously favored sudden growth as a causative factor. Despite these methodological shortcomings, the authors conclude that "There is no association between this type of striae distensae and any chronic medical condition, bacterial infection, or exogenous steroid use. Thus, a careful review of systems and counseling *without further medical testing* is reasonable management" (emphasis added). This study obviously has several methodological flaws, and the conclusion is not supported by the methods or results of the study.

The most reliable research concerning these skin lesions (and *Bartonella* in general) comes from the Intracellular Pathogens Research Laboratory, Comparative Medicine Institute, College of Veterinary Medicine at the North Carolina State University. In one study of thirty-three patients with neuropsychiatric symptoms, twenty-nine were found to have serologic evidence (IFA or PCR) of *Bartonella* species infection.[132] The study included both males *and* females ages 12–58. Twenty-four of the twenty-nine patients with positive serology reported classic *Bartonella* skin lesions which appeared *at the same time* that their neurologic symptoms started. Only one patient in this study had rapid weight gain. Only five reported steroid use, four of whom were treated for less than one month. Of note, the testing demonstrated antibody titers to several different species of *Bartonella*, including *Bartonella vinsonii berkhoffii* (types 1,2,3), *Bartonella henselae*, *Bartonella koehlerae*, and *Bartonella quintana*. The authors of this paper[132] make an interesting statement at the end of the Discussion section, where they state:

> Mechanistically, could long-standing microvascular injury induced by this endotheliotropic bacteria result in chronic vascular inflammation, local mast cell activation, collagen injury, and the development of a spectrum of BACL?

They also mention resolution of skin lesions following antibiotic therapy in a child with PANS, which was noted in another case report.[133] Other case reports describe *Bartonella* isolation from biopsies of striae lesions directly using several advanced imaging techniques.[132,134] *Bartonella* associated skin lesions are often vertical and in areas other than the low back, which further differentiates them from classic striae distensae. The previously cited paper contains multiple excellent, high-quality images of *Bartonella* associated cutaneous lesions for clinical reference.[132]

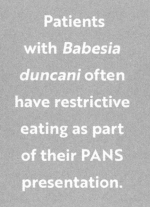

Patients with *Babesia duncani* often have restrictive eating as part of their PANS presentation.

Testing for *Bartonella* species

Conventional IgG and IgM testing for *Bartonella henselae* and *Bartonella quintana* can be obtained through conventional labs like LabCorp, Quest, or hospital laboratories. Medical Diagnostic Laboratories (MDL) has IgG and IgM testing for *Bartonella henselae* only.

IGeneX laboratories has IgG and IgM immunoblot testing for *B. henselae*, *B. quintana*, *B. elizabethae*, and *B. vinsonii*. Immunoblotting is considered more sensitive than conventional ELISA or Western blot tests.

We also use Infectolab testing for *Bartonella henselae*. This test measures IFN-γ and Interleukin 2 (IL-2) levels to the organism. Elevated levels suggest that the immune system is dealing with an active infection. This test is useful in practice since it typically becomes negative when patients improve clinically, suggesting resolution of the active infection. Infectolab does not test for other types of *Bartonella* at this time.

Since *Bartonella* has the capability to evade the immune system and seronegative infections may occur,[129,132] a multifaceted testing strategy may be required for definitive diagnosis. One such strategy uses serology and PCR of a special enriched culture media called BAPGM. This greatly increases sensitivity of the testing to detect *Bartonella*. This testing is available from Galaxy Labs (www.galaxydx.com). The panels available from Galaxy Labs test for *B. henselae, B. quintana, B. vinsonii berkhoffii,* and *B. koehlerae*. This testing is the most expensive of the methods described to test for *Bartonella* species, but it is very accurate. After payment, the company will file with insurance, but reimbursement is variable.

> *Babesia* species stimulate release of interferon γ from T-cells in the body.

BABESIA SPECIES

Babesia species (*B. microti, B. duncani,* and *B. divergens*) are malaria-like parasites which are transmitted to humans in the United States via the bite of the *Ixodes scapularis* tick. They inhabit host red blood cells like *Falciparum*[135] species and cause a spectrum of illness.

Some patients remain asymptomatic. Others may develop a flu-like illness. In severe cases, hemolytic anemia may develop. In splenectomized patients, the disease can lead to multisystem organ failure and death. Patients with more mild infections may complain of transient air hunger and night sweats.

There are reports of *Babesia* infections causing neurologic symptoms in older patients.[136,137] The connection to neuropsychiatric complications is not as strong as is seen with *Borrelia* and *Bartonella*. We have seen multiple patients in our practice with PANS and *Babesia spp.* infections. We have also noted that, similar to *Mycoplasma* infections, patients with *Babesia duncani* often have restrictive eating as part of their PANS presentation.

It is important to note that *Babesia* species exist as coinfections commonly with *Borrelia* and other tick-borne illnesses such as *Ehrlichia* and *Anaplasma*.[98–105] The incidence of babesiosis seems to be increasing at a greater rate than borreliosis in New England.[138] Although infections usually last weeks to months, some patients may develop prolonged infections which last up to a year, especially when occurring as a coinfection with Lyme disease.[139,140] *Babesia microti* is endemic in the eastern United States while *Babeisa divergens* and *Babesia duncani* are found in the Midwest and western United States, respectively. *Babesia* infection has been spread perinatally[141,142] and through blood transfusion.[143,144]

The gold standard for diagnosis of *Babesia* species is microscopy of a thick and thin blood smear which can identify intra-erythrocytic parasites. PCR amplification is also reliable. Serum IgG and IgM titers may be obtained from standard labs. In our practice we find IGeneX testing very sensitive. Babesia species stimulate release of interferon γ from T-cells in the body.[138]

We also use Infectolab testing for *Babesia microti*. This test measures IFN-γ and Interleukin 2 (IL-2) levels to the organism. Elevated levels suggest that the immune system is dealing with an active infection. This test is useful in practice since it typically becomes negative when patients improve clinically, suggesting resolution of the active infection. At this time, Infectolab only tests for *Babesia microti* and not *Babesia duncani,* which we see quite often in our patient population in the Midwest. If the patient has severe illness, conventional blood testing may demonstrate hemolytic anemia, with elevated indirect bilirubin and LDH.

TICK-BORNE RELAPSING FEVER (TBRF)

Borrelia miyamotoi is an infectious agent (along with *B. hermsii*, *B. turicatae*, and *B. parkerii*) which is responsible for a group of diseases called "tick-borne relapsing fever" (TBRF). These disorders present like Lyme disease, but relapsing fever as a symptom is only seen in about 10% of cases.[145–147]

Tick-borne relapsing fever is caused by several different strains of *Borrelia* distinct from *Borrelia burgdorferi*. Initially described as being spread by the bite of soft-bodied ticks, recent evidence shows that hard-bodied ticks transmit this disease as well.[145,146] This disease is found in North America (in the Northeast, Midwest, and western states), Europe, and Asia.

The taxonomy of TBRF is a bit complex. It is generally recognized that the relapsing fever agents are split into two groups. One group are the pathogens responsible for *traditional* relapsing fever (*B. hermsii*, *B. parkerii*, and *Borrelia turicate*). *Borrelia miyamotoi* is a separate species "complex" and not generally considered a "true" relapsing fever species.[147]

Additional relapsing fever species are found in Europe and Asia. One reason that *B. miyamotoi* is not lumped in with the other TBRF species is that the clinical presentation is different. The *traditional* species noted above produce a relapsing fever (usually two or more episodes of fever ≥102°F) and more severe disease with hypotension, splenomegaly, and jaundice being common signs,[147] while patients with *B. miyamotoi* infection may recall an episode of headache and body aches (like a typical viral illness) either with or without a fever.

Borrelia miyamotoi can be a coinfection with

> *Borrelia miyamotoi* has probably been an endemic infection which coexisted with *Borrelia burgdorferi* since the 1970s.

other tick-borne illnesses and may be confused with Lyme disease, *Ehrlichia*, or *Anaplasma*. For this reason, when a tick-borne illness is suspected, testing should be performed for all of the pathogens. Experts have stated that *Borrelia miyamotoi* has probably been an endemic infection which coexisted with *Borrelia burgdorferi* since the 1970s; subclinical infections are suspected based upon cross-sectional serosurveys.[146,147]

We have seen several cases of *Borrelia miyamotoi* in our patients with PANS. A tick bite is seldom recalled, again as it is often transmitted by nymphal ticks. No rash is typically seen with *Borrelia miyamotoi*. It should be noted that, although now considered an endemic coinfection with *Borrelia*, *Anaplasma*, and *Babesia*, current infectious disease texts contain sparse information about TBRF pathogens in general and specifically *B. miyamotoi*.[148]

TBRF species may sometimes be seen on microscopy of a thick blood smear. PCR amplification is also reliable. Serum IgG and IgM titers for *Borrelia miyamotoi* are not available from most standard labs. In our practice, we use IGeneX, as it offers PCR and IgG/IgM tests for *Borrelia miyamotoi* with speciation, which can identify exposure to other TBRF spirochetes in the traditional group, such as *B. hermsii* and *B. turicatae*. IGeneX TBRF testing has been approved by the state health department in New York.[149] We also use Infectolab testing for *Borrelia miyamotoi*. This test measures IFN-γ and Interleukin 2 (IL-2) levels to the organism. Elevated levels suggest that the immune system is dealing with an active infection. This test is useful in practice since it typically becomes negative when patients improve clinically, suggesting resolution of the active infection. Infectolab only tests for *Borrelia miyamotoi* and not other organisms in the TBRF family.

ANAPLASMA AND EHRLICHIA

Ehrlichia species (*Ehrlichia chaffeensis* and *Ehrlichia ewingii*) and *Anaplasma phagocytophilum* are intracellular gram-negative bacteria. They are both spread by tick bites. *Ehrlichia* species can be found in Lone Star ticks and dog ticks, while *Anaplasma* is found in deer ticks like *Ixodes scapularis*. Initially discovered in the 1980s,[150] these infections have steadily increased in prevalence, likely due to increased awareness of the diseases. What we now call *Ehrlichia chaffensis* was once referred to as "human monocytic ehrlichiosis." *Ehrlichia ewingii* and *Anaplasma* were once grouped together as "human granulocytic ehrlichiosis." Now *Anaplasma phagocytophilium* is known as a separate, although related, entity.

Most cases of *Anaplasma* have symptoms such as fever, headache, fatigue, and flu-like symptoms, although some patients may have a more serious presentation with elevated liver transaminases, leukopenia, and thrombocytopenia.[151] Confusion has been reported as well. There is a case report of a patient with anaplasmosis who presented with trigeminal neuralgia[152] and another case report of a patient who presented with brachial plexopathy.[153] In some cases, such as in immunocompromised patients or patients of advanced age, anaplasmosis can be fatal.[154] The incubation period from tick bite to clinical symptoms is usually 1–2 weeks.

Seroprevalence of *Anaplasma* antibodies in patients with tick bites ranges from 8.9% to 36%.[155] Seroprevalence of *Anaplasma* in healthy patients in the midwestern United States has been found to be 14.9%.[156] The rate is somewhat higher in Connecticut. Anaplasmosis has been identified after tick bites in Europe as well. One case of perinatal transmission of anaplasmosis has been reported[157] and several cases among patients who had butchered white-tailed deer have been noted.[158]

There is no literature which has linked *Anaplasma* to PANS, but we have identified prior infections with *Anaplasma* in a small number of our patients. In these cases, it was in concert with concomitant infection with *Borrelia* or *Bartonella* species. PCR testing for *Anaplasma* can be performed from most conventional labs, although in our practice we use IGeneX as it offers PCR and IgG/ IgM tests for *Anaplasma*. Infectolab testing is not available for *Anaplasma*.

Ehrlichiosis has a very similar presentation and similar complications to *Anaplasma* infection.

Symptom presentation, lab abnormalities, and the possibility of progression to fulminant multisystem organ failure and death mirror *Anaplasma* infections. Rash is present in about 10% of patients. The disease is found mainly in the southeastern and south central United States.[159]

There is no literature which has linked *Ehrlichia* to PANS, but we have identified prior infections with *Ehrlichia* in a small number of our patients. In these cases, it was usually in concert with concomitant infection with *Borrelia* or *Bartonella* species. Testing for antibodies to HME (*Ehrlichia chafeensis*), HGE (*Ehrlichia ewingii*), and PCR testing is available from LabCorp. We also use Infectolab testing for *Ehrlichia*. This test measures IFN-γ and Interleukin 2 (IL-2) levels to the organism. Elevated levels suggest that the immune system is dealing with an active infection. This test is useful in practice since it typically becomes negative when patients improve clinically, suggesting resolution of the active infection. The company does not specify which species of *Ehrlichia* is tested.

Unlike *Borrelia*, there is no evidence to date which has shown that persistent infection or symptoms occur with *Anaplasma* or *Ehrlichia*. Relatively little information is present in current infectious disease texts about either ehrlichiosis or anaplasmosis.[159] We test for these infections as it may be a clue to coinfection if Lyme testing remains nondiagnostic.

RICKETTSIA, TULAREMIA, TICK-BORNE VIRUSES

There are various other illnesses carried by ticks. Some of the infectious agents carry significant

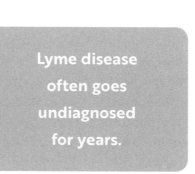

Lyme disease often goes undiagnosed for years.

morbidity and mortality. In some cases, these disorders may be fatal. There are no links established in the peer-reviewed literature which connect these infections with PANS. They are not known to have chronic persistence of symptoms like *Borrelia*.

We have tested for these agents in the past and have not had any PANS patients with positive serology. We do not consider these tests necessary for the majority of patients with PANS unless specific circumstances warrant consideration.

It is disappointing to think how many patients with symptoms compatible with tick-borne illnesses (fatigue, persistent headaches, strange neurologic symptoms, anxiety, mood disorders) are dismissed due to failure to test at all, failure to use a test with high enough sensitivity, or failure to test for organisms like *Borrelia miyamotoi*, *Babesia*, and *Bartonella*.

We see these patients every day. Parents of some of these children are told that they just have mental illness, and symptom management (mopping up the floor) is the best they could hope for. Seeing these patients recover after treatment for tick-borne infections is truly inspiring.

Question 6: What about "chronic Lyme disease"?

Many patients with Lyme disease develop symptoms which persist, even after what may be considered appropriate antimicrobial therapy. These patients often present with a host of nonspecific complaints such as fatigue, paresthesias, brain fog, and muscle and joint pains. This constellation of symptoms in patients who have been previously treated is known as "chronic Lyme disease" or sometimes as "post-treatment Lyme disease" (PTLD).

It should be noted that Lyme disease often goes undiagnosed for years. In this case, it should be referred to as "late-disseminated Lyme disease" or "latent Lyme disease." These patients don't have "chronic Lyme disease." They are just previously undiagnosed.

In most medical reference texts, chronic Lyme disease or post-treatment Lyme disease are discounted, much like chronic fatigue syndrome or fibromyalgia.[160] However, chronic neurologic manifestations have been reported in patients who had been treated for Lyme disease with a course of IV antibiotics.[161] Patients described in this reference[161] were found to have varied neurologic syndromes, including polyneuropathy

In another study from researchers at Boston University, Cornell University, and New York Medical College, anti-neuronal antibodies were significantly elevated in patients with post-Lyme treatment symptoms as compared to a group of post-Lyme treated patients with no symptoms, and healthy patients with no previous history of Lyme disease.[162] Another arm of this study contained patients with a lupus diagnosis. Similar elevations of anti-neuronal antibodies were noted in this group. It should be noted that the anti-neuronal antibody measured in this study was anti-tubulin antibody, which is also associated with Sydenham chorea[163–168] and PANDAS.[169–171]

Genetic mutations and immune system dysregulation have been found in some patients with antibiotic-refractory arthritis post-treatment for Lyme disease.[172–174]

> Anti-neuronal antibodies were significantly elevated in patients with post-Lyme treatment symptoms as compared to a group of post-Lyme treated patients with no symptoms, and healthy patients with no previous history of Lyme disease.

with radicular pain or distal paresthesias (70% of the study group), mild encephalopathy with memory loss/mood changes/sleep disturbance (89%), EMG evidence of axonal polyneuropathy (59%), and elevated intrathecal protein or CSF antibody production to Lyme (67%). Of the patients above reporting mild encephalopathy, 58% had measurable abnormalities on neuropsychological testing. These patients also reported fatigue, headache, and persistent arthritis.

The concepts of PTLD or chronic Lyme disease remain controversial despite substantial evidence from peer-reviewed journals from several academic institutions, such as Johns Hopkins, that patients with Lyme disease, with or without standard treatment, may experience chronic disabling symptoms for years following infection.[175–177]

But do recurrent courses of antibiotics lead to improvement of PTLD symptoms? In a prospective study from 2001, patients with positive Lyme disease diagnosis who had been treated with antibiotics and had persistent symptoms consistent with PTLD were given both IV and oral antibiotics.[178] The study demonstrated no improvement in the treatment group. The materials and methods section of this paper notes that the patients in the study had previously been treated with a "recommended antibiotic regimen." The treatment recommendations

> Persistence of viable *Borrelia* organisms inside human fibroblasts has been demonstrated following antibiotic treatment.

at the time the paper was written would have been 14–21 days of a tetracycline antibiotic like doxycycline.

Careful analysis of the data from this study indicates that the average length of treatment was between 57–71 days. The average number of courses of antibiotics between all groups (including controls) was about three courses. The specific agents used for prior treatment were not listed in the study.

Additional studies[179,180] have also failed to demonstrate the efficacy of additional courses of antibiotics to improve symptoms of PTLD. Based upon these studies, many physicians have concluded that persistent infection does not occur and that PTLD is not a real phenomenon.

But are we asking the right questions?

Considering what we know about coinfections, it is possible that patients with persistent symptoms may have had other unidentified infections such as *Babesia* or *Borrelia miyamotoi*, which are known to produce more severe or persistent disease when coupled with Lyme.

More importantly, there is good evidence that antibiotic-tolerant persistent infections can occur, which may require additional antibiotics, pulsed dose antibiotics, and/or biofilm disruption[181,182] (see Chapter 14). Atypical and cystic forms of the Lyme spirochete have been found in studies of neuroborreliosis.[183–185] Persistent infection after antibiotic treatment has been noted in dogs,[186] mice,[187] and monkeys.[188]

Interestingly, the CDC held a webinar on *Borrelia* persisters which highlighted several of the references cited in the above paragraph, thereby lending credence to the concept.[189] Persistence of viable *Borrelia* organisms inside human fibroblasts has been demonstrated following antibiotic treatment.[190] This intracellular migration may also contribute to antibiotic resistance.

The vast majority of adult patients who present to our practice with long-term symptoms suggesting Lyme disease have not been previously treated. Those who subsequently test positive should not be considered PTLD, and the term "chronic Lyme" should not be used. As previously noted, *late-disseminated Lyme disease* is a more appropriate term.

In our practice, 14–21 days of antibiotic treatment is seldom sufficient to treat adults with tick-borne illness. Longer courses, pulsed antibiotics, and the addition of herbal agents and biofilm disruptors to prescription antimicrobials is most effective. See Chapter 16 for details on the treatment of Lyme disease and tick-borne coinfections in children with PANS and PANDAS.

There is no existing data on post-treatment symptoms in children with Lyme disease, but the majority of the children we diagnose and treat for tick-borne illnesses, including Lyme, have resolution of their symptoms with initial treatment. They do not seem to suffer the chronic sequelae some adults experience.

CHAPTER 9 REFERENCES

1. Mast WE, Burrows WM. Erythema chronicum migrans and "lyme arthritis." *JAMA*. 1976;236(21):2392

2. Hazard GW, Leland K, Mathewson HO. Erythema chronicum migrans and "Lyme arthritis." *JAMA*. 1976;236(21):2392

3. Steere AC, Malawista SE, Snydman DR, et al. Lyme arthritis: an epidemic of oligoarticular arthritis in children and adults in three Connecticut communities. *Arthritis and Rheumatism*. 1977;20(1):7–17

4. Burgdorfer W. Discovery of the Lyme disease spirochete and its relation to tick vectors. *Yale J Biol Med*. 1984;57(4):515–520

5. Steere AC, Hutchinson GJ, Rahn DW, et al. Treatment of the early manifestations of Lyme disease. *Annals of Internal Medicine*. 1983;99(1):22–6

6. www.web.archive.org/web/20111019172457/http:/ngm.nationalgeographic.com/2011/11/iceman--autopsy/hall-text, accessed 6/1/2022

7. Mead PS. Epidemiology of Lyme disease. *Infect Dis Clin North Am*. 2015;29(2):187–210

8. www.cdc.gov/lyme/stats/humancases.html, accessed 6/22/22

9. Steere AC. Lyme disease (Lyme borreliosis) due to *Borrelia burgdorferi*. In Bennett J, Dolin R, Blaser M, editors. *Mandell, Douglas, and Bennett's Principles and Practice of Infectious Diseases*. 9th ed. Philadelphia, PA. Elsevier. 2020;2:2911–2922

10. Steere AC, Bartenhagen NH, Craft JE, et al. The early clinical manifestations of Lyme disease. *Ann Intern Med*. 1983;99(1):76–82

11. Tibbles CD, Edlow JA. Does this patient have erythema migrans? *JAMA*. 2007;297(23):2617–2627

12. Shapiro ED. Clinical practice: Lyme disease. *N Engl J Med*. 2014;370(18):1724–1731

13. www.cdc.gov/lyme/signs_symptoms/index.html#:~:text=Erythema%20migrans%20(EM)%20rash%20(,average%20is%20about%207%20days), accessed 6/22/2022

14. Pachner AR, Steere AC. The triad of neurologic manifestations of Lyme disease: meningitis, cranial neuritis, and radiculoneuritis. *Neurology*. 1985;35(1):47–53

15. Steere AC, Batsford WP, Weinberg M, et al. Lyme carditis: cardiac abnormalities of Lyme disease. *Ann Intern Med*. 1980;93(1):8–16

16. Nagi KS, Joshi R, Thakur RK. Cardiac manifestations of Lyme disease: a review. *Can J Cardiol*. 1996;12(5):503–506

17. Jones KL, McHugh GA, Glickstein LJ, et al. Analysis of *Borrelia burgdorferi* genotypes in patients with Lyme arthritis: high frequency of ribosomal RNA intergenic spacer type 1 strains in antibiotic-refractory arthritis. *Arthritis Rheum.* 2009;60(7):2174–2182

18. Logigian EL, Kaplan RF, Steere AC. Chronic neurologic manifestations of Lyme disease. *N Engl J Med.* 1990;323(21):1438–1444

19. Logigian EL, Steere AC. Clinical and electrophysiologic findings in chronic neuropathy of Lyme disease. *Neurology.* 1992;42(2):303–311

20. Weder B, Wiedersheim P, Matter L, et al. Chronic progressive neurological involvement in *Borrelia burgdorferi* infection. *J Neurol.* 1987;234(1):40–43

21. Zhang Y, Lafontant G, Bonner FJ. Lyme neuroborreliosis mimics stroke: a case report. *Archives of Physical Medicine and Rehabilitation.* 2000;81(4):519 – 521

22. Kohler J, Kern U, Kasper J, et al. Chronic central nervous system involvement in Lyme borreliosis. *Neurology.* 1988;38(6):863–867

23. Garkowski A, Zajkowska J, Zajkowska A, et al. Cerebrovascular manifestations of Lyme neuroborreliosis: a systematic review of published cases. *Front Neurol.* 2017;8:146:1–8

24. Murray R, Morawetz R, Kepes J, et al. Lyme neuroborreliosis manifesting as an intracranial mass lesion. *Neurosurgery.* 1992;30(5):769–773

25. Moses JM, Riseberg RS, Mansbach JM. Lyme disease presenting with persistent headache. *Pediatrics.* 2003;112:477–449

26. Belman AL, Iyer M, Coyle PK, et al. Neurologic manifestations in children with North American Lyme disease. *Neurology.* 1993;43(12):2609–14

27. Brinck T, Hansen K, Olesen J. Headache resembling tension-type headache as the single manifestation of Lyme neuroborreliosis. *Cephalalgia.* 1993;13(3):207–209

28. Quinn SJ, Boucher BJ, Booth JB. Reversible sensorineural hearing loss in Lyme disease. *J Laryngol Otol.* 1997;111(6):562–564

29. Reik L Jr, Smith L, Khan A, et al. Demyelinating encephalopathy in Lyme disease. *Neurology.* 1985;35(2):267–269

30. Maimone D, Villanova M, Stanta G, et al. Detection of *Borrelia burgdorferi* DNA and complement membrane attack complex deposits in the sural nerve of a patient with chronic polyneuropathy and tertiary Lyme disease. *Muscle & Nerve.* 1997;20(8):969–975

31. Burakgazi AZ. Lyme disease-induced polyradiculopathy mimicking amyotrophic lateral sclerosis. *Int J Neurosci.* 2014;124(11):859–62

32. Pachner AR. *Borrelia burgdorferi* in the nervous system: the new "great imitator." *Ann NY Acad Sci.* 1988;539:56–64

33. Kaiser, R. Neuroborreliosis. *J Neurol.* 1998;245(5):247–255

34. Benke T, Gasse T, Hittmair-Delazer M, et al. Lyme encephalopathy: long-term neuropsychological deficits years after acute neuroborreliosis. *Acta Neurol Scand.* 1995;91(5):353–357

35. Kaplan RF, Jones-Woodward L, Workman K, et al. Neuropsychological deficits in Lyme disease patients with and without other evidence of central nervous system pathology. *Appl Neuropsychol.* 1999;6(1):3–11

36. Bloom B, Wyckoff P, Meissner H, et al. Neurocognitive abnormalities in children after classic manifestations of Lyme disease. *Pediatr Infect Dis J.* 1998;17(3):189–196

37. Tager FA, Fallon BA, Keilp J, et al. A controlled study of cognitive deficits in children with chronic Lyme disease. *Journal of Neuropsychiatry and Clinical Neurosciences.* 2001;13(4):500–507

38. Engman M, Lindstrom K, Sallamba M, et al. One-year follow-up of tick-borne central nervous system infections in childhood. *Pediatr Infect Dis J.* 2012;31(6):570–574

39. Fallon BA, Nields JA. Lyme disease: a neuropsychiatric illness. *Am J Psychiatry.* 1994;151(11):1571–83

40. Fallon BA, Nields JA, Parsons B, et al. Psychiatric manifestations of Lyme borreliosis. *J Clin Psychiatry.* 1993;54(7):263–268

41. Fallon BA, Kochevar JM, Gaito A, Nields JA. The underdiagnosis of neuropsychiatric Lyme disease in children and adults. *Psychiatr Clin North Am.* 1998;21:693–703

42. Roelcke U, Barnett W, Wilder-Smith E, et al. Untreated neuroborreliosis: Bannwarth's syndrome evolving into acute schizophrenia-like psychosis: a case report. *J Neurol.* 1992 Mar;239(3):129–131

43. Hess A, Buchmann J, Zettl UK, et al. *Borrelia burgdorferi* central nervous system infection presenting as an organic schizophrenia like disorder. *Biol Psychiatry.* 1999;45(6):795

44. Johnco C, Kugler BB, Murphy TK, et al. Obsessive-compulsive symptoms in adults with Lyme disease. *Gen Hosp Psychiatry.* 2018;51:85–89

45. Riedel M, Straube A, Schwarz MJ, et al. Lyme disease presenting as Tourette's syndrome. *Lancet.* 1998;351(9100):418–9

46. Stricker RB, Winger EE. Musical hallucinations in patients with Lyme disease. *South Med J.* 2003;96(7):711–715

47. Binalsheikh IM, Griesemer D, Wang S, et al. Lyme neuroborreliosis presenting as Alice in Wonderland syndrome. *Pediatr Neurol.* 2012;46:185–186

48. Garakani A, Mitton AG. New-onset panic, depression with suicidal thoughts, and somatic symptoms in a patient with a history of Lyme disease. *Case Rep Psychiatry.* 2015;2015:457947:1–5

49. Rhee H, Cameron DJ. Lyme disease and pediatric autoimmune neuropsychiatric disorders associated with streptococcal infections (PANDAS): an overview. *Int J Gen Med.* 2012;5:163–174

50. Alaedini A, Latov N. Antibodies against OspA epitopes of *Borrelia burgdorferi* cross- react with neural tissue. *J Neuroimmunol.* 2005;159(1–2):192–5

51. Chandra A et al. Anti-neural antibody reactivity in patients with a history of Lyme borreliosis and persistent symptoms. *Brain Behav Immun.* 2010;24(6):1018–1024

52. Oksi J, Kalimo H, Marttila RJ, et al. Inflammatory brain changes in Lyme borreliosis. A report on three patients and review of literature. *Brain.*1996;119(6):2143–2154

53. Fallon BA, Levin ES, Schweitzer PJ, et al. Inflammation and central nervous system Lyme disease. *Neurobiol Dis.* 2010;37(3):534–41

54. Pachne AR, Steiner I. Lyme neuroborreliosis: infection, immunity and inflammation. *Lancet Neurol.* 2007;6(6):544–52

55. Ramesh G, Didier PJ, England JD, et al. Inflammation in the pathogenesis of Lyme neuroborreliosis. *Am J Pathol.* 2015;185(5):1344–60

56. Ramesh R, Borda JT, Dufor J, et al. Interaction of the Lyme disease spirochete *Borrelia burgdorferi* with brain parenchyma elicits inflammatory mediators from glial cells as well as glial and neuronal apoptosis. *Am J Pathol.* 2008;173 (5):1415–27

57. Bransfield RC. Relationship of inflammation and autoimmunity to psychiatric sequelae in Lyme disease. *Psychiatric Ann*. 2012;42(9):337–41

58. Bransfield RC. The psychoimmunology of Lyme/tick-borne diseases and its association with neuropsychiatric symptoms. *Open Neurol J*. 2012;6:88–93

59. Luft BJ, Steinman CR, Neimark HC, et al. Invasion of the CNS by *Borrelia burgdorferi* in acute disseminated infection. *JAMA*. 1992;267:1364–1367

60. Livengood JA, Gilmore RD Jr. Invasion of human neuronal and glial cells by an infectious strain of *Borrelia burgdorferi*. *Microbes and Infection*. 2006;8:2832–2840

61. Garcia-Monco JC, Villar BF, Alen JC, et al. *Borrelia burgdorferi* in the central nervous system: experimental and clinical evidence for early invasion. *J Infect Dis*. 1990;161(6):1187–93

62. Giedd JN, Rapoport JL, Kruesi MJ, et al. Sydenham's chorea: magnetic resonance imaging of the basal ganglia. *Neurology*. 1995;45(12):2199–2202

63. Traill Z, Pike M, Byrne J. Sydenham's chorea: a case showing reversible striatal abnormalities on CT and MRI. *Dev Med Child Neurol*. 1995;37(3):270–273

64. Aron AM. Sydenham's chorea: positron emission tomographic (PET) scan studies. *J Child Neurol*. 2005;20(10):832–833

65. Goldman S, Amrom D, Szliwowski HB, et al. Reversible striatal hypermetabolism in a case of Sydenham's chorea. *Mov Disord*. 1993;8(3):355–358

66. Giedd JN, Rapoport JL, Garvey MA, et al. MRI assessment of children with obsessive-compulsive disorder or tics associated with streptococcal infection. *American Journal of Psychiatry*. 2000;157(2):281–283

67. Fallon BA, Das S, Plutchok JJ, et al. Functional brain imaging and neuropsychological testing in Lyme disease. *Clin Infect Dis*. 1997;25(suppl 1):S57–S63

68. Donta ST, Noto RB, Vento JA. SPECT brain imaging in chronic Lyme disease. *Clin Nucl Med*. 2012;37(9):e219–e222

69. Farshad-Amacker NA, Scheffel H, Frauenfelder T, et al. Brainstem abnormalities and vestibular nerve enhancement in acute neuroborreliosis. *BMC Research Notes*. 2013;6:551

70. Hildenbrand P, Craven DE, Jone R, et al. Lyme neuroborreliosis: manifestations of a rapidly emerging zoonosis. *Am J Neuroradiol*. 2009;30:1079–87

71. www.cdc.gov/lyme/stats/tables.html, accessed 6/25/2022

72. Shapiro ED, Gerber MA. Lyme disease. *Clinical Infectious Diseases*. 2000;31(2): 533–542

73. Watson SC, Liu Y, Lund RB, et al. A Bayesian spatio-temporal model for forecasting the prevalence of antibodies to *Borrelia burgdorferi*, causative agent of Lyme disease, in domestic dogs within the contiguous United States. *PLoS One*. 2017;12(5): e0174428:1–22

74. Alby K, Capraro GA. Alternatives to serologic testing for diagnosis of Lyme disease. *Clin Lab Med*. 2015;35(4):815–825

75. Halperin JJ, Logigian EL, Finkel MF, et al. Practice parameters for the diagnosis of patients with nervous system Lyme borreliosis (Lyme disease). Quality standards subcommittee of the American Academy of Neurology. *Neurology*. 1996;46:619–627

76. www.cdc.gov/lyme/index.html, accessed 7/22/2022

77. www.cdc.gov/lyme/treatment/erythema-migrans-rash.html, accessed 7/22/2022

78. www.columbia-lyme.org/diagnosis, accessed 7/22/2022

79. Lantos PM, Rumbaugh J, Bockenstedt LK, et al. Clinical practice guidelines by the Infectious Diseases Society of America (IDSA), American Academy of Neurology (AAN), and American College of Rheumatology (ACR): 2020 guidelines for the prevention, diagnosis, and treatment of Lyme disease. *Arthritis Care Res* (Hoboken). 2021;73(1):1–9

80. www.cdc.gov/lyme/diagnosistesting/index.html, accessed 7/24/2022

81. www.cdc.gov/mmwr/volumes/68/wr/mm6832a4.htm?s_cid=mm6832a4_w, accessed 7/24/2022

82. Kodym P, Kurzová Z, Berenová D, et al. Serological diagnostics of Lyme borreliosis: comparison of universal and *Borrelia* species–specific tests based on whole-cell and recombinant antigens. *J Clin Microbiol*. 2018;56(11):e00601–18

83. Leeflang MM, Ang CW, Berkhout J, et al. The diagnostic accuracy of serological tests for Lyme borreliosis in Europe: a systematic review and meta-analysis. *BMC Infect Dis*. 2016;16:140:1–26

84. Waddell LA, Greig J, Mascarenhas M, et al. The accuracy of diagnostic tests for Lyme disease in humans, a systematic review and meta-analysis of North American research. *PLoS One*. 2016;11(12):e0168613:1–23

85. Wormser GP, Liveris D, Hanincová K, et al. Effect of *Borrelia burgdorferi* genotype on the sensitivity of C6 and 2-tier testing in North American patients with culture-confirmed Lyme disease. *Clin Infect Dis*. 2008;47(7):910–914

86. Feder HM Jr., Gerber MA, Luger SW, et al. Persistence of serum antibodies to *Borrelia burgdorferi* in patients treated for Lyme disease. *Clinical Infectious Diseases*. 1992;15(5):788–93

87. Seriburi N, Ndukwe Z, Chang ME, et al. High frequency of false positive IgM immunoblots for *Borrelia burgdorferi* in clinical practice. *Clinical Microbiology and Infection*. 2012;18(12):1236–1240

88. Pritt BS, Mead PS, Johnson DKH, et al. Identification of a novel pathogenic *Borrelia* species causing Lyme borreliosis with unusually high spirochaetaemia: a descriptive study. *Lancet Infect Dis*. 2016;16(5):556–564

89. Siy PN, Larson RT, Zembsch TE, et al. High prevalence of *Borrelia mayonii* (*Spirochaetales: Spirochaetaceae*) in field-caught *Tamias striatus* (*Rodentia: Sciuridae*) from Northern Wisconsin. *Journal of Medical Entomology*. 2021;58(6):2504–2507

90. www.ndc.services.cdc.gov/case-definitions/lyme-disease-2022, accessed 7/25/2022

91. www.igenex.com/press-release/igenex-inc-introduces-new-diagnostic-tests-for-lyme-disease-and-tick--borne-relapsing-fever, accessed 7/25/2022

92. www.aha.org/news/headline/2020–08–21-hhs-laboratory-developed-tests-do-not-require-fda-approval-or#:~:text=HHS%3A%20Laboratory%20developed%20tests%20do%20not%20require%20FDA%20approval%20or%20authorization,-Aug%2021%2C%202020, accessed 7/25/2022

93. www.aacc.org/advocacy-and-outreach/position-statements/2020/oversight-of-laboratory-developed--tests, accessed 7/25/2022

94. www.igenex.com/licenses-certifications, accessed 7/25/2022

95. Stricker RB, Burrascano J, Winger E. Long term decrease in the CD57 lymphocyte subset in a patient with chronic Lyme disease. *Ann Agric Environ Med*. 2002;9(1):111–3

96. Stricker RB, Winger EE. Decreased CD57 lymphocyte subset in patients with chronic Lyme disease. *Immunol Lett*. 2001;76(1):43–48

97. Marques A, Brown MR, Fleisher TA. Natural killer cell counts are not different between patients with post-Lyme disease syndrome and controls. *Clin Vaccine Immunol*. 2009;16(8):1249–1250

98. Belongia EA. Epidemiology and impact of coinfections acquired from Ixodes ticks. *Vector Borne Zoonotic Dis*. 2002;2(4):265–73

99. Moutailler S, Valiente Moro C, Vaumourin E, et al. Co-infection of ticks: the rule rather than the exception. *PLoS Negl Trop Dis*. 2016;10(3):e0004539:1–17

100. Swanson SJ, Neitzel D, Reed KD, et al. Coinfections acquired from ixodes ticks. *Clin Microbiol Rev*. 2006;19(4):708–27

101. Magnarelli, LA, Dumler JS, Anderson JF, et al. Coexistence of antibodies to tick-borne pathogens of babesiosis, ehrlichiosis, and Lyme borreliosis in human sera. *J. Clin. Microbiol*. 1995;33:3054–3057

102. Mitchell PD, Reed KD, Hofkes JM. Immunoserologic evidence of coinfection with *Borrelia burgdorferi*, *Babesia microti*, and human granulocytic *Ehrlichia* species in residents of Wisconsin and Minnesota. *J. Clin. Microbiol*. 1996;34:724–727

103. Thompson C, Spielman A, Krause PJ. Coinfecting deer-associated zoonoses: Lyme disease, babesiosis, and ehrlichiosis. *Clin Infect Dis*. 2001;33(5):676–85

104. Kinderlehrer DA. Anorexia nervosa caused by polymicrobial tick-borne infections: a case study. *Int Med Case Rep J*. 2021;14:279–287

105. Caulfield AJ, Pritt BS. Lyme disease coinfections in the United States. *Clin Lab Med*. 2015;35(4):827–46

106. Maurin M, Birtles R, Raoult D. Current knowledge of *Bartonella* species. *Eur. J. Clin. Microbiol. Infect. Dis*. 1997;16(7):487–506

107. Rose SR, Koehler JE. *Bartonella*, including cat-scratch disease. In Bennett J, Dolin R, Blaser M, editors. *Mandell, Douglas, and Bennett's Principles and Practice of Infectious Diseases*. 9th ed. Philadelphia, PA. Elsevier. 2020;2:2824–2843

108. Carithers HA, Margileth AM. Cat-scratch disease: acute encephalopathy and other neurologic manifestations. *Am J Dis Child*. 1991;145(1):98–101

109. Breitschwerdt EB, Sontakke S, Hopkins S. Neurological manifestations of bartonellosis in immunocompetent patients: a composite of reports from 2005–2012. *J Neuroparasitol*. 2012;3(235640):1–15

110. Revol A, Vighetto A, Jouvet A, et al. Encephalitis in cat scratch disease with persistent dementia. *J Neurol Neurosurg Psychiatry*. 1992;55:133–135

111. Breitschwerdt EB, Maggi RG, Nicholson WL, et al. Bartonella sp. bacteremia in patients with neurological and neurocognitive dysfunction. *J Clin Microbiol*. 2008;46(9):2856–2861

112. Breitschwerdt EB, Kordick DL. Bartonella infection in animals: carriership, reservoir potential, pathogenicity, and zoonotic potential for human infection. *Clinical Microbiology Reviews*. 2000;13(3):428–38

113. www.cdc.gov/bartonella/faq.html, accessed 10/10/2022

114. Telford SR, Wormser GP. Bartonella spp. Transmission by ticks not established. *Emerg Infect Dis*. 2010;16(3):379–84

115. www.bestpractice.bmj.com/topics/en-us/1152, accessed 10/30/2022

116. Chang CC, Hayashidani H, Pusterla N, et al. Investigation of Bartonella infection in Ixodid ticks from California. *Comp Immunol Microbiol Infect Dis*. 2002;25:229–236

117. Adelson ME, Rao RV, Tilton RC, et al. Prevalence of *Borrelia burgdorferi, Bartonella spp., Babesia microti,* and *Anaplasma phagocytophila* in *Ixodes scapularis* ticks collected in northern New Jersey. *J Clin Microbiol.* 2004;42:2799–2801

118. Sanogo YO, Zeaiter Z, Caruso G, et al. Bartonella henselae in Ixodes ricinus ticks (Acari: Ixodida) removed from humans, Belluno province, Italy. *Emerg Infect Dis.* 2003;9:329–332

119. Holden K, Boothby JT, Kasten RW, et al. Co-detection of *Bartonella henselae, Borrelia burgdorferi,* and *Anaplasma phago- cytophilum* in *Ixodes pacificus* ticks from California, USA. *Vector Borne Zoonotic Dis.* 2006;6:99–102

120. Morozova OV, Cabello FC, Dobrotvorsky AK. Semi-nested PCR detection of *Bartonella henselae* in *Ixodes persulcatus* ticks from Western Siberia, Russia. *Vector Borne Zoonotic Dis.* 2004;4:306–9

121. Schouls LM, van de Pol I, Rijpkema SG, et al. Detection and identification of *Ehrlichia, Borrelia burgdorferi* sensu lato, and *Bartonella* species in Dutch *Ixodes ricinus* ticks. *J Clin Microbiol.* 1999;37:2215–22

122. Cotté V, Bonnet S, Le Rhun D, et al. Transmission of Bartonella henselae by Ixodes ricinus. *Emerg Infect Dis.* 2008;14(7):1074–1080

123. Billeter SA, Miller MK, Breitschwerdt EB, et al. Detection of two Bartonella tamiae-like sequences in Amblyomma americanum (Acari: Ixodidae) using 16S-23S intergenic spacer region-specific primers. *J Med Entomol.* 2008;45:176–179

124. McQuiston JH, Childs JE, Chamberland ME, et al. Transmission of tick-borne agents of disease by blood transfusion: a review of known and potential risks in the United States. *Transfusion.* 2000;40:274–284

125. Lin JW, Chen CM, Chang CC. Unknown fever and back pain caused by Bartonella henselae in a veterinarian after a needle puncture: a case report and literature review. *Vector Borne Zoonotic Dis.* 2011;11:589–591

126. Oliveira AM, Maggi RG, Woods CW, et al. Suspected needle stick transmission of Bartonella vinsonii subspecies berkhoffii to a veterinarian. *J Vet Intern Med.* 2010;24:1229–1232

127. Breitschwerdt EB, Maggi RG, Lantos PM, et al. Bartonella vinsonii subsp. berkhoffii and Bartonella henselae bacteremia in a father and daughter with neurological disease. *Parasit Vectors.* 2010;3(1):1–9

128. Eskow E, Rao RV, Mordechai E. Concurrent infection of the central nervous system by *Borrelia burgdorferi* and *Bartonella henselae*: evidence for a novel tick-borne disease complex. *Arch Neurol.* 2001;58(9):1357–63

129. Maggi RG, Ericson M, Mascarelli PE, et al. Bartonella henselae bacteremia in a mother and son potentially associated with tick exposure. *Parasites & Vectors.* 2013 Dec;6(1):1–9

130. www.aad.org/dw/dw-insights-and-inquiries/dermatopathology/striae-due-to-bartonella-is-a-stretch, accessed 10/31/2022

131. Boozalis E, Grossberg A, Puttgen K, et al. Demographic characteristics of teenage boys with horizontal striae distensae of the lower back. *Pediatric Dermatology.* 2017;35(1):59–63

132. Breitschwerdt EB, Bradley JM, Maggi RG, et al. *Bartonella* associated cutaneous lesions (bacl) in people with neuropsychiatric symptoms. *Pathogens.* 2020;9(12):1023

133. Breitschwerdt EB, Greenberg R, Maggi RG, et al. *Bartonella henselae* Bloodstream Infection in a Boy With Pediatric Acute-Onset Neuropsychiatric Syndrome. *J Cent Nerv Syst Dis.* 2019;11:1–8

134. Maluki A, Breitschwerdt E, Bemis L, et al. Imaging analysis of Bartonella species in the skin using single-photon and multi-photon (second harmonic generation) laser scanning microscopy. *Clin Case Rep*. 2020;8:1564–1570

135. Clark IA, Jacobson LS. Do babesiosis and malaria share a common disease process? *Annals of Tropical Medicine & Parasitology*. 1998;92(4):483–489

136. Usmani-Brown S, Halperin J, Krause P. Neurological manifestations of human babesiosis. *Handbook of Clinical Neurology*. 2013;114:199–203

137. Venigalla T, Adekayode C, Doreswamy S, et al. Atypical presentation of babesiosis with neurological manifestations as well as hematological manifestations. *Cureus*. 2022;14(7): e26811:1–7

138. Vannier E, Krause PJ. Human babesiosis. *N Engl J Med*. 2012;366:2397–2407

139. Knapp KL, Rice NA. Human coinfection with *Borrelia burgdorferi* and *Babesia microti* in the United States. *Journal of Parasitology Research*. 2015;587131:1–11

140. Krause PJ, Telford SR 3rd, Spielman A, et al. Concurrent Lyme disease and babesiosis: evidence for increased severity and duration of illness. *JAMA*. 1996;275(21):1657–60

141. Esernio-Jenssen D, Scimeca PG, Benach JL, et al. Transplacental/perinatal babesiosis. *J Pediatr*. 1987;110(4):570–2

142. Fox LM, Wingerter S, Ahmed A, et al. Neonatal babesiosis: case report and review of the literature. *Pediatr Infect Dis J*. 2006;25(2):169–73

143. Herwaldt BL, Neitzel DF, Gorlin JB, et al. Transmission of Babesia microti in Minnesota through four blood donations from the same donor over a 6-month period. *Transfusion*. 2002;42(9):1154–8

144. Leiby DA. Babesiosis and blood transfusion: flying under the radar. *Vox Sang*. 2006;90(3):157–65

145. Jakab Á, Kahlig P, Kuenzli E, et al. Tick-borne relapsing fever—a systematic review and analysis of the literature. *PLoS Negl Trop Dis*. 2022;16(2): e0010212:1–41

146. Hoornstra D, Azagi T, van Eck JA, et al. Prevalence and clinical manifestation of *Borrelia miyamotoi* in Ixodes ticks and humans in the northern hemisphere: a systematic review and meta-analysis. *Lancet Microbe*. 2022;(10):e772–e786

147. Telford SR 3rd, Goethert HK, Molloy PJ, et al. *Borrelia miyamotoi* disease: neither Lyme disease nor relapsing fever. *Clin Lab Med*. 2015;35(4):867–82

148. Levitt A, Messonnier N, Jernigan D, et al. Emerging and reemerging infectious disease threats. In Bennett J, Dolin R, Blaser M, editors. *Mandell, Douglas, and Bennett's Principles and Practice of Infectious Diseases*. 9th ed. Philadelphia, PA. Elsevier. 2020;1:177–178

149. www.360dx.com/immunoassays/igenex-gets-new-york-state-approval-tick-borne-relapsing-fever--immunoblot-tests#.Yt7x1-zMK84, accessed 7/25/2022

150. www.cdc.gov/ehrlichiosis/stats/index.html, accessed 11/7/2022

151. Bakken JS, Dumler JS. Human granulocytic anaplasmosis. *Infect Dis Clin North Am*. 2015;29(2):341–55

152. LeDonne M, Ahmed Sultan, Keeney S, et al. Trigeminal neuralgia as the principal manifestation of anaplasmosis: a case report. *Cureus*. 2022;14(1):e21668

153. Horowitz HW, Marks SJ, Weintraub M, et al. Brachial plexopathy associated with human granulocytic ehrlichiosis. *Neurology*.1996;46(4):1026–1029

154. Bakken JS, Dumler JS. Clinical diagnosis and treatment of human granulocytotropic anaplasmosis. *Ann NY Acad Sci*. 2006;1078:236–47

155. Aguero-Rosenfeld ME, Donnarumma L, Zentmaier L, et al. Seroprevalence of antibodies that react with *Anaplasma phagocytophila*, the agent of human granulocytic ehrlichiosis, in different populations in Westchester County, New York. *J Clin Microbiol.* 2002;40:2612–5

156. Bakken JS, Goellner P, VanEtten M, et al. Seroprevalence of human granulocytic ehrlichiosis among permanent residents of northwestern Wisconsin. *Clin Infect Dis.* 1998;27:1491–6

157. Horowitz HW, Kilchevsky E, Haber S, et al. Perinatal transmission of the agent of human granulocytic ehrlichiosis. *N Engl J Med.* 1998;339:375–8

158. Bakken JS ,Krueth JK, Lund T, et al. Exposure to deer blood may be a cause of human granulocytic ehrlichiosis. *Clin Infect Dis.* 1996;23:198

159. Dumler JS, Walker DH. *Ehrlichia chaffeensis* (human monocytotropic ehrlichiosis), *anaplasma phagocytophilium* (human granulocytotropic anaplasmosis), and other anaplasmataceae. In Bennett J, Dolin R, Blaser M, editors. *Mandell, Douglas, and Bennett's Principles and Practice of Infectious Diseases.* 9th ed. Philadelphia, PA. Elsevier. 2020;2:177–178

160. Steere AC. Lyme Disease (Lyme borreliosis) due to *Borrelia burgdorferi*. In Bennett J, Dolin R, Blaser M, editors. *Mandell, Douglas, and Bennett's Principles and Practice of Infectious Diseases.* 9th ed. Philadelphia, PA. Elsevier. 2020;2:2917

161. Logigian EL, Kaplan RF, Steere AC. Chronic neurologic manifestations of Lyme disease. *N Engl J Med.* 1990;323(21):1438–44

162. Chandra A, Wormser GP, Klempner MS, et al. Anti-neural antibody reactivity in patients with a history of Lyme borreliosis and persistent symptoms. *Brain, Behavior, and Immunity.* 2010;24(6):1018–1024

163. Kirvan CA, Swedo SE, Heuser JS, et al. Mimicry and autoantibody-mediated neuronal cell signaling in Sydenham chorea. *Nat Med.* 2003;9(7):914–920

164. Church AJ, Dale RC, Cardoso F, et al. CSF and serum immune parameters in Sydenham's chorea: evidence of an autoimmune syndrome? *J Neuroimmunol.* 2003;136(1–2):149–153

165. Church AJ, Cardoso F, Dale RC, et al. Anti-basal ganglia antibodies in acute and persistent Sydenham's chorea. *Neurology.* 2002;59(2):227–231

166. Kotby AA, El Badawy N, El Sokkary S, et al. Antineuronal antibodies in rheumatic chorea. *Clin Diagn Lab Immunol.* 1998;5(6):836–839

167. Kirvan CA, Cox CJ, Swedo SE, et al. Tubulin is a neuronal target of autoantibodies in Sydenham's chorea. *J Immunol.* 2007;178(11):7412–21

168. Husby G, van de Rijn I, Zabriskie JB, et al. Antibodies reacting with cytoplasm of subthalamic and caudate nuclei neurons in chorea and acute rheumatic fever. *J Exp Med.* 1976;144(4):1094–1110

169. Swedo SE, Leonard HL, Kiessling LS. Speculations on antineuronal antibody-mediated neuropsychiatric disorders of childhood. *Pediatrics.* 1994;93(2):323–326

170. Swedo SE, Leonard HL, Mittleman BB, et al. Identification of children with pediatric autoimmune neuropsychiatric disorders associated with streptococcal infections by a marker associated with rheumatic fever. *American Journal of Psychiatry.* 1997;154(1):110–112

171. Frick LR, Rapanelli M, Jindachomthong K, et al. Differential binding of antibodies in PANDAS patients to cholinergic interneurons in the striatum. *Brain, Behavior, and Immunity.* 2018;69:304–311

172. Strle K, Shin JJ, Glickstein LJ, et al. Association of a toll-like receptor 1 polymorphism with heightened Th1 inflammatory responses and antibiotic-refractory Lyme arthritis. *Arthritis Rheum*. 2012;64(5):1497–507

173. Steere AC, Klitz W, Drouin EE, et al. Antibiotic-refractory Lyme arthritis is associated with HLA-DR molecules that bind a *Borrelia burgdorferi* peptide. *J Exp Med*. 2006;203(4):961–71

174. Vudattu NK, Strle K, Steere AC, et al. Dysregulation of CD4+CD25(high) T cells in the synovial fluid of patients with antibiotic-refractory Lyme arthritis. *Arthritis Rheum*. 2013;65(6):1643–53

175. Rebman AW, Aucott JN. Post-treatment Lyme disease as a model for persistent symptoms in Lyme disease. *Front Med* (Lausanne). 2020;7(57):1–43

176. Asch ES, Bujak DI, Weiss M, et al. Lyme disease: an infectious and postinfectious syndrome. *J Rheumatol*. 1994;21(3):454–61

177. Shadick NA, Phillips CB, Logigian EL, et al. The long-term clinical outcomes of Lyme disease: a population-based retrospective cohort study. *Annals of Internal Medicine*. 1994;121(8):560–7

178. Klempner MS, Hu LT, Evans J, et al. Two controlled trials of antibiotic treatment in patients with persistent symptoms and a history of Lyme disease. *N Engl J Med*. 2001;345(2):85–92

179. Kaplan RF, Trevino RP, Johnson GM, et al. Cognitive function in post-treatment Lyme disease: do additional antibiotics help? *Neurology*. 2003;60:1916–22

180. Fallon BA, Keilp JG, Corbera KM, et al. A randomized, placebo-controlled trial of repeated IV antibiotic therapy for Lyme encephalopathy. *Neurology*. 2008;70:992–1003

181. Sharma B, Brown AV, Matluck NE, et al. *Borrelia burgdorferi*, the causative agent of Lyme disease, forms drug-tolerant persister cells. *Antimicrob Agents Chemother*. 2015;59:4616–24

182. Feng J, Li T, Yee R, et al. Stationary phase persister/biofilm microcolony of *Borrelia burgdorferi* causes more severe disease in a mouse model of Lyme arthritis: implications for understanding persistence, post-treatment Lyme disease syndrome (PTLDS), and treatment failure. *Discov Med*. 2019;27:125–38

183. Miklossy J, Kasas S, Zurn AD, et al. Persisting atypical and cystic forms of *Borrelia burgdorferi* and local inflammation in Lyme neuroborreliosis. *J Neuroinflammation*. 2008;5(40):1–23

184. Merilainen L, Brander H, Herranen A, et al. Pleomorphic forms of *Borrelia burgdorferi* induce distinct immune responses. *Microbes Infect*. 2016;18(7–8):484–495

185. Rudenko N, Golovchenko M, Kybicova K. *et al*. Metamorphoses of Lyme disease spirochetes: phenomenon of *Borrelia* persisters. *Parasites Vectors*. 2019;12(237):1–10

186. Straubinger RK, Summers BA, Chang YF, et al. Persistence of *Borrelia burgdorferi* in experimentally infected dogs after antibiotic treatment. *J Clin Microbiol*. 1997;35(1):111–116

187. Hodzic E, Imai D, Feng S, et al. Resurgence of persisting non-cultivable *Borrelia burgdorferi* following antibiotic treatment in mice. *PLoS One*. 2014;9(1):e86907:1–11

188. Crossland NA, Alvarez X, Embers ME. Late disseminated Lyme disease: associated pathology and spirochete persistence posttreatment in Rhesus Macaques. *Am J Pathol*. 2018;188:672–82

189. www.cdc.gov/lyme/pdfs/PersistenceWebinarSlides.pdf, accessed 11/10/2022

190. Klempner MS, Noring R, Rogers RA. Invasion of human skin fibroblasts by the Lyme disease spirochete, *Borrelia burgdorferi*. *Journal of Infectious Diseases*. 1993;167(5):1074–1081

REDUCE: SYMPTOMS

Trying to suppress or eradicate symptoms on the physical level can be extremely important, but there's more to healing than that; dealing with psychological, emotional and spiritual issues involved in treating sickness is equally important.
~ **MARIANNE WILLIAMSON**

KEY POINTS

▸ Reducing symptoms in PANS and PANDAS is best accomplished by using a wide range of therapeutics, including prescription medications, supplements, mindfulness, and cognitive-behavioral therapy

▸ Cognitive-behavioral therapy and exposure-response prevention often outperform medications and have a more favorable side effect profile

▸ Other adjunctive therapies such as NLP, hypnosis, neurofeedback, and smartphone apps may be helpful for managing or resolving symptoms

Although the long-term solution to PANS and PANDAS requires a root cause approach which focuses on what is in the hose and what is in the flowerpot to achieve the best clinical outcome, patients come to us to help first with what is in the puddle—symptoms, in other words.

The signs and symptoms of PANS and PANDAS are oppressive and heartbreaking. It's not enough to wait for the antibiotic, IVIG, or home remediation to solve the problem over weeks or months. From the first time we see our patients in person, we provide real, practical solutions to these challenges.

In this chapter you will find information on the basic science and clinical evidence for what we have found to be most helpful for these difficult symptoms. As always, I will temper what I know from the literature with my clinical experience in treating hundreds of these children. This satisfies the original definition of evidence-based medicine (EBM), which defines EBM as having three components: patient (parent) preference, the best available published evidence, and clinical experience.[1,2]

NOTE: Dosages for medications and supplements that we commonly use in patients with PANS and PANDAS can be found in Appendix B.

REDUCE: OCD

Obsessive-compulsive disorder (OCD) is defined by obsessions (continuous intrusive thoughts) and compulsive behaviors or rituals. OCD is one of the two primary symptoms listed in the case definition of PANS and PANDAS. Pop culture often uses the term *OCD* to describe a situation when people double-check their work or check their clock twice before going to bed to make sure they don't oversleep.

In contrast, the intrusive thoughts and compulsive behaviors in PANS and PANDAS are severe and overwhelming. These thoughts and behaviors significantly impact many aspects of life.

> As many as 50–60% of patients remain symptomatic when treated with SSRIs.

Conventional treatment guidelines for OCD currently recommend SSRI medication, some form of cognitive behavioral therapy (CBT), or both.[3–5]

Medications for OCD - the evidence

The most effective group of psychiatric medications for OCD are the serotonin reuptake inhibitor (SRI) clomipramine and selective serotonin reuptake inhibitors (SSRIs). Clomipramine and four SSRIs (sertraline, fluoxetine, fluvoxamine, paroxetine) are FDA approved for OCD.[4,6]

Meta-analyses of double-blind, placebo-controlled studies have demonstrated that SSRIs are superior to placebo for the treatment of OCD.[7,8] Although medications are often cited in guidelines as "first-line" treatments, they are characterized in several studies (including a 2009 Cochrane review) as merely offering a moderate improvement in patient symptoms.[7,9]

In fact, as many as 50–60% of patients remain symptomatic when treated with SSRIs.[3,4] Initially it was thought that clomipramine was superior to the SSRIs, but a subsequent meta-analysis showed that SSRIs are just as effective and have a lower side effect profile.[7] No differences have been seen among the various SSRIs in terms of efficacy.[7]

In contrast to depression and anxiety treatment, where improvements are seen within a few weeks, improvements in OCD symptoms with SSRIs may not be seen until 10–12 weeks after initiation of treatment at the maximum tolerated dose.[3,9,10]

Maintenance of medication dosage for 1–2 years is usually recommended to prevent recurrence of OCD symptoms, which may be seen with early discontinuation.[3,4,6,10] If SSRI treatment does not result in adequate reduction of symptoms, many clinicians add atypical antipsychotics, although there are currently no approved antipsychotic medications for the treatment of OCD.[9] Unpleasant withdrawal symptoms, including dizziness, nausea, vomiting, headache, lethargy, agitation, insomnia, myoclonic jerks, and paresthesias, may also be seen if SSRIs are stopped suddenly rather than slowly tapered.[3,4]

Inadequate response to SSRI treatment for OCD has been correlated with concomitant depression, poor insight (which is common in PANS and PANDAS patients), hoarding behaviors, and in patients with tic disorders and Tourette syndrome.[3,5,9,10] In patients with tic disorders, some SSRIs can increase tics.[10]

> **In patients with tic disorders, some SSRIs can increase tics.**

Significant side effects may be seen when using SSRIs, even at therapeutic dosages. These side effects may include gastrointestinal symptoms (often early in the treatment course), insomnia, somnolence, agitation, and increased sweating.[3,5] SSRI medications contain a black box warning for increased risks of suicide and suicidal ideation in children and adolescents.[3,4,8]

There are also concerns with some SSRIs and atypical antipsychotics due to potential QTc prolongation.[5] This becomes an issue if patients on these medications require azithromycin, since prolongation of the QTc may be seen when azithromycin is used in concert with other drugs, including SSRIs and/or antipsychotics.

In a published case series of thirty-eight children with OCD and PANDAS who had a history of SSRI use, the medications were discontinued in fourteen (37%) due to behavioral activation symptoms, including mania, hyperactivity, disinhibition, aggression, worsening OCD/ compulsive behavior, and suicidality/self harm.[11] Many patients report symptoms of behavioral activation with more than one SSRI.

Numerous anecdotal reports from physicians who treat PANS and PANDAS have noted that these patients may be more sensitive to adverse effects such as dystonia, catatonia, or agitation when placed on psychotropic medications.[12] This has been confirmed by our own clinical experience.

A survey of families of children with PANS and PANDAS[13] indicated that SSRIs are discontinued due to side effects in about 25% of treated children. In this same study, parents noted that SSRIs were "very effective" in only 17% of patients and "somewhat effective" an additional 27% of the time. Since this was a survey, this response was not linked to rating scales, so it is not clear whether "improved" met the accepted definition of symptom scale reduction used in other studies. These medications were discontinued between 21–32% of the time (depending on the medication) and were discontinued due to lack of efficacy in 16–28% of the cases.

Some clinicians have used serotonin norepinephrine reuptake inhibitors (SNRIs) like venlafaxine or duloxetine, but there is no evidence that they are more effective than SSRIs.

As noted in Chapter 7, there is evidence that antidepressants have antimicrobial activity which may affect the gut microbiome.[14,15] We believe that manipulation of the microbiome

> ERP is recognized as a first-line treatment appropriate for monotherapy in current professional guidelines for patients with OCD.

may be the reason that they are sometimes effective in patients. It may also be the reason that parents sometimes report that these medications immediately worsen symptoms. Future studies may shed light on the role of microbiome manipulation as a therapeutic intervention in patients with mental illnesses.

In our practice, we do not recommend SSRI medications, SNRIs, antipsychotics, or benzodiazepines as a primary treatment option. For this reason, we do not prescribe these medications. If patients are already on these medications when they come to our office, we usually instruct them to continue the medications until symptoms are stabilized by addressing infections, toxins, immune dysregulation, and neural loops (management of OCD). Once this is done, we taper medications very slowly over a few months. If patients are on multiple psychiatric medications, we usually consult their primary psychiatrist to come up with a weaning plan.

We also check for medication interactions when patients come to us on multiple medications or before we add a new prescription medication. If interactions are found, we advise them to let their primary prescriber know about the interactions so they can change the regimen if the interactions are deemed clinically significant.

Many interaction checking programs for physicians are available. We commonly use Epocrates (www.epocrates.com). A printout of interactions by severity level is available on the website. There is a membership charge for this service. Epocrates also provides details about common dosages for most medications. A good source of information on supplements (including dosage), herbals, and other natural medicines as well as supplement/medication interactions can be found here: www.naturalmedicines.therapeuticresearch.com

Cognitive behavioral therapy for OCD - the evidence

The most common type of cognitive behavioral therapy (CBT) used is exposure response prevention (ERP) therapy. In ERP, patients are exposed to the stimulus (a situation or object) that usually triggers them to perform a ritual (for example, compulsive handwashing). Patients are instructed to refrain from performing the ritual. Subjective anxiety levels are measured initially and after some measured period of time. Through gradual desensitization and repetition, anxiety levels decrease and the need for the ritual is *disconnected* from the stimulus.[16]

ERP is recognized as a first-line treatment appropriate for monotherapy in current professional guidelines for patients with OCD.[3,5] Multiple studies and meta-analyses have shown that ERP is more effective than progressive relaxation and pill placebo.[3,5,6,17]

Several meta-analyses have shown that CBT outperforms medications for the treatment of OCD in children and adolescents.[18–21] The meta-analysis by Öst et al. contains the best summary of the studies comparing SRI medications to CBT/ERP.[18] In this study, the authors took particular care to standardize measures across thirty-nine studies with 1,990 patients. The authors found that the response rate for CBT was 70%. The response rate for CBT plus SRI was 66%, SRI alone was 49%, placebo pill was 29%, and wait list control (who received no treatment contact at all) was 13%. Remission rates were 53% for CBT, 49% for the combination of SRI and CBT, 24% for SRI alone, 15% for placebo, and 10% for the wait list control group. No evidence was found that moderate to severe cases require SRI and CBT over CBT alone.

Additional research has confirmed that the addition of SRI medication does not increase response rates in patients over CBT alone, although adding CBT to SRIs when incomplete recovery is seen is helpful.[22,23]

Another review of the clinical evidence for all treatment modalities for pediatric OCD lists ERP as "beneficial," while it lists SRIs (SSRI and clomipramine) as a "trade off between benefit and harm."[7] The American Academy of Child and

> **CBT outperforms medications for the treatment of OCD in children and adolescents.**

Adolescent Psychiatry[24] and the Royal College of Psychiatrists (UK)[25] both maintain that CBT is the first-line treatment (and thus should be viewed as the standard of care) for child and adolescent OCD.

This mirrors our own clinical experience. The single most effective treatment we have found in our practice for OCD ("neural loops") in PANS and PANDAS is ERP. Patients presenting on prescription medications are seldom well controlled in terms of OCD. In this regard, the addition of ERP to the treatment regimen is often life-changing.

The techniques and specific methods for instituting ERP are beyond the scope of this book. It is best to establish a referral network for ERP and counseling in your area prior to seeing patients with PANS and PANDAS. One online ERP program that our patients have found helpful is www.treatmyocd.com.

Interested readers can find more information about ERP here:

Grebe SC, Bergez KC, Lee EB, et al: Evidence-based treatment of pediatric obsessive-compulsive and related disorders; in *Handbook of Evidence-Based Therapies for Children and Adolescents. Issues in Clinical Child Psychology*. Edited by Steele RG, Roberts MC. New York, Springer, 2020

Tompkins MA, Owen DJ, Shiloff NH, et al: *Cognitive Behavior Therapy for OCD in Youth: A Step-By-Step Guide*. Washington, DC, American Psychological Association, 2020

It's very important to support the parents and instruct them not to participate in OCD rituals, as this will reinforce OCD behaviors and the hold it has on the child.[26] Instead, parents should be instructed to reward desired behaviors, establish reward systems, and set clear limits with consequences for extreme behaviors.

Supplements for OCD

NOTE: Appendix B provides a guide to supplement and medication dosages we commonly use.

Reducing anxiety helps patients better deal with OCD. For this reason, many of the supplements we use for the treatment of anxiety (see below) can demonstrate a benefit for OCD symptoms. Although we always stress the importance of a healthy diet, it is virtually impossible to achieve therapeutic doses of nutrients through diet alone (especially in children with PANS and PANDAS who may have an aversion to healthy foods).

N-acetyl cysteine

N-acetyl cysteine (NAC) has been well studied for OCD. A growing body of literature supports the fact that hyperactivity in the cortico-striatal-thalamic-cortical (CSTC) region and abnormal glutamate metabolism are operative in OCD.[27–29] Excess glutamate levels lead to excitotoxicity of the neurons in this region, which correlates with increased symptoms of OCD.[30] Higher levels of glutamate have been found in the CSF of patients with OCD.[30–32] There is also evidence that oxidative stress (specifically lipid peroxidation) in the brain is linked to OCD.[33–34]

NAC is a precursor to glutathione. Studies have shown that NAC reduces the synaptic

> It's very important to support the parents and instruct them not to participate in OCD rituals, as this will reinforce OCD behaviors.

release of glutamate through an exchange mechanism.[31,35–37] In this way, NAC can be viewed as a glutamate modulator. As a precursor to glutathione, it also stimulates oxidative defenses in the body.

Adult studies of NAC supplementation in adults with OCD have shown that it is safe, well-tolerated, and effective.[31,35–38] Trials have typically been twelve weeks in duration and have used doses of NAC ranging from 2400–3000 mg (divided Q12 hours). There is one small trial which used NAC in children (ages 8–17) with OCD.[39] The children were administered NAC in effervescent tablet form. The original dose was 900 mg once daily and was titrated each week to a target dose of 2700 mg daily (900 mg TID). This dose was continued for twelve weeks. NAC was noted to be safe, well-tolerated, and effective in this trial as well. In both adult trials and the pediatric trial cited above, NAC was used as monotherapy and as an adjunct to prescription medications.

Oral or IV NAC is an effective treatment for acetaminophen overdose. It functions as a powerful hepatic protection compound by making glutathione, which removes toxic metabolites of the ingested drug. Since PANS and PANDAS patients commonly have an increased mycotoxin burden, it makes sense that NAC administration (with resultant increases in glutathione) can lead to a reduction in symptoms.

One theoretical contraindication to NAC use is known as cystinuria, as NAC use could possibly

> Studies have shown lower levels of vitamin D in patients who have OCD and a direct correlation between symptom severity and deficiency.

increase the chance of nephrolithiasis. Another caution would be an increase in agitation in patients (seen much more commonly with glutathione) due to the rapid liberation of toxins.

Vitamin D

As noted earlier, Vitamin D is not actually a vitamin but is a neurosteroid hormone.[40] It is required for proper brain development and homeostasis, immune modulation, antioxidant processes, and the inflammatory response.[40,41] Studies have shown lower levels of vitamin D in patients who have OCD[42,43] and a direct

correlation between symptom severity and deficiency. There are no studies currently which have examined the effects of vitamin D supplementation on symptoms in OCD patients.

The evidence for vitamin D supplementation is much stronger for depression and anxiety.

Selenium

Selenium is a trace mineral which plays a role in antioxidant defenses as a vital constituent of glutathione peroxidase.[41] One study showed that lower levels of selenium were present in patients with OCD.[44] Another study showed that supplementation with 200 mcg of selenium significantly improved symptoms in adult patients with OCD who were on SSRIs at baseline.[45]

We do not separately supplement with selenium, as it is included in the multivitamin we use.

Zinc

Zinc plays many vital roles in the body, including modulation of GABA (inhibitory) and NDMA (excitatory) neural transmission.[46] Specifically, it lessens NMDA mediated neurotoxicity.[46] In a placebo-controlled, randomized trial in adults, the addition of zinc to fluoxetine showed a statistically significant reduction in OCD symptoms compared to fluoxetine plus placebo.[47] The zinc dosage was unusually high in this trial (440 mg daily). Dosages over 50 mg, however, cause significant nausea (especially on an empty stomach). In our practice, we prescribe a multivitamin with zinc, but the dosages of zinc are much lower. If taken separately, zinc should always be taken with food or it may cause nausea.

B12 and folate

Low B12 and folate stores can lead to neuropsychiatric issues as these deficiencies can change neurotransmitter levels due to abnormal mono-amine metabolism.[48] B12 and folate deficiencies with hyperhomocysteinemia have been found in patients with OCD more often than control populations.[49,50]

There are no trials investigating methyl-folate (the most helpful form of folate supplementation) or B12 in patients with isolated OCD. The evidence for B12 and folate supplementation is much stronger for depression and anxiety.

Palmitoylethanolamide (PEA)

Although some physicians report positive results anecdotally with PEA (+/- luteolin) in OCD patients, we have not noted a dramatic improvement with this supplement in our patients and there is no published literature on PEA use in OCD patients.

Neurolinguistic programming (NLP) for OCD

See Chapter 21 for a detailed discussion of NLP and its utility in PANS and PANDAS.

Hypnosis for OCD

See Chapter 21 for a detailed discussion of hypnosis and its utility in PANS and PANDAS.

REDUCE: ANXIETY

Anxiety is a universal symptom in patients with PANS and PANDAS. It can be argued that much of what is called "defiance" in these patients is actually fear and anxiety driven by intrusive thoughts and compulsions. This can be quite difficult to manage for the child and their family.

Medications for anxiety - the evidence

The American Academy of Child and Adolescent Psychiatry recommends SSRI medication as a first-line treatment for various types of anxiety in children from 6–18 years of age.[51] The academy also lists SNRI medication as a possible option and acknowledges the risks, side effects, and withdrawal symptoms associated with discontinuation of SSRIs and SNRIs (as discussed in the previous section on OCD).

A randomized, controlled trial of 488 patients with anxiety between 7–17 years of age which compared CBT to sertraline to a combination of both to pill placebo was published in the *New England Journal of Medicine* in 2008.[52] The study showed that improve-

> **B12 and folate deficiencies with hyperhomocysteinemia have been found in patients with OCD more often than control populations.**

ment with sertraline was seen in 54.9%, while improvement with CBT was 59.7%. The combination yielded improvement in 80.7% of cases, and the placebo experienced improvement 23.7% of the time. There was less fatigue, sedation, insomnia, and restlessness in the CBT group compared to the sertraline group. Patients receiving CBT alone were much less likely to withdraw from the study than those in the sertraline group. The patients in the combination group (medication plus CBT) actually knew they were treated with active sertraline. It is unclear whether or how this might have impacted results. It would have helped if the study also had a pill placebo plus CBT group to see if the increase in effectiveness of the combination was truly attributable to sertraline.

An excellent systematic review and meta-analysis comparing CBT and pharmacotherapy for pediatric anxiety was published in *JAMA Pediatrics* in 2017.[53] The analysis reviewed 115 studies with a total of 7,719 patients. The mean age of the children was 9.2 years. SSRIs and SNRIs were found to be effective. Benzodiazepines and tricyclic antidepressants were not found to be effective in reducing symptoms. CBT reduced primary anxiety symptoms more than fluoxetine. Adverse events were seen with medications but not with CBT. Interestingly, CBT was associated with less dropout from studies than medications or pill placebo. The report stated that superiority of SSRIs over placebo was not seen in child reporting. In addition to being ineffective at reducing anxiety, benzodiazepines are very addictive, disrupt sleep architecture, worsen sleep-disordered breathing, and can lead to daytime sleepiness and adverse cognitive effects.[54]

Please see this chapter's earlier section on SSRI medications for OCD treatment for a complete discussion of side effects (particularly in patients with PANS and PANDAS), efficacy, and drug interactions. In our practice, we do not prescribe SSRIs for anxiety in children with PANS and PANDAS. As supported by the literature, we consider CBT to be a superior intervention when coupled with the adjunctive treatments that follow.

In cases of severe agitation, depression, or aggression, we obtain urgent psychiatric input. In these cases, pharmacotherapy may be instituted to try to stabilize the situation acutely. Later in the course of treatment, patients are often able to taper off these medications slowly.

Breathwork for anxiety

Deep breathing, changing breathing patterns, and breathing exercises (collectively known as "breathwork") as treatments for anxiety have been studied extensively. These techniques are safe, easy to teach, easy to learn, and effective. A meta-analysis of the effects of slow breathing demonstrated that this type of voluntary breathing exercise causes profound, favorable physiologic and behavioral changes.[55] The authors noted increased heart rate variability, increased alpha brain waves (also seen with meditation), a shift to the parasympathetic state (relaxation), and decreased symptoms of arousal, depression, anxiety, anger, and confusion.

Another prospective, randomized study showed that eight weeks of a diaphragmatic breathing intervention led to a decrease in negative affect, an increase in sustained attention, and, most importantly, significantly lower cortisol levels compared with the control group.[56]

Two studies showed that diaphragmatic breathing exercises lowered anxiety, fear, self-reported pain, and sympathetic activation in children undergoing dental treatments, including intraoral injections of local anesthetics for dental procedures.[57,58]

Easy and effective breathing exercises

"4-7-8 breathing": This is a type of diaphragmatic breathing which works well for adults and older children. To do it, breathe in for a count of four, hold for a count of seven, and exhale for a count of eight. Repeat this 5–10 times in a row. It is best to repeat this pattern 2–3 times a day.

Box breathing: This works well for younger children or adults who may get distracted counting 4-7-8. To perform this exercise, breathe in for a count of four, hold your breath for a count of four, breathe out for a count of four, and hold your breath for a count of four. Repeat this 5–10 times in a row. It is best to repeat this pattern 2–3 times a day.

Mindfulness for anxiety

Mindfulness can be thought of as a specific type of CBT. It is separate and distinct from simple meditative practices. The practice of mindfulness involves patients increasing their attention to experiences using their senses (visual, auditory, kinesthetic) and acknowledging their thoughts and feelings as they have them. It is not meditation per se but has some similarities. The exercises involved are usually called "mindfulness-based

> **The practice of mindfulness is associated with increased psychological well-being.**

interventions" or MBIs. This category may be further broken into mindfulness-based stress reduction (MBSR) and mindfulness-based cognitive therapy (MBCT).

The process of MBI involves becoming aware of bodily sensations, thoughts, environment, and consciousness. These things are brought to awareness without judgment, but with openness, acceptance, and curiosity.[59–61] This requires self-regulation and staying in the present moment.

Most of our time is not spent in the present moment observing our environment but is spent dissociated from our experience with a wandering mind. One study showed that approximately 47% of our waking existence is spent in

a state of mind-wandering. The study also found that increasing the amount of time we spend in this state is associated with subsequent unhappiness.[62] Meanwhile, the practice of mindfulness is associated with increased psychological well-being.[63] When children with PANS and PANDAS focus on internal thoughts (as is seen in mind wandering), they are often riddled with obsessions, rituals, anxiety, and self-criticism.

The evidence for the effectiveness of MBIs for both immediate and long-term improvement in patients with anxiety is robust.[64–67] A great summary of the evidence for mindfulness in the treatment of anxiety, depression (including prevention of relapse), stress, chronic pain, emotional distress, drug addiction, and quality of life can be found in two excellent references.[66,67]

Mindfulness-based programs have been specifically shown to be effective in both healthcare workers experiencing stress[68] and in children with anxiety.[69] Physiologically, in patients with generalized anxiety disorder, using MBSR programs has been shown to reduce adrenocorticotropic hormone (ACTH) and proinflammatory cytokines compared to controls.[70]

The original MBSR program has been credited to the work of Jon Kabat-Zinn, PhD, in the 1980s. His program is still followed by therapists in many locations across the country today. It involves eight weekly sessions of training in mindfulness, daily practice at home, and a daylong retreat. This program is not specifically directed at sick children and is not likely to be feasible for most children with PANS and PANDAS. It would, however, be beneficial for parents of children with PANS and PANDAS. Group (versus individual) MBSR programs also exist in many places. There are several online manuals with directions for establishing MBSR groups, but this is best accomplished by dedicated and trained therapists.

Although MBSR may not be possible for children with PANS and PANDAS and their families, there are some easy exercises based upon the program that can be used with older children and their families anytime. Here are four easy examples parents can use.

1. Focusing attentively on an object or food (parents can help facilitate this exercise):
   A. Take an object like a leaf or a piece of food and notice everything about it.
   B. Notice how the object looks. What color is it? Is there any contrast, pattern, or gradient or is it all one color? Can you name some other items with this color or pattern?
   C. Notice how it feels: What is the texture? Is it soft or hard? Is it fuzzy or smooth?
   D. Is there a sound associated with it when you touch it?
   E. Does the object have a smell?
   F. If it is a food, how does it taste and feel when it is in your mouth?

2. Perform a body scan:
   A. Lay down in a comfortable position and close your eyes.
   B. Notice how your toes and feet feel. Do you have socks on? What kind of socks?
   C. Feel your calves and thighs.
   D. Notice how your body feels lying on what you are lying on. Feel the support. Is it soft or hard? Is it warm or cold?
   E. Notice how your fingers and hands feel.
   F. This exercise goes on highlighting each body part and draws the child's attention to each area.

3. Mindful seeing:
   A. Find a comfortable seat near a window.
   B. Look out the window and notice colors, patterns, and shapes.
   C. Don't label the objects; just notice things about them as noted above.
   D. Describe what you see.

4. The five senses exercise:
   A. Name five things you can see.
   B. Name four things that you can feel.
   C. Name three things that you can hear.
   D. Name two things that you can smell.
   E. Name one thing you can taste. The child can actually try this with a food that they have on hand.

Additional examples of easy mindfulness exercises and prompts can be found online.[71]

Meditation or prayer for anxiety

Meditation and prayer are contemplative practices which have been around for thousands of years. Like prayer, meditation is considered by some to have a spiritual dimension. There are not many high-quality studies done on meditation practices. One study in *JAMA* showed positive effects of meditation on depression, anxiety, stress, and pain.[72] Unlike mindfulness, meditation tends to focus on emptying the mind or concentrating on one specific thing (such as a mantra or repeated prayer) to induce calmness.

Due to the heterogeneous nature of prayer techniques, there are limited studies of the effects of prayer on psychological complaints. On a personal note, we have found prayer transformative, calming, healing, and inspiring both in our lives and in those of our patients.

Neurofeedback for anxiety

Numerous investigations over the last thirty years have demonstrated that patients with anxiety, OCD, ADHD, and depression have distinct electroencephalographic brain wave patterns as compared to controls.[73–76]

Since that time, quantitative EEG (qEEG) devices have been developed to gather EEG data on patients with these disorders which can be used to construct a report comparing their measurements to healthy controls. If abnormalities are noted, a computer interface device is used to teach the patient neurofeedback, which is a form of biofeedback. EEG leads are applied to the regions of the scalp where abnormal readings have previously been found. Those leads then go into the computer interface, which is connected to a computer screen. The screen may display visual patterns or even video games.

The machine is set to monitor ongoing brain activity and programmed for desired changes in areas where abnormalities are seen. The patient is instructed to concentrate on the screen. When the brain waves are normalized to the desired pattern in the monitored area, the video screen becomes clear or a pleasant tone sounds. At first this positive brain wave change may be transitory. However, with continued training sessions, the normalization of the brain waves becomes more consistent and is maintained well after therapy is over.[75]

> Patients with anxiety, OCD, ADHD, and depression have distinct electroencephalographic brain wave patterns as compared to controls.

This is an advanced form of operant conditioning. Most of the time, sessions are conducted in a medical office, but there are some home units which may be used between sessions. Research in adults has shown that qEEG neurofeedback is very effective in treating anxiety disorders, ADHD, mood disorders, addiction, PTSD, and brain injury.[76] There is not as much research in children and adolescents, but in our practice, we have seen similar benefits in children when using this treatment modality.

In one large review of eleven randomized trials of patients with ADHD, personalized qEEG neurofeedback yielded "superior clinical effectiveness relative to medication."[77] In addition, qEEG can be used to differentiate monopolar from bipolar depression and can be used to predict medication responsiveness.[76]

In an editorial published in the journal *Clinical Electroencephalography* in 2000, Dr. Frank Duffy (a pediatric neurologist from Harvard) wrote that neurofeedback "should play a major therapeutic role in many difficult areas."[78] He further states, "In my opinion, if any medication had demonstrated such a wide spectrum of efficacy, it would be universally accepted and widely used."

Supplements for anxiety
Vitamin D

Since vitamin D is involved in brain development and other neuropsychiatric disorders, we consider optimization of vitamin D levels essential when treating PANS and PANDAS. As previously noted, vitamin D is a neurosteroid hormone.[40] It is required for proper brain development and homeostasis, immune modulation, antioxidant processes, and the inflammatory response.[40,41]

Studies investigating the role of vitamin D deficiency and vitamin D supplementation in patients with anxiety and depression have shown a direct relationship between vitamin D deficiency and worsening symptoms of anxiety and depression.[79-82] These studies have also shown that supplementation with vitamin D improves these symptoms.

In one poorly researched commentary, vitamin D was referred to as the "Charlie Brown of supplements" after several studies had been done which did not show any difference in clinical outcomes for various diseases when vitamin D supplementation was compared to placebo.[83] Careful analysis of the materials and methods sections of these studies (including the study which sparked this commentary) shows that serum vitamin D levels were not checked before or after supplementation and that the doses of vitamin D given (usually below 1,000 IU daily) are not high enough to increase levels or change clinical outcomes.

Due to genetic differences in vitamin D receptors, the dosage of vitamin D must be individualized based upon blood levels. Vitamin D receptor mutations can result in vitamin D deficiencies, even in sunny areas.[84,85]

> Vitamin D should be given as vitamin D3, as it is absorbed better than vitamin D2.

The US National Institute of Health lists the RDA for vitamin D in adults and children over the age of one as 600 IU.[87] In the same reference, normal levels of vitamin D are listed as >20 ng/mL.

The RDA was based upon calculations by the Institute of Medicine. Subsequently, researchers found that the IOM had made a statistical error in their math which grossly underestimated the amount of vitamin D needed to produce adequate blood levels.[87-89] When corrected for the math error, the actual vitamin D intake to achieve optimum blood levels (50–70 ng/mL) is as high as 3,000 IU for children and 5,000–8,000 IU for adults daily. Dosing is ultimately based upon testing.

Vitamin D should be given as vitamin D3, as it is absorbed better than vitamin D2.[90] Vitamin K is given with vitamin D3 to support bone health.[91] The K2MK7 form of Vitamin K is usually given as it is a vital nutrient for mitochondrial health.[92]

Magnesium

Although there is evidence that magnesium supplementation helps with anxiety, the evidence is not of high quality. Clinically, in our practice, we have noted that magnesium supplementation helps reduce anxiety and depression. Studies which use dietary surveys or serum magnesium levels (instead of the more accurate RBC magnesium levels) are difficult to interpret.[93,94]

Magnesium exists in several forms. Magnesium sulfate is given IV for various medical indications in the hospital setting. The most common forms of magnesium given orally are magnesium oxide and magnesium citrate. Magnesium citrate has been shown to increase magnesium levels better than magnesium oxide.[95] Both magnesium citrate and magnesium oxide have the lowest bioavailability of all the magnesium supplements, while magnesium malate has the highest.[96]

There is some evidence that magnesium malate may be particularly helpful in fibromyalgia as it provides malic acid, which is an intermediate compound in the Krebs cycle. This can increase energy production and helps in exercise recovery.[97] Magnesium glycinate is a good general-purpose formulation of magnesium. In animal models, magnesium L-threonate increases CSF magnesium levels more than magnesium sulfate.[98] Studies show that magnesium L-threonate is very efficient at crossing the blood-brain barrier.[99]

In our practice, we use magnesium citrate for constipation, magnesium glycinate for general repletion, and combination supplements with mixtures of magnesium malate, threonate, and glycinate for various reasons in children with PANS and PANDAS.

Myo-inositol

Myo-inositol, once referred to as vitamin B8, is not a vitamin but a caroboxylic sugar. It is often used to treat polycystic ovarian syndrome (PCOS). There is quite a bit of evidence that it can be used to treat OCD and anxiety.

Double-blind, placebo-controlled trials have shown that it is significantly more effective in panic disorder than placebo.[100–103] Studies have shown it to be as effective as imipramine[100] and more effective than fluvoxamine[103] for the treatment of panic disorders.

In addition, studies have shown that inositol levels are low in depression, and that it can be effective as the sole agent used for treament.[100] The drug has been shown to be safe and non-toxic at doses of 12–18 grams daily.[101–103] It can be effective for OCD as well.[102] No benefit was seen when it was administered to treat Alzheimer's disease or schizophrenia, and it can make ADHD behaviors worse.[102]

L-theanine

This nonprotein amino acid is found in green tea.

> Studies have shown that inositol levels are low in depression, and that it can be effective as the sole agent used for treament.

A systematic review of the literature regarding the anxiolytic effects of L-theanine was published in 2020.[104] This paper reviews nine peer-reviewed studies where L-theanine was compared to controls (270 participants total). The studies demonstrated that 200–400 mg of oral L-theanine provided stress and anxiety reduction without causing drowsiness.

The review also notes that L-theanine suppressed excess cortisol production in response to stressful stimuli. The effects of L-theanine are likely due to reduction of glutaminergic transmission via suppression of glutamine to glutamate conversion and/or competitive binding of L-theanine to various receptors which blocks glutamate binding. In our experience, L-theanine also helps to combat insomnia.

GABA

γ-aminobutyric acid (GABA) is the chief inhibitory neurotransmitter in the CNS and helps inhibit neuronal excitability. It actually counterbalances the excitatory neurotransmitter glutamate. Studies have shown decreased levels of GABA in patients with anxiety disorders.[105] Prescription GABA-ergic agents include agents that increase GABA release like gabapentin and agents that inhibit GABA reuptake like tiagabine. Benzodiazepines act as GABA agonists. It has been shown that patients with anxiety disorders have decreased benzodiazepine binding sites in the brain.[105]

GABA supplements are usually marketed as GABA or PharmaGABA. The difference is that GABA is synthesized from chemical precursors while PharmaGABA is produced through fermentation by a specific strain of lactobacillus. Although various supplement companies and blogs report that supplements containing PharmaGABA are better absorbed, more effective, and safer than GABA supplements, there is no high-quality data to support these claims.

Although there is contradictory evidence as to whether orally administered GABA supplements can cross the blood-brain barrier, multiple studies have shown anxiolytic effects of GABA supplementation.[106] We use GABA supplements and combination products which contain GABA in our practice.

Cannabidiol (CBD)

CBD oil comes from the cannabis plant. Numerous CBD products have emerged over the last ten years with various dosage forms. Appropriate preparations for pediatric use are organic and contain no significant levels of tetrahydrocannabinol (THC). CBD should not be confused with medical cannabis ("medical marijuana"), which is a topic that is beyond the scope of this textbook.

There are no large-scale randomized studies on CBD oil for anxiety, but several reviews and case series[107–109] have established the fact that CBD is effective for the treatment of anxiety. In our practice, we have seen anxiolytic effects and improvements in insomnia with CBD.

Additional electronic modalities for anxiety

One excellent review provides lists of smartphone apps for relaxation, breathwork, and mind-body work.[110] This article also contains additional information about cranial electrical stimulation and other useful devices. We also recommend the Alpha-Stim device (www.alpha-stim.com) for our patients with anxiety. The

> γ-aminobutyric acid (GABA) is the chief inhibitory neurotransmitter in the CNS and helps inhibit neuronal excitability.

Alpha-Stim device uses earlobe clips and helps induce an alpha brain wave state that helps alleviate anxiety.

Homeopathy

Homeopathic remedies are minute doses of substances which would normally cause symptoms in healthy people. The remedies are usually supplied in the form of very small, round, candy-like tablets a bit larger than the ball of a ballpoint pen. These remedies are widely available online without a prescription. The substances in the tablets are reportedly so dilute that no trace of the original substance remains. Proponents argue that the *spiritual* essence of the original substance remains. Spectroscopic analysis of homeopathic compounds has demonstrated that the remedies tested had no differences in signature as compared to placebo.[111]

Systematic reviews and double-blind placebo-controlled studies (including a systematic review published in a homeopathy journal) have failed to show any benefit of homeopathic remedies when compared to controls in patients with anxiety.[112–114]

Although some practitioners claim (mainly online) that homeopathy is close to a miracle cure for PANS and PANDAS, there is no supportive scientific evidence in the literature. We have used some homeopathic remedies in patients with PANS and PANDAS (and have seen patients who have consulted with homeopathic specialists) and have not consistently seen a measurable improvement in any symptoms. For this reason, we seldom recommend homeopathic remedies in our patients with PANS or PANDAS.

Neurolinguistic programming (NLP) for anxiety

Chapter 21 contains a detailed discussion of NLP in general and NLP approaches to anxiety reduction in PANS and PANDAS.

Hypnosis for anxiety

Chapter 21 contains a detailed discussion of hypnosis in general and the utility of hypnosis for anxiety reduction in PANS and PANDAS.

Vagus nerve exercises for anxiety

See Chapter 20 for a detailed discussion of the autonomic nervous system and vagus nerve exercises to cut down sympathetic overactivation. These exercises, like heart rate variability training, help reduce sympathetic tone, which helps reduce anxiety.

REDUCE: TICS

Tics are repetitive motor movements (motor tics) and/or repetitive sounds (phonic tics). The term

> Tourette disorder (or syndrome) is defined as the presence of both motor and phonic tics for more than a year.

"phonic" is preferred to the older term "vocal" since some of the sounds produced don't involve the vocal cords. There are various tic disorders described in the literature.

If tics are present for less than one year, the term *provisional tic disorder* is used (formerly called *transient tic disorder*). If tics are present for more than a year and contain only motor tics, this is known as *persistent motor tic disorder*. If only phonic tics are present, this is known as *persistent vocal tic disorder*.

Tourette disorder (or syndrome) is defined as the presence of both motor and phonic tics for more than a year.[115] Complex phonic/vocal tics may contain words or sentences. They may take the form of echolalia (repeating the words of others), repeating one's own words or syllables (palilalia), or coprolalia (obscene or vulgar words or phrases). Coprolalia, animal sounds, and loud outbursts and motor tics are the hallmarks of Tourette syndrome. There is some evidence that most, if not all, patients with chronic tic disorders are somewhere on a spectrum which includes Tourette syndrome.[116]

Tics are distinct from chorea since movements[115] in chorea are quick, jerking, and non-repetitive. The movements in chorea also typically involve proximal joints and flow from joint to joint.

Tics are often seen in children with PANS and PANDAS. There is currently some discussion among PANDAS physicians as to whether the acute onset of tics should be considered one of the primary diagnostic criteria (with OCD and food restriction) rather than just one of the secondary criteria.

The most common tics we see in cases of PANS and PANDAS are grimacing, mouth opening/ stretching, repetitive blinking (blepharospasm), eye rolling (oculogyric tics), sniffing, shoulder shrugs, head jerks, and frequent throat clearing. All tic disorders tend to have a waxing and waning course, and the location of tics and their magnitude may change. This variability is seen with PANS and PANDAS.

Neuroimaging and pathology studies have shown that patients with Tourette syndrome have abnormalities in the basal ganglia.[115,117] Similar changes in this area of the brain were found on MRI, CT, and PET scans in patients with Sydenham chorea (an autoimmune condition which may occur after *Strep* infection) and in patients with PANDAS.[118–122]

Studies in mice have shown that damaging cholinergic interneurons of the striatum leads to tic-like behaviors.[123] A small but interesting study in mice showed that the sera of children with PANDAS binds to the cholinergic interneurons of the striatum.[124] The study showed that if sera was injected after the children had received IVIG, the binding in the mouse brain tissue returned to normal levels.

> About 96% of patients with Tourette syndrome have an onset before the age of eleven.

The diagnostic criteria for Tourette syndrome also require that the onset of tics begin before age twenty-one. About 96% of patients with Tourette syndrome have an onset before the age of eleven.[125]

Tics are the only movement disorder in which movements can be voluntarily suppressed,[115–117,126,127] although this may require intense mental effort. This fact makes it difficult to precisely label these movements as involuntary. Tics may increase in frequency when patients are stressed, tired, bored, fatigued, excited, or exposed to heat. Patients with PANS and PANDAS may experience new tics or increased frequency or amplitude of tics when they have a flare or experience illness. In some patients, SSRIs can exacerbate tics.[115] Focused activities can decrease the frequency of tics.

Concomitant psychopathology is commonly seen with tic disorders. The most common concomitant disorder is ADHD, which is seen in 50–80% of patients with chronic tic disorders.[115] This combination may lead to frustration and disruptive behaviors in school.[115] We have frequently seen a worsening of tics in patients who were placed on stimulants for ADHD before establishing care with us.

OCD is seen in approximately 20–60% of children and adults with chronic tic disorders.[115] A further connection between patients with tics and OCD/intrusive thoughts is the fact that most patients with tic disorders report an urge or sensory feeling which seems to compel them to perform a tic.[115–117,126,127] Patients often state that the tics must be repeated to make them feel "just right." OCD is present in 82% of patients with Sydenham chorea overall and is present in 100% of patients who have a recurrence of chorea.[128,129]

> **Children with chronic tic disorders have lower levels of vitamin D and a higher incidence of vitamin D deficiency than controls.**

Guidelines[115] for the treatment of tics from the American Academy of Child and Adolescent Psychiatry state that behavioral interventions are an effective treatment strategy for moderate tics if they cause impairment of the patient's life. The training program with the most evidence is called habit reversal training (HRT) or comprehensive behavioral intervention for tics (CBIT). This is typically an 8–10 week training program with parental involvement.

The guidelines[115] also recommend medications for patients with severe tics or tics with comorbid psychiatric disorders. When patients with tics arrive at our office for their initial appointment, they have often been prescribed alpha-adrenergic agonists such as clonidine or guanfacine for tic control. Meta-analyses have shown that these medications may be useful in patients with both tics and comorbid ADHD but have no significant effect on tic reduction in patients without ADHD.[130]

A comprehensive, systematic review of treatment recommendations for Tourette syndrome and chronic tic disorders, which was published in the journal *Neurology*, states that there is high-quality evidence that patients with tics receiving CBIT are more likely than those receiving psychotherapy to have reduced tic severity.[131]

There is moderate-quality evidence, however, that people receiving clonidine or some antipsychotics are "probably more likely" than patients receiving placebos to have decreased tic severity. There is low-quality evidence that patients on guanfacine are "possibly more likely" than patients receiving placebos to have decreased tic severity. A randomized controlled trial published in *JAMA* also affirmed the effectiveness of behavioral therapy for children with Tourette syndrome and chronic tic disorder.[132]

Supplements for tics

One study showed that children with chronic tic disorders have lower levels of vitamin D and a higher incidence of vitamin D deficiency than controls.[133] A study of 120 children with tic disorders confirmed the fact that children with tics had lower levels of vitamin D as compared to controls and showed that vitamin D supplementation resulted in significant improvement.[134] The combination of L-theanine and vitamin B6 was shown in one study to significantly reduce the severity of tics in the treatment group compared to controls.[135]

Hypnosis for tics

Teaching patients self-hypnosis is an effective treatment method to improve or eliminate tics in children.[136] We have found hypnosis to be effective in reducing tics in patients with PANS and PANDAS. Hypnosis is discussed further in Chapter 21.

> **Randomized, placebo-controlled studies have shown that folate (specifically L-methylfolate) is helpful in patients with depression.**

REDUCE: DEPRESSION

Labile mood (sudden mood changes) is a common symptom in children with PANS and PANDAS. Their mood can shift very suddenly from a calm state to screaming or crying. Depressive thoughts are very common.

Many of these children will make statements like they "wished they would die" or that they "don't deserve to live." True suicide attempts are exceedingly rare. We have not seen a serious attempt in our patient population to date. These children do sometimes threaten to jump out of a window or a moving vehicle and may unbuckle the seat belt while parents are driving. All such statements should be viewed cautiously and investigated; however, the motivation for the child in these situations is often to relieve stress or create parental conflict. Worrying about having thoughts of suicide is also a common OCD theme. In this case it is the "thought about the thought" that disturbs them.

Obviously, any child who is actively suicidal or who attempts suicide should immediately be taken to the nearest emergency department for urgent evaluation.

Since labile mood and depressive thoughts are usually secondary to anxiety and OCD in these children, managing anxiety, intrusive thoughts, sleep, and family dynamics, coupled with counseling, is the best approach for these thoughts.

SSRI medications are not usually effective at reducing labile mood in patients with PANS and PANDAS and have their own side effects and risks.

Supplements for depression
Folate

Randomized, placebo-controlled studies have shown that folate (specifically L-methylfolate) is helpful in patients with depression.[137] The relationship is supported by the fact that elevated homocysteine (due to poor methylation and homozygous MTHFR C677T genetic mutations) is associated with depressive disorders.[138–143] Patients with elevated homocysteine and depression also have low folate levels, and low 5-HT, dopamine, and norepinephrine metabolites in the CSF.[144]

Folate as a monotherapy was equal to amitriptyline in one study[145] and performed better than trazodone in another.[146] Both studies were composed of patients with mostly normal folate levels. Folate provides substantial benefit as an adjunct to antidepressants versus placebo.[147–149]

Methylfolate is a vital regulator of the synthesis of dopamine, serotonin, and norepinephrine.[150] A review by Menezo et al. compares and contrasts the efficacy and safety of folic acid, folinic acid, and 5-methyl-tetrahydrofolate (5-MTHF) in patients with methylation issues such as MTHFR.[151] The review establishes 5-MTHF as the safest effective treatment in these patients. It also provides evidence that unmetabolized folic acid (a synthetic product) may be harmful in the body.

We use 5-MTHF in our patients with significant MTHFR mutations, especially if they have elevated homocysteine levels.

S-adenosylmethionine (SAMe)

SAMe is a molecule made from the essential amino acid methionine, and is involved in the process of methylation. In fact, it is the principal methyl donor, is a key molecule for the normal structure and function of cell membranes, and is a precursor of glutathione.[152,153] SAMe serves as a cofactor for almost as many biochemical reactions as ATP.[152]

SAMe administration has been proven to be helpful in patients with depression both as a monotherapy and as an adjunct to traditional pharmacotherapy.[137] It is as effective as tricyclic antidepressants and is superior to placebo when used as an adjunct to SSRIs and SNRIs.[137,154] Reduction of aggressive behavior and improved quality of life in patients with schizophrenia was seen in one small study.[155]

We use SAMe in our practice with patients who demonstrate significant depressive symptoms or aggression. There is another genetic mutation (SNP) that can affect how methylating agents like methylfolate and SAMe work in the body. It is called catechol-O-methyltransferase (COMT). If present, depending on the genotype (heterozygous vs. homozygous), SAMe or folate administration may cause agitation. The relationship between methylating agents and COMT is complex, and the literature is not consistent.

REDUCE: INSOMNIA

Insomnia is very common in children with PANS and PANDAS. So much so that the lack of insomnia warrants careful reappraisal of the

> SAMe serves as a cofactor for almost as many biochemical reactions as ATP.

presentation to make sure the patient's symptoms are not a result of another neuropsychiatric condition. Sleep delays are often due to hyperarousal and increased sympathetic autonomic tone.

Both early waking and difficulty getting to sleep may be seen. Occasionally, sleep inversion may take place whereby the child stays up all night and sleeps during the day. Keeping a sleep diary to log sleep patterns often provides valuable clinical information and helps assess whether interventions are helping.

The first thing to look for are signs of sleep-disordered breathing such as snoring, open-mouth breathing, periods of apparent apnea, and excessive daytime sleepiness. Any of the above warrants a formal pediatric sleep study.

Next, careful attention should be paid to proper sleep hygiene. A fixed protocol or routine will help your child develop proper habits and an expectation for sleep. The bedroom should be quiet, cool, and dark during sleep hours. White noise can be helpful, but music with lyrics or TV should not be used as these modalities may stimulate the brain and prevent restful sleep. Children may develop complex rituals related to getting to sleep. Parents should not participate in rituals as this may cement the OCD patterns and make them harder to overcome.

The use of blue screens (TV, computer monitors or laptops, phones, video games) should not occur for two hours prior to attempting to get to sleep. Short-wave blue light (which is emitted from screens of electronic devices) has been shown to adversely affect sleep quality and sleep timing.[156,157] There are several types of blue-blocking glasses available to purchase online which may help support sleep if screens are used close to bedtime.[156] Some electronic devices may have a feature that changes the colors on the screen to eliminate or reduce blue light.

We have also found cranial electrotherapy stimulation devices like the Alpha-Stim device helpful to reduce insomnia. Mindfulness practices and breathing exercises (see the section of this chapter on anxiety) can also be helpful. Vagus nerve exercises to decrease sympathetic tone can help as well (see Chapter 20).

We do not recommend prescription medications for sleep (especially benzodiazepines), as they tend to disturb sleep architecture and potentially worsen sleep-disordered breathing.[158]

We teach parents a simple exercise (below) which they can use to help their children settle in for sleep. Adults can also use this exercise.

A simple sleep countdown exercise:
1. Invite the child to get comfortable where they will sleep.

2. Using the same words or phrases may help.
3. When the child is settled, ask them to imagine seeing "ten yellow bananas" and then "nine orange carrots." Slowly count down in the pattern of a number and a color and an object. Take a very short pause on each fruit or vegetable (or whatever objects you are using). Ask them to imagine what it would be like to smell it or bite into it.
4. The exercise does not have to be food related, but objects that you can feel, smell, taste, see, and hear yield best results.
5. The natural countdown is something our brains associate with an ending or relaxing.

Self-hypnosis can be very helpful with sleep issues. (See Chapter 21 for details on hypnosis.)

> Children may develop complex rituals related to getting to sleep. Parents should not participate in rituals as this may cement the OCD patterns and make them harder to overcome.

Supplements for insomnia
Melatonin
Melatonin is an indole hormone that is produced from tryptophan in the pineal gland in the brain

in response to darkness. It helps control the sleep-wake cycle. Blue light exposure at night can result in decreased amounts of melatonin, which may affect sleep. Melatonin is a chronobiotic (a substance which helps with sleep), an antioxidant, and an analgesic. Commercial mela-

> L-theanine has been shown to improve sleep quality through anxiolysis and it is not sedating.

tonin preparations are used by many adults and in children to aid sleep.

Studies have shown melatonin produces benefits in sleep architecture in patients with ADHD, autism spectrum disorders, and developmental disorders.[159,160] There are not many studies of melatonin in children with primary sleep issues who do not have one of these disorders. There are no studies in children with PANS and PANDAS. One randomized, placebo-controlled study of children who were given 5 mg of melatonin showed that it was significantly more effective than placebo.[161] Melatonin is generally considered safe in children.[159–161] Very few side effects have been seen in children who take melatonin. Additional studies are needed to confirm the appropriate dose for children. We do not routinely use melatonin for insomnia in children with PANS and PANDAS.

Magnesium

We have observed clinically that magnesium malate, magnesium threonate, and magnesium glycinate can help with insomnia in our adult and pediatric patients.

L-theanine

L-theanine has been shown to improve sleep quality through anxiolysis and it is not sedating.[162,163] We use L-theanine in our patients as it also helps with anxiety.

GABA

At least one study in adults showed that GABA supplements are safe and effective at improving subjective sleep quality and improving objective sleep efficacy compared to controls.[164] We use GABA supplementation both separately and in a combination product in children with PANS and PANDAS.

REDUCE: DEFIANCE

Although defiance is listed in the symptom groups that can establish the diagnosis of PANS and PANDAS, the behaviors defined as defiance are most often due to OCD and severe anxiety.

We tell parents to imagine they are in a large office building which caught on fire. As they are running through the lobby to get outside to safety, a security guard in the lobby yells that they may not run in the lobby. They continue running undeterred for fear that they may die if they stay in the building. Even if the security guard threatened to subject them to some form of citation or reporting, they would not likely stop.

This is representative of the battle parents have with children with PANS and PANDAS when they try to enforce rules. In this case it is a matter of extreme fear and OCD, not defiance for defiance's sake. Of course, there must be some rules of the house for the family to exist in peace and safety. But we tell parents to keep their own anxiety barometer on alert so that they can remain attentive to times when they may be asking something that the child feels is simply impossible.

REDUCE: CONCENTRATION ISSUES AND EXECUTIVE FUNCTIONING DEFICITS

Many children with PANS and PANDAS are diagnosed with ADHD. We hesitate to say "misdiagnosed" as they may meet published DSM criteria for the disorder. It is more accurate to say they are *incompletely* diagnosed, as the ADHD criteria are just symptoms when PANS or PANDAS may actually be the root cause. This is especially true if the concentration issues are of sudden onset. We do not favor stimulants in these cases as they can make anxiety, OCD, and agitation worse.

The techniques and supplements mentioned in the earlier section on anxiety can help decrease distractibility in these children.

In recent years, inflammation and increased oxidative stress have been recognized as significant in the pathophysiology of ADHD.[165–167] Polyphenols are plant-based compounds rich in antioxidants. Dietary polyphenol levels have been noted to be lower in children with ADHD.[168] Supplementation of antioxidants, particularly supplementation of the polyphenolic substance Pycnogenol has been associated with increases in glutathione, reduction of oxidative stress markers like 8-OHdG, reduction of catecholamine levels, and improved symptoms.[169–171] Pycnogenol is made from pine bark extract.

Although supplements containing only Pycnogenol are available, we use a product which contains turmeric extract (an anti-inflammatory substance), pine bark extract, various other antioxidant polyphenols, and EGCG (from green tea). We have seen clinical improvements in attention and a decrease in hyperactivity in our patients taking this supplement.

Issues with fine motor control or executive functioning can be improved with occupational therapy and supportive services at school or at home. An early IEP or 504 plan is advisable. (See Appendix D.)

Persistent memory loss, disorientation, or progressive loss of attention with a rapid progression should prompt urgent evaluation. In these cases, neuroimaging and more intensive testing such as a lumbar puncture should be considered. This pattern is not consistent with PANS and PANDAS and suggests an alternative diagnosis until proven otherwise.

REDUCE: PAIN

Pain in muscles and joints can be seen in PANS

> Inflammation and increased oxidative stress have been recognized as significant in the pathophysiology of ADHD.

and PANDAS cases. It can be due to infections, especially tick-borne infections like Lyme disease. At other times, the pain may result from an autoimmune process. In these cases, elevation of the serum ANA, rheumatoid factor, or anti-CCP antibodies may be seen. These laboratory changes and symptoms often disappear with re-regulation of the immune system, healing the gut (decreasing intestinal permeability), and the removal of triggers (infections and/or toxins). Studies have documented autoimmune joint pain (sometimes referred to as enthesitis) in about 28% of PANS and PANDAS cases.[172]

Intermittent courses of NSAIDs (ibuprofen or naproxen) can be used for pain relief. Severe pain may require referral to a pediatric rheumatologist.

REDUCE: URINARY FREQUENCY AND ENURESIS

Changes in urination are common in PANS and PANDAS. Sudden frequent urges are often seen, which are likely due to autonomic imbalances. Urinary tract infection should be ruled out if the changes are sudden in onset. Vagus nerve exercises (see Chapter 20) can be helpful in treating the symptoms of urinary frequency or urgency in the absence of UTI.

Nocturnal enuresis or daytime wetting may be seen as well. While buzzing monitors with moisture sensors are sometimes used in children with nocturnal enuresis as a form of training, we do not recommend these monitors for use in children with PANS and PANDAS. They can cause agitation and may further exacerbate sleep issues.

Teaching children self-hypnosis is very effective in reducing or eradicating nocturnal enuresis. A helpful online program can be found at www.keepingthebeddry.com.

REDUCE: CONSTIPATION OR DIARRHEA

Constipation may be seen in these patients due to imbalance of the autonomic nervous system. In addition, constipation can be due to dehydration, poor oral intake, or anatomic issues unrelated to PANS and PANDAS. If concerns for obstruction or more serious issues are noted on the physical exam, referral for an urgent evaluation in the emergency department is warranted. Normal bowel movements should occur 1–2 times per day.

Treatment of constipation should begin with increased oral intake of fluids and higher-fiber foods. If not sufficient, magnesium citrate can be helpful to normalize bowel movements. Vagus nerve exercises (see Chapter 20) can help restore autonomic balance.

Diarrhea may also be due to autonomic imbalance. Additional causes may include parasitic infections, *C. difficile* infection, food allergies, and food sensitivities. There is no specific treatment, but vagus nerve exercises may help normalize bowel function. If dehydration is noted, assisted oral rehydration or IV fluids may be necessary.

CHAPTER 10 REFERENCES

1. Sackett, DL, Rosenberg WMC, Muir Gray JA, et al. Evidence based medicine: what it is and what it isn't. *BMJ*. 1996;312(7023):71–72

2. Haynes RB, Devereaux PJ, and Guyatt GH. Clinical expertise in the era of evidence-based medicine and patient choice. *BMJ Evidence-Based Medicine*. 2002;7(2):36–38

3. Koran LM, Hanna GL, Hollander E, et al. American Psychiatric Association: Practice guideline for the treatment of patients with obsessive-compulsive disorder. *Am J Psychiatry*. 2007;164(suppl):5–53

4. Stein DJ, Koen N, Fineberg N, et al. A 2012 evidence-based algorithm for the pharmacotherapy for obsessive-compulsive disorder. *Curr Psychiatry Rep*. 2012;14(3):211–9

5. Koran LM, Simpson HB. *Guideline watch (March 2013): Practice Guideline for the Treatment of Patients with Obsessive-Compulsive Disorder*. Arlington, VA: American Psychiatric Association

6. Sassano-Higgins S, Pato M. Obsessive-compulsive disorder: diagnosis, epidemiology, etiology, and treatment. *Focus*. 2015;13:129–141

7. Soomro GM, Altman D, Rajagopal S, Oakley-Browne M. Selective serotonin re-uptake inhibitors (SSRIs) versus placebo for obsessive compulsive disorder (OCD). *Cochrane Database Syst Rev*. 2008 Jan 23;2008(1):CD001765:1–56

8. Geller DA, Biederman J, Stewart SE, et al. Which SSRI? A meta-analysis of pharmacotherapy trials in pediatric obsessive-compulsive disorder. *Am J Psychiatry*. 2003;160(11):1919–28

9. Del Casale A, Sorice S, Padovano A, et al. Psychopharmacological treatment of obsessive-compulsive disorder (OCD). *Curr Neuropharmacol*. 2019;17(8):710–736

10. Blier P, Habib R, Flament MF. Pharmacotherapies in the management of obsessive-compulsive disorder. *Canadian Journal of Psychiatry*. 2006;51(7):417–30

11. Murphy TK, Storch EA, Strawser MS: Selective serotonin reuptake inhibitor-induced behavioral activation in the PANDAS subtype. *Primary Psychiatry*. 2006;13:87–89

12. Thienemann M, Murphy T, Leckman J. Clinical management of pediatric acute-onset neuropsychiatric syndrome: part I: psychiatric and behavioral interventions. *J Child Adolesc Psychopharmacol*. 2017;27(7):566–573

13. Calaprice D, Tona J. Treatment of pediatric acute-onset neuropsychiatric disorder in a large survey population. J. *Child Adolesc. Psychopharmacol*. 2017;28(2):92–103

14. Shoubridge AP, Choo JM, Martin AM, et al. The gut microbiome and mental health: advances in research and emerging priorities. *Mol Psychiatry*. 2022;27(4):1908–1919

15. Butler MI, Mörkl S, Sandhu KV, et al. The gut microbiome and mental health: what should we tell our patients?: Le microbiote Intestinal et la Santé Mentale: que Devrions-Nous dire à nos Patients? *Can J Psychiatry*. 2019;64(11):747–760

16. Abramowitz JS. The psychological treatment of obsessive-compulsive disorder. *Can J Psychiatry*. 2006;51(7):407–16

17. Van Noppen B, Sassano-Higgins S, Appasani R, et al. Cognitive-behavioral therapy for obsessive-compulsive disorder: 2021 update. *Focus*. 2021;19(4):430–43

18. Öst LG, Riise EN, Wergeland GJ, et al. Cognitive behavioral and pharmacological treatments of OCD in children: a systematic review and meta-analysis. *J Anxiety Disord*. 2016;43:58–69

19. McGuire JF, Piacentini J, Lewin AB, et al. A meta-analysis of cognitive behavior therapy and medication for child obsessive-compulsive disorder: moderators of treatment efficacy, response, and remission. *Depress Anxiety*. 2015 Aug;32(8):580–93

20. Ivarsson T, Skarphedinsson G, Kornør H, et al. Accreditation task force of the Canadian Institute for Obsessive Compulsive Disorders: the place of and evidence for serotonin reuptake inhibitors (SRIs) for obsessive compulsive disorder (OCD) in children and adolescents: views based on a systematic review and meta-analysis. *Psychiatry Res*. 2015;227(1):93–103

21. Sánchez-Meca J, Rosa-Alcázar AI, Iniesta-Sepúlveda M, et al. Differential efficacy of cognitive-behavioral therapy and pharmacological treatments for pediatric obsessive-compulsive disorder: a meta-analysis. *J Anxiety Disord*. 2014;28(1):31–44

22. Foa EB, Liebowitz MR, Kozak MJ, et al. Randomized, placebo-controlled trial of exposure and ritual prevention, clomipramine, and their combination in the treatment of obsessive-compulsive disorder. *Am J Psychiatry*. 2005;162(1):151–61

23. Simpson HB, Foa EB, Liebowitz MR, et al. A randomized, controlled trial of cognitive-behavioral therapy for augmenting pharmacotherapy in obsessive-compulsive disorder. *Am J Psychiatry*. 2008;165(5):621–30

24. Practice parameter for the assessment and treatment of children and adolescents with obsessive-compulsive disorder. *J Am Acad Child Adolesc Psychiatry*. 2012;51(1):98–113

25. National Institute for Health and Clinical Excellence. Obsessive-compulsive disorder: core interventions in the treatment of obsessive-compulsive disorder and body dysmorphic disorder. www.nice.org.uk/guidance/cg31, accessed 1/11/2023

26. Lebowitz ER, Vitulano LA, Mataix-Cols D, Leckman JF: Editorial perspective: when OCD takes over the family! Coercive and disruptive behaviours in paediatric obsessive-compulsive disorder. *J Child Psychol Psychiatry*. 52:1249–1250, 2011

27. Kariuki-Nyuthe C, Gomez-Mancilla B, Stein DJ. Obsessive compulsive disorder and the glutamatergic system. *Current Opinion in Psychiatry* 2014;27(1):32–37

28. Pittenger C, Bloch MH, Williams K. Glutamate abnormalities in obsessive compulsive disorder: neurobiology, pathophysiology, and treatment. *Pharmacology & Therapeutics*. 2011;132(3):314–332

29. Adler CM, McDonough-Ryan P, Sax KW, et al. fMRI of neuronal activation with symptom provocation in unmedicated patients with obsessive compulsive disorder. *J Psychiatr Res*. 2000;34:317–324

30. Yücel M, Wood SJ, Wellard RM, et al. Anterior cingulate glutamate-glutamine levels predict symptom severity in women with obsessive- compulsive disorder. *Aust N Z J Psychiatry*. 2008;42:467–477

31. Oliver G, Dean O, Camfield D, et al. N-acetyl cysteine in the treatment of obsessive compulsive and related disorders: a systematic review. *Clin Psychopharmacol Neurosci*. 2015;13(1):12–24

32. Bhattacharyya S, Khanna S, Chakrabarty K, et al. Anti-brain autoantibodies and altered excitatory neurotransmitters in obsessive-compulsive disorder. *Neuropsychopharmacology*. 2009;34:2489–2496

33. Ersan S, Bakir S, Erdal Ersan E, et al. Examination of free radical metabolism and antioxidant defence system elements in patients with obsessive-compulsive disorder. *Prog Neuropsychopharmacol Biol Psychiatry*. 2006;30:1039–1042

34. Ozdemir E, Cetinkaya S, Ersan S, et al. Serum selenium and plasma malondialdehyde levels and antioxidant enzyme activities in patients with obsessive-compulsive disorder. *Prog Neuropsychopharmacol Biol Psychiatry*. 2009;33:62–65

35. Afshar H, Roohafza H, Mohammad-Beigi H. N-acetylcysteine add-on treatment in refractory obsessive-compulsive disorder: a randomized, double-blind, placebo-controlled trial. *Journal of Clinical Psychopharmacology*. 2012;32(6):797–803

36. Ghanizadeh A, Mohammadi MR, Bahraini S, et al. Efficacy of N-acetylcysteine augmentation on obsessive compulsive disorder: a multicenter randomized double-blind, placebo-controlled clinical trial. *Iran J Psychiatry*. 2017;12(2):134–141

37. Sarris J, Oliver G, Camfield DA, et al. N-acetyl cysteine (NAC) in the treatment of obsessive-compulsive disorder: a 16-week, double-blind, randomised, placebo-controlled study. *CNS Drugs*. 2015;29(9):801–809

38. Paydary K, Akamaloo A, Ahmadipour A, et al. N-acetylcysteine augmentation therapy for moderate-to-severe obsessive-compulsive disorder: randomized, double-blind, placebo-controlled trial. *J Clin Pharm Ther*. 2016;41:214–219

39. Li F, Welling MC, Johnson JA, et al. N-acetylcysteine for pediatric obsessive-compulsive disorder: a small pilot study. *Journal of Child and Adolescent Psychopharmacology*. 2020;30(1):32–37

40. Eyles DW, Burne TH, McGrath JJ. Vitamin D, effects on brain development, adult brain function and the links between low levels of vitamin D and neuropsychiatric disease. *Front Neuroendocrinol*. 2013;34(1):47–64

41. Kuygun KC, Gül CG. Nutritional and herbal supplements in the treatment of obsessive-compulsive disorder. *Gen Psychiatr*. 2020;33(2):e100159:1–6

42. Esnafoğlu E, Yaman E. Vitamin B12, folic acid, homocysteine and vitamin D levels in children and adolescents with obsessive compulsive disorder. *Psychiatry Res*. 2017;254:232–237

43. Soyak HM, Karakükcü Ç. Investıgation of vitamin D levels in obsessive-compulsive disorder. *Indian J Psychiatry*. 2022;64(4):349–353

44. Ozdemir E, Cetinkaya S, Ersan S, et al. Serum selenium and plasma malondialdehyde levels and antioxidant enzyme activities in patients with obsessive-compulsive disorder. *Prog Neuropsychopharmacol Biol Psychiatry*. 2009;33(1):62–5

45. Sayyah M, Andishmand M, Ganji R. Effect of selenium as an adjunctive therapy in patients with treatment-resistant obsessive- compulsive disorder: a pilot randomized double blind placebo-controlled clinical trial. *Arch Psych Psych* 2018;20:57–65

46. Peters S, Koh J, Choi DW. Zinc selectively blocks the action of N-methyl-D-aspartate on cortical neurons. *Science*. 1987;236(4801):589–93

47. Sayyah M, Olapour A, Saeedabad Y. Evaluation of oral zinc sulfate effect on obsessive-compulsive disorder: a randomized placebo-controlled clinical trial. *Nutrition*. 2012;28(9):892–5

48. Bottiglieri T. Homocysteine and folate metabolism in depression. *Prog Neuropsychopharmacol Biol Psychiatry*. 2005;29(7):1103–12

49. Atmaca M, Tezcan E, Kuloglu M, et al. Serum folate and homocysteine levels in patients with obsessive-compulsive disorder. *Psychiatry Clin Neurosci*. 2005 Oct;59(5):616–20

50. Türksoy N, Bilici R, Yalçıner A, et al. Vitamin B12, folate, and homocysteine levels in patients with obsessive-compulsive disorder. *Neuropsychiatr Dis Treat*. 2014;10:1671–5

51. Walter HJ, Bukstein OG, Abright AR, et al. Clinical practice guideline for the assessment and treatment of children and adolescents with anxiety disorders. *J Am Acad Child Adolesc Psychiatry*. 2020;59(10):1107–1124

52. Walkup JT, Albano AM, Piacentini J, et al. Cognitive behavioral therapy, sertraline, or a combination in childhood anxiety. *New England Journal of Medicine*. 2008;359(26):2753–66

53. Wang Z, Whiteside SPH, Sim L, et al. Comparative effectiveness and safety of cognitive behavioral therapy and pharmacotherapy for childhood anxiety disorders: a systematic review and meta-analysis. *JAMA Pediatr*. 2017;171(11):1049–1056

54. Lewandowski AS, Ward TM, Palermo TM. Sleep problems in children and adolescents with common medical conditions. *Pediatr Clin North Am*. 2011;58(3):699–713

55. Zaccaro A, Piarulli A, Laurino M, et al. How breath-control can change your life: a systematic review on psycho-physiological correlates of slow breathing. *Front Hum Neurosci*. 2018;12:353:1–16

56. Ma X, Yue ZQ, Gong ZQ, et al. The effect of diaphragmatic breathing on attention, negative affect and stress in healthy adults. *Front Psychol*. 2017;8:874:1–23

57. Levi M, Bossù M, Luzzi V, et al. Breathing out dental fear: a feasibility crossover study on the effectiveness of diaphragmatic breathing in children sitting on the dentist's chair. *Int J Paediatr Dent*. 2022;32(6):801–811

58. Bahrololoomi Z, Sadeghiyeh T, Rezaei M, et al. The effect of breathing exercise using bubble blower on anxiety and pain during inferior alveolar nerve block in children aged 7 to 10 years: a crossover randomized clinical trial. *Pain Res Manag*. 2022;7817267:1–8

59. Bishop SR. Mindfulness: a proposed operational definition. *Clinical Psychology: Science and Practice*. 2004;11(3):230–241

60. Kabat-Zinn J. Mindfulness-based interventions in context: past, present, and future. *Clinical Psychology: Science and Practice*. 2003;10(2):144–156

61. Melbourne Academic Mindfulness Interest Group. Mindfulness-based psychotherapies: a review of conceptual foundations, empirical evidence and practical considerations. *Aust N Z J Psychiatry*. 2006;40(4):285–29

62. Killingsworth MA, Gilbert DT. A wandering mind is an unhappy mind. *Science*. 2010;330(6006):932

63. Brown KW, Ryan RM. The benefits of being present: mindfulness and its role in psychological well-being. *J Pers Soc Psychol*. 2003;84(4):822–48

64. Miller JJ, Fletcher K, Kabat-Zinn J. Three-year follow-up and clinical implications of a mindfulness meditation-based stress reduction intervention in the treatment of anxiety disorders. *Gen Hosp Psychiatry*. 1995;17(3):192–200

65. Kabat-Zinn J, Massion AO, Kristeller J, et al. Effectiveness of a meditation-based stress reduction program in the treatment of anxiety disorders. *Am J Psychiatry*. 1992;149(7):936–43

66. Hofmann SG, Gómez AF. Mindfulness-based interventions for anxiety and depression. *Psychiatr Clin North Am*. 2017;40(4):739–749

67. Khoury B, Lecomte T, Fortin G, et al. Mindfulness-based therapy: a comprehensive meta-analysis. *Clin Psychol Rev*. 2013;33(6):763–71

68. Spinelli C, Wisener M, Khoury B. Mindfulness training for healthcare professionals and trainees: a meta-analysis of randomized controlled trials. *J Psychosom Res*. 2019;120:29–38

69. Semple RJ, Reid EF, Miller L. Treating anxiety with mindfulness: an open trial of mindfulness training for anxious children. *Journal of Cognitive Psychotherapy*. 2005;19(4):379–392

70. Hoge EA, Bui E, Palitz SA, et al. The effect of mindfulness meditation training on biological acute stress responses in generalized anxiety disorder. *Psychiatry Res*. 2018;262:328–332

71. www.positivepsychology.com/mindfulness-exercises-techniques-activities, accessed 1/22/2023

72. Goyal M, Singh S, Sibinga EM, et al. Meditation programs for psychological stress and well-being: a systematic review and meta-analysis. *JAMA Intern Med*. 2014;174(3):357–68

73. Chabot RJ, di Michele F, Prichep L. The role of quantitative electroencephalography in child and adolescent psychiatric disorders. *Child and Adolescent Psychiatric Clinics of North America*. 2005;14(1):21–53

74. Gruzelier J, Egner T. Critical validation studies of neurofeedback. *Child and Adolescent Psychiatric Clinics of North America*. 2005;14(1):83–104

75. Hammond DC. Neurofeedback with anxiety and affective disorders. *Child and Adolescent Psychiatric Clinics of North America*. 2005;14(1):105–123

76. Simkin DR, Thatcher RW, Lubar J. Quantitative EEG and neurofeedback in children and adolescents: anxiety disorders, depressive disorders, comorbid addiction and attention-deficit/hyperactivity disorder, and brain injury. *Child and Adolescent Psychiatric Clinics*. 2014;23(3):427–6

77. Garcia Pimenta M, Brown T, Arns M, et al. Treatment efficacy and clinical effectiveness of EEG neurofeedback as a personalized and multimodal treatment in ADHD: a critical review. *Neuropsychiatr Dis Treat*. 2021;17:637–648

78. Duffy FH. The state of EEG biofeedback therapy (EEG operant conditioning) in 2000: an editor's opinion. *Clin Electroencephalogr*. 2000 Jan;31(1):V–VII

79. Cheng YC, Huang YC, Huang WL. The effect of vitamin D supplement on negative emotions: a systematic review and meta-analysis. *Depress Anxiety*. 2020;37(6):549–564

80. Eid A, Khoja S, AlGhamdi S, et al. Vitamin D supplementation ameliorates severity of generalized anxiety disorder (GAD). *Metab Brain Dis*. 20219;34:1781–1786

81. Kouba BR, Camargo A, Gil-Mohapel J, Rodrigues ALS. Molecular basis underlying the therapeutic potential of vitamin D for the treatment of depression and anxiety. *International Journal of Molecular Sciences*. 2022;23(13):7077

82. Casseb GAS, Kaster MP, Rodrigues ALS. Potential role of vitamin D for the management of depression and anxiety. *CNS Drugs*. 2019;33:619–637

83. www.medscape.com/viewarticle/920520, accessed 1/22/2023

84. Divanoglou N, Komninou D, Stea EA, et al. Association of vitamin D receptor gene polymorphisms with serum vitamin D levels in a Greek rural population (Velestino study). *Lifestyle Genom*. 2021;14(3):81–90

85. Redenšek S, Kristanc T, Blagus T, Trošt M, Dolžan V. Genetic variability of the vitamin D Receptor affects susceptibility to parkinson's disease and dopaminergic treatment adverse events. *Front Aging Neurosci*. 2022;14:853277:1–16

86. www.ods.od.nih.gov/factsheets/VitaminD-HealthProfessional, accessed 1/22/2023

87. Papadimitriou DT. The big vitamin D mistake. *J Prev Med Public Health*. 2017;50(4):278–281

88. Veugelers PJ, Ekwaru JP. A statistical error in the estimation of the recommended dietary allowance for vitamin D. *Nutrients*. 2014;6(10):4472–4475

89. Heaney R, Garland C, Baggerly C, et al. Letter to Veugelers PJ and Ekwaru JP: a statistical error in the estimation of the recommended dietary allowance for vitamin D. *Nutrients*. 2014, 6, 4472–4475

90. Shieh A, Chun RF, Ma C, et al. Effects of high-dose vitamin D2 versus D3 on total and free 25-hydroxyvitamin D and markers of calcium balance. *J Clin Endocrinol Metab*. 2016;101(8):3070–8

91. Weber P. Vitamin K and bone health. *Nutrition*. 2001;17(10):880–7

92. Bhalerao S, Clandinin TR. Cell biology: vitamin K2 takes charge. *Science*. 2012;336(6086):1241–2

93. Razzaque MS. Magnesium: are we consuming enough? *Nutrients*. 2018;10(12):1863:1–8

94. Cox IM, Campbell MJ, Dowson D. Red blood cell magnesium and chronic fatigue syndrome. *Lancet*.1991;337(8744):757–760

95. Lindberg JS, Zobitz MM, Poindexter JR, et al. Magnesium bioavailability from magnesium citrate and magnesium oxide. *Journal of the American College of Nutrition*. 1990;9(1):48–55

96. Uysal N, Kizildag S, Yuce Z, et al. Timeline (bioavailability) of magnesium compounds in hours: which magnesium compound works best? *Biological Trace Element Research*. 2019;187(1):128–36

97. Abraham GE, Flechas JD. Management of fibromyalgia: rationale for the use of magnesium and malic acid. *Journal of Nutritional Medicine*. 1992;3(1):49–59

98. Shen Y, Dai L, Tian H, et al. Treatment of magnesium-L-threonate elevates the magnesium level in the cerebrospinal fluid and attenuates motor deficits and dopamine neuron loss in a mouse model of Parkinson's disease. *Neuropsychiatric Disease and Treatment*. 2019;15:3143

99. Mathew AA, Panonnummal R. A mini review on the various facets affecting brain delivery of magnesium and its role in neurological disorders. *Biological Trace Element Research*. 2022; Dec:1–6

100. Benjamin J, Agam G, Levine J, et al. Inositol treatment in psychiatry. *Psychopharmacology bulletin*. 1995;31(1):167–175

101. Benjamin J, Levine J, Fux M, et al. Double-blind, placebo-controlled, crossover trial of inositol treatment for panic disorder. *American Journal of Psychiatry*. 1995;152(7):1084–6

102. Levine J. Controlled trials of inositol in psychiatry. *European Neuropsychopharmacology*. 1997;7(2):147–55

103. Palatnik A, Frolov K, Fux M, et al. Double-blind, controlled, crossover trial of inositol versus fluvoxamine for the treatment of panic disorder. *Journal of Clinical Psychopharmacology*. 2001;21(3):335–9

104. Williams JL, Everett JM, D'Cunha NM, et al. The effects of green tea amino acid L-theanine consumption on the ability to manage stress and anxiety levels: a systematic review. *Plant Foods for Human Nutrition*. 2020;75(1):12–23

105. Lydiard RB. The role of GABA in anxiety disorders. *Journal of Clinical Psychiatry*. 2003;64:21–7

106. Boonstra E, De Kleijn R, Colzato LS, et al. Neurotransmitters as food supplements: the effects of GABA on brain and behavior. *Frontiers in Psychology*. 2015;6:1520:(1–6)

107. Blessing EM, Steenkamp MM, Manzanares J et al. Cannabidiol as a potential treatment for anxiety disorders. *Neurotherapeutics*. 2015;12(4):825–36

108. Shannon S, Lewis N, Lee H, et al. Cannabidiol in anxiety and sleep: a large case series. *Permanente Journal*. 2019;23:108–111

109. García-Gutiérrez MS, Navarrete F, Gasparyan A, et al. Cannabidiol: a potential new alternative for the treatment of anxiety, depression, and psychotic disorders. *Biomolecules*. 2020;10(11):1575:1–34

110. Culbert T. Perspectives on technology-assisted relaxation approaches to support mind-body skills practice in children and teens: clinical experience and commentary. *Children* (Basel). 2017;4(4):20:1–15

111. Anick DJ. High sensitivity ^{1}H-NMR spectroscopy of homeopathic remedies made in water. *BMC Complement Altern Med*. 2004;4:15:1–24

112. Davidson JR, Crawford C, Ives JA, et al. Homeopathic treatments in psychiatry: a systematic review of randomized placebo-controlled studies. *Journal of Clinical Psychiatry*. 2011;72(6):8318

113. Bonne O, Shemer Y, Gorali Y, et al. A randomized, double-blind, placebo-controlled study of classical homeopathy in generalized anxiety disorder. *Journal of Clinical Psychiatry*. 2003;64(3):282–7

114. Pilkington K, Kirkwood G, Rampes H, et al. Homeopathy for anxiety and anxiety disorders: a systematic review of the research. *Homeopathy*. 2006;95(03):151–62

115. Murphy TK, Lewin AB, Storch EA, et al. Practice parameter for the assessment and treatment of children and adolescents with tic disorders. *Journal of the American Academy of Child & Adolescent Psychiatry*. 2013;52(12):1341–59

116. Jankovic J. Phenomenology and classification of tics. *Neurologic Clinics*. 1997;15(2):267–75

117. Ganos C. Tics and Tourette's: update on pathophysiology and tic control. *Current Opinion in Neurology*. 2016;29(4):513–8

118. Giedd JN, Rapoport JL, Kruesi MJ, et al. Sydenham's chorea: magnetic resonance imaging of the basal ganglia. *Neurology*. 1995;45(12):2199

119. Traill Z, Pike M, Byrne J. Sydenham's chorea: a case showing reversible striatal abnormalities on CT and MRI. *Dev Med Child Neurol*. 1995;37(3):270

120. Aron AM. Sydenham's chorea: positron emission tomographic (PET) scan studies. *J Child Neurol*. 2005;20(10):832

121. Goldman S, Amrom D, Szliwowski HB, et al. Reversible striatal hypermetabolism in a case of Sydenham's chorea. *Mov Disord*. 1993;8(3):355

122. Giedd JN, Rapoport JL, Garvey MA, et al. MRI assessment of children with obsessive-compulsive disorder or tics associated with streptococcal infection. *American Journal of Psychiatry*. 2000;157(2):281–283

123. Xu M, Kobets A, Du JC, et al. Targeted ablation of cholinergic interneurons in the dorsolateral striatum produces behavioral manifestations of Tourette syndrome. *Proc Natl Acad Sci U S A*. 2015;112(3):893–8

124. Frick LR, Rapanelli M, Jindachomthong K, et al. Differential binding of antibodies in PANDAS patients to cholinergic interneurons in the striatum. B*rain, behavior, and immunity*. 2018;69:304–311

125. Robertson MM. The Gilles de la Tourette syndrome: the current status. *Br J Psychiatry*. 1989;154:147–69

126. Coffey BJ, Park KS. Behavioral and emotional aspects of Tourette syndrome. *Neurol Clin*. 1997;15(2):277–89

127. Ganos C, Münchau A, Bhatia KP. The semiology of tics, Tourette's, and their associations. *Mov Disord Clin Pract*. 2014;1(3):145–153

128. Maia DP, Teixeira AL, Cunningham MC, et al. Obsessive-compulsive behavior, hyperactivity, and attention deficit disorder in Sydenham chorea. *Neurology*. 2005;64(10):1799

129. Swedo SE, Leonard HL, Casey BJ, et al. Sydenham's chorea: physical and psychological symptoms of St. Vitus dance. *Pediatrics*. 1993;91(4):706–713

130. Weisman H, Qureshi IA, Leckman JF, et al. Systematic review: pharmacological treatment of tic disorders: efficacy of antipsychotic and alpha-2 adrenergic agonist agents. *Neurosci Biobehav Rev*. 2013;37(6):1162–71

131. Pringsheim T, Holler-Managan Y, Okun MS, et al. Comprehensive systematic review summary: treatment of tics in people with Tourette syndrome and chronic tic disorders. *Neurology*. 2019;92(19):907–915

132. Piacentini J, Woods DW, Scahill L, et al. Behavior therapy for children with Tourette disorder: a randomized controlled trial. *JAMA*. 2010;303(19):1929–37

133. Li HH, Wang B, Shan L, et al. Serum levels of 25-hydroxyvitamin D in children with tic disorders. *Chinese Journal of Contemporary Pediatrics*. 2017;19(11):1165–8

134. Li HH, Xu ZD, Wang B, Feng JY, Dong HY, Jia FY. Clinical improvement following vitamin D3 supplementation in children with chronic tic disorders. *Neuropsychiatr Dis Treat*. 2019;15:2443–2450

135. Rizzo R, Prato A, Scerbo M, et al. Use of nutritional supplements based on L-theanine and vitamin B6 in children with Tourette syndrome, with anxiety disorders: a pilot study. *Nutrients*. 2022;14(4):852

136. Lazarus JE, Klein SK. Nonpharmacological treatment of tics in Tourette syndrome adding videotape training to self-hypnosis. *J Dev Behav Pediatr*. 2010;31(6):498–504

137. Papakostas GI, Cassiello CF, Iovieno N. Folates and S-adenosylmethionine for major depressive disorder. *Can J Psychiatry*. 2012;57(7):406–13

138. Tiemeier H, van Tuijl HR, Hofman A, et al. Vitamin B12, folate, and homocysteine in depression: the Rotterdam study. *Am J Psychiatry*. 2002;159(12):2099–2101

139. Bjelland I, Tell GS, Vollset SE, et al. Folate, vitamin B12, homocysteine, and the MTHFR 677C->T polymorphism in anxiety and depression: the Hordaland Homocysteine Study. *Arch Gen Psychiatry*. 2003;60(6):618–626

140. Lewis SJ, Lawlor DA, Davey Smith G, et al. The thermolabile variant of MTHFR is associated with depression in the British Women's Heart and Health Study and a meta-analysis. *Mol Psychiatry*. 2006;11(4):352–360

141. Gilbody S, Lewis S, Lightfoot T. Methylenetetrahydrofolate reductase (MTHFR) genetic polymorphisms and psychiatric disorders: a HuGE review. *Am J Epidemiol*. 2007;165(1):1–13

142. Almeida OP, McCaul K, Hankey GJ, et al. Homocysteine and depression in later life. *Arch Gen Psychiatry*. 2008;65(11):1286–1294

143. López-León S, Janssens AC, González-Zuloeta Ladd AM, et al. Meta-analyses of genetic studies on major depressive disorder. *Mol Psychiatry*. 2008;13(8):772–785

144. Bottiglieri T, Laundry M, Crellin R, et al. Homocysteine, folate, methylation, and monoamine metabolism in depression. *J Neurol Neurosurg Psychiatry*. 2000;69:228–232

145. Crellin R, Bottiglieri T, Reynolds EH. Folates and psychiatric disorders: clinical potential. *Drugs*. 1993;45(5):623–636

146. Passeri M, Cucinotta D, Abate G, et al. Oral 5'-methyltetrahydrofolic acid in senile organic mental disorders with depression: results of a double-blind multicenter study. *Aging* (Milano). 1993;5(1):63–71

147. Resler G, Lavie R, Campos J, et al. Effect of folic acid combined with fluoxetine in patients with major depression on plasma homocysteine and vitamin B12, and serotonin levels in lymphocytes. *Neuroimmunomodulation*. 2008;15(3):145–152

148. Coppen A, Bailey J. Enhancement of the antidepressant action of fluoxetine by folic acid: a randomised, placebo-controlled trial. *J Affect Disord*. 2000;60(2):121–130

149. Godfrey PSA, Toone BK, Carney MWP, et al. Enhancement of recovery from psychiatric illness by methylfolate. *Lancet*. 1990;336(8712):392–395

150. Stahl SM. L-methylfolate: a vitamin for your monoamines. *J Clin Psychiatry*. 2008;69(9):1352–3

151. Menezo Y, Elder K, Clement A, et al. Folic acid, folinic acid, 5 methyl tetrahydrofolate supplementation for mutations that affect epigenesis through the folate and one-carbon cycles. *Biomolecules*. 2022;12(2):197:1–14

152. Lu SC. S-adenosylmethionine. *International Journal of Biochemistry & Cell Biology*. 2000;32(4):391–5

153. Lieber CS, Packer L. S-adenosylmethionine: molecular, biological, and clinical aspects: an introduction. *American Journal of Clinical Nutrition*. 2002;76(5):1148S–50S

154. Kagan BL, Sultzer DL, Rosenlicht N, et al. Oral S-adenosylmethionine in depression: a randomized, double-blind, placebo-controlled trial. *American Journal of Psychiatry*. 1990;147(5):591–595

155. Strous RD, Ritsner MS, Adler S, et al. Improvement of aggressive behavior and quality of life impairment following S-adenosyl-methionine (SAM-e) augmentation in schizophrenia. *European Neuropsychopharmacology*. 2009;19(1):14–22

156. Shechter A, Quispe KA, Mizhquiri Barbecho JS, et al. Interventions to reduce short-wavelength ("blue") light exposure at night and their effects on sleep: a systematic review and meta-analysis. *Sleep Advances*. 2020;1(1):1–13

157. Burgess HJ, Molina TA. Home lighting before usual bedtime impacts circadian timing: a field study. *Photochem Photobiol*. 2014;90(3):723–6

158. Lewandowski AS, Ward TM, Palermo TM. Sleep problems in children and adolescents with common medical conditions. *Pediatr Clin North Am*. 2011;58(3):699–713

159. Esposito S, Laino D, D'Alonzo R, et al. Pediatric sleep disturbances and treatment with melatonin. *Journal of Translational Medicine*. 2019;17(1):1–8

160. Sánchez-Barceló EJ, Mediavilla MD, Reiter RJ. Clinical uses of melatonin in pediatrics. *International Journal of Pediatrics*. 2011;2011:1–12

161. Smits MG, Nagtegaal EE, van der Heijden J, et al. Melatonin for chronic sleep onset insomnia in children: a randomized placebo-controlled trial. *J Child Neurol*. 2001;16(2):86–92

162. Rao TP, Ozeki M, Juneja LR. In search of a safe natural sleep aid. *Journal of the American College of Nutrition*. 2015;34(5):436–47

163. Lyon MR, Kapoor MP, Juneja LR. The effects of L-theanine (Suntheanine) on objective sleep quality in boys with attention deficit hyperactivity disorder (ADHD): a randomized, double-blind, placebo--controlled clinical trial. *Alternative Medicine Review*. 2011;16(4):348–354

164. Byun JI, Shin YY, Chung SE, et al. Safety and efficacy of gamma-aminobutyric acid from fermented rice germ in patients with insomnia symptoms: a randomized, double-blind trial. *Journal of Clinical Neurology*. 2018;14(3):291–5

165. A. Sezen H, Kandemir H, Savik E, et al. Increased oxidative stress in children with attention deficit hyperactivity disorder. *Redox Report*. 2016;21(6):248–53

166. Verlaet AA, Breynaert A, Ceulemans B, et al. Oxidative stress and immune aberrancies in attention-deficit/hyperactivity disorder (ADHD): a case-control comparison. *European Child & Adolescent Psychiatry*. 2019;28:719–29

167. Alvarez-Arellano L, González-García N, Salazar-García M, et al. Antioxidants as a potential target against inflammation and oxidative stress in attention-deficit/hyperactivity disorder. *Antioxidants*. 2020;9(2):176

168. Darzi M, Abbasi K, Ghiasvand R, et al. The association between dietary polyphenol intake and attention-deficit hyperactivity disorder: a case-control study. *BMC Pediatrics*. 2022;22(1):700

169. Dvořáková M, Sivoňová M, Trebatická J, et al. The effect of polyphenolic extract from pine bark, Pycnogenol on the level of glutathione in children suffering from attention deficit hyperactivity disorder (ADHD). *Redox Report*. 2006;11(4):163–72

170. Chovanová Z, Muchová J, Sivoňová M, et al. Effect of polyphenolic extract, Pycnogenol, on the level of 8-oxoguanine in children suffering from attention deficit/hyperactivity disorder. *Free Radical Research*. 2006;40(9):1003–10

171. Dvořáková M, Ježová D, Blažíček P, et al. Urinary catecholamines in children with attention deficit hyperactivity disorder (ADHD): modulation by a polyphenolic extract from pine bark (Pycnogenol). *Nutritional Neuroscience*. 2007;10(3–4):151–7

172. Frankovich J, Thienemann M, Pearlstein J, et al. Multidisciplinary clinic dedicated to treating youth with pediatric acute-onset neuropsychiatric syndrome: presenting characteristics of the first 47 consecutive patients. *J Child Adolesc Psychopharmacol*. 2015;25(1):38–47

REDUCE: ENVIRONMENTAL TOXINS AND TOXICANTS

It is, of course, one of the miracles of science that the germs that used to be in our food have been replaced by poisons.
~ **WENDELL BERRY**

KEY POINTS

▸ Reduction of environmental toxins and toxicants (including inflammatory foods) is an important part of restoring proper immune system function

▸ Patients spending time in a toxic environment are not likely to fully recover

▸ Mold remediation is a complicated process and best handled by a professional

In the IDENTIFY chapters, we identified what was in the hose (the "overload"), what was in the flowerpot (the "overwhelm"), and what was in the puddle (the "overflow"). Once we have IDENTIFIED these three vital pieces of information, we proceed to methodically REDUCE anything we have IDENTIFIED that is adversely affecting our patients' health.

The chapters in the textbook on REDUCING, OPTIMIZING, SUPPORTING, and PERSONALIZING reflect the approach we have found to be consistently effective in the management of these challenging patients.

A vital part of the REDUCE pillar in the Fully Functional process involves reducing what is in the hose. And that usually starts with food.

REDUCING INFLAMMATORY FOODS

As long as the patient has no food restrictive behaviors, reduction of inflammatory foods can be prescribed. If there is any history of food restriction, dietary modification should be delayed until this symptom is completely absent, the patient is of optimal weight, and the patient has had significant reduction in OCD and anxiety.

We place foods into a conceptual list, with the most inflammatory foods at the top. That way, if parents are very stressed due to their child's illness, we can tell them to eliminate foods slowly, one group at a time, with the most inflammatory being removed first. Details concerning the science behind why these foods contribute to human disease are outlined in Chapter 5.

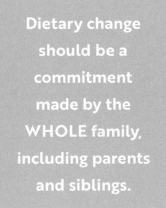

Dietary change should be a commitment made by the WHOLE family, including parents and siblings.

Foods that are highly processed, have additives, or foods that may contain pesticide residues (often seen with GMOs) cause inflammation, oxidative stress, or other issues. We tell our patients to be cautious with anything in a box, bag, or can. Foods should be organic, and meats should be free-range and pasture raised. Fish should be small and wild-caught to avoid potential heavy metal and chemical contamination.

The next food on the inflammatory list is food with high sugar content. Highly processed sugars such as high-fructose corn syrup or white sugar are particularly inflammatory. Sugar addiction is difficult to overcome. A good tactic is to make "this not that" food choices initially. Even if foods with higher than optimal sugar content remain in the diet, switching from processed to more natural sugars like maple syrup or honey can be a helpful first step.

This is a good place to note that dietary change should be a commitment made by the WHOLE family, including parents and siblings. It is impossible (and rather unfair) to explain to a defiant, ill child why they have to avoid foods if Mom, Dad, and siblings can still eat them in the home. Having the family embrace healthy dietary changes is one way that, in the midst of a mighty struggle, the whole family can become healthier.

Next on the list is gluten. We have outlined the issues with gluten in Chapter 5. Patients should be educated on hidden sources of gluten, including soy sauce, many barbecue sauces, and spice mixtures and coatings used on meat or french fries. In addition, other grains like oats are not guaranteed to be gluten free unless specifically labeled. Licorice and other chewy candies usually contain wheat. Just because foods are labeled gluten free does not mean they are healthy. Many of the most popular gluten free snacks have a very high sugar content and may contain other preservatives and additives.

Dairy would be next on the list of inflammatory foods for some patients. This includes milk products, ice cream, cheese, and yogurt. Many dairy-free nut milks, yogurts, and ice creams are available, but high sugar content can be an issue.

Although some patients with autoimmune conditions such as rheumatoid arthritis find relief by eliminating all grains (gluten, rice, corn, oats), we do not recommend eliminating these foods for most children as significant weight loss can occur. Non-gluten grains may be the only source of fiber in children who do not have adequate vegetable intake.

If patients have IgE food reactions noted on lab testing, these foods should be avoided completely, even if no prior anaphylaxis has been noted. Repeat testing can be done after 6–12 months to see if immunity has shifted from Th2 dominance and gut healing has improved tolerance. If IgG food reactions are noted, these foods are often rotated, but elimination of all IgG foods is not usually necessary.

Semantically, it is better in both pediatric and adult patients to refer to this as an "anti-inflammatory diet" rather than an "elimination diet."

REDUCING STRESS INPUTS

As noted in Chapter 5, stress is a leading cause of preventable illness. Stress has the capacity to magnify symptoms or worsen other illnesses. Stress reduction is very helpful in treating a variety of diseases and is a vital starting point for maintaining optimal health.

Reducing stress in patients with PANS and PANDAS initially begins with having parents address their own stress. In Appendix D, we will discuss caring for the caregiver. This appendix contains valuable information to help reduce parental stress, which will help modulate the stress of the sick child.

Establishing an IEP (see Appendix D) can help reduce stressful situations at school. Explaining PANS and PANDAS to family members can help reduce conflicts for the child as well.

For the remainder of the REDUCE chapters as well as the OPTIMIZE and SUPPORT chapters, we will discuss prescription medications, supplements, and herbal remedies. You will find the rationale, literature support, and our clinical experience in the descriptions of each of these therapies. In Appendix B, you will find common dosages for the agents we use by age or weight.

> Stress has the capacity to magnify symptoms or worsen other illnesses.

REDUCE: TOXINS IN PERSONAL CARE PRODUCTS

Cosmetic products such as toothpaste, shampoo, and soaps often have chemicals that have not been tested in animals or humans. In fact, the FDA requires that chemicals in personal care products be "safe for human use" but does not require or undertake any specific testing prior to these products being brought to market.[1] Harmful chemicals found in some cosmetics may include heavy metals, formaldehyde, parabens (which are known endocrine disruptors), and some chemicals that are known carcinogens.

> Failure to address mold properly and completely in the home or the body can result in continued flares of illness for years to come.

Some skin creams actually contain steroids and hormones like progesterone. The Environmental Working Group (EWG) provides helpful guidance[2] on avoiding these chemicals.

REDUCE: ENVIRONMENTAL TOXINS IN WATER AND PARTICULATES IN THE AIR

Various devices are available for water filtration. We recommend reverse osmosis as the best option for most homes. Using bottled water is not as beneficial since some bottled water comes from municipal sources and contamination with plastics is possible. Testing water for bacterial contaminants and heavy metals is recommended, especially for well water. SimpleLab (www.gosimplelab.com) provides an array of testing for tap water in the home. Filtering water tends to remove beneficial minerals along with toxins, so minerals should be added to water or taken in supplement form.

High-quality HEPA air filtration devices to improve indoor air quality are available from several companies including IQAir (www.iqair.com/us), Molekule (www.molekule.com), Austin Air (www.austinair.com), and Honeywell (www.honeywellstore.com/store/category/air-purifiers.htm).

REDUCE: HUMIDITY, WATER DAMAGE, MOLD, AND MYCOTOXINS

In Chapter 5, we described the significant health consequences of mold, mycotoxins, and *Actinomyces* exposures. We also outlined the utility of various testing options for homes and explained what type of inspection should be conducted by a qualified indoor environmental professional (IEP). An online database that may be useful to help patients locate an IEP is www.iseai.org/find-a-professional. It is always best to get personal referrals from satisfied customers.

All home modification work should be done by licensed, insured contractors. Remediation, if needed, should be left to a qualified IEP and contractors familiar with safe mold remediation. We have had patients become much sicker by using inexperienced general contractors or family members in an attempt to save money.

The long-term health risks of continued mold/mycotoxin exposure for the whole family are not worth the money saved in the short term. It is very important to understand, as previously noted, that mycotoxins and other debris from mold exposures are a major cause of immune dysregulation. Failure to address mold properly and completely in the home or the body can result in continued flares of illness for years to come. Remediating a water-damaged home is often the single most important thing patients can do to start to heal from complex chronic illness.

MOLD REMEDIATION ACTION STEPS
Water outside the home
The slope of the ground should be graded or sloped away from the home. If low spots are noted near the foundation, foundation drains may need to be installed with sump pumps in the basement or crawl space. Sump pumps take water away from these areas. The best sump pumps have a battery backup in case of power failure and many now come with notification systems such as audible alarms in case of pump failure or high water levels.

Some pumps also contain transmitters which will provide text or email alerts in the case of power failure. Power outages are the most common cause of sump pump failure and basement flooding. All downspouts should remove water at least six feet from the outer walls of the home. Cleanouts on downspouts to remove leaves will help prevent blockage and downspout failure. Home generators can keep furnaces, sump pumps, dehumidifiers, and air filters running in the event of an electrical power failure.

Water intrusion
If water continues to enter a home (from basement walls, the roof or chimney, or from windows), microbial growth and mycotoxin production will continue. These should be the first thing to be fixed to address water intrusion problems. A house cannot be made safe with active water intrusion. If roof repair is required, it is very important to deal with dead valleys and to apply an ice and water shield and high-quality composite shingles (with a warranty). Wooden shingles are not recommended.

High humidity
Dehumidifiers should be installed to keep the humidity below 50% year-round. Whole-home dehumidifiers exist but may be expensive. Portable dehumidifiers are widely available. Some models have a pump feature and hose coupling to allow drainage to a sump pit or some other area outside the home. Models with a bucket are not as convenient since they typi-

> **Whole-home humidifiers and even small vaporizers can lead to issues with microbial growth and should not be used.**

cally need to be emptied every 3–4 hours in a humid home. Whole-home humidifiers and even small vaporizers can lead to issues with microbial growth and should not be used.

Bathroom fans
All bathroom fans should drain to the outside of the home. Unfortunately, these fans are often vented to the attic and humidity from these fans over time can lead to microbial growth.

Portable air conditioners

Drain lines and filters in portable window-mounted air conditioners can harbor microbial growth and may need to be cleaned or repaired.

Contaminated building materials

Any building materials that are noted to have possible or confirmed microbial growth need to be removed under "encapsulated conditions." A qualified IEP understands how to tape and cordon off an area so that contaminated materials can be wrapped and removed without spreading mold/mycotoxin contamination all over the rest of the home.

If there is an acute water intrusion event like a bathtub leak or a sump failure, immediate removal of wet building materials and aggressive drying with industrial fans may prevent microbial growth if drying starts within twenty-four hours. Wet drywall behind wood trim can be hard to dry without removing the trim.

In general, all drywall that becomes wet will need removal. Drying with fans is fine for wood and composite, which usually does not have to be removed if completely dry. The IEP can take serial measurements of building materials with a two-prong professional hygrometer to define the extent of wet drywall or provide a benchmark for when it is safe to stop drying and rebuild the living space. Bleach should never be poured on suspected areas of mold since it may result in a sudden release of mycotoxins.

> **Bleach should never be poured on suspected areas of mold since it may result in a sudden release of mycotoxins.**

Duct cleaning

Any home with detectable mold, mycotoxins, actinomyces, or water intrusion should have a professional duct cleaning. Fogging the system with safe anti-mold/mycotoxin cleaning products after duct cleaning is recommended. High MERV rated filters should be used in all air handlers. MERV 13–16 products have the highest filtration efficiency. Patients should check with an HVAC professional before installing a new filter since some systems cannot function with high MERV filters due to airflow restriction.

Fogging

Some companies use commercial foggers to rid the air of mold and mycotoxins. Following this fogging, surfaces are wiped down and vacuumed. Various products are used. While any remediation activity occurs, especially fogging, the family should not be in the house and should stay away for several hours after the work is completed. Duct cleaning and fogging are always important. Even if mold was only found on one level, the air register intakes can return contaminated air to the furnace, from which it can be spread throughout the rest of the home.

Air filtration

As noted above, high-quality portable air filtration devices are made by IQAir (www.iqair.com/us), Air Doctor (www.airdoctorpro.com), and Austin Air (www.austinair.com). The IEP will have access to commercial grade air scrubbers during remediation.

Belongings

This is one of the most common questions we get but also one of the most difficult to answer. Nonporous surfaces (plastic or metal items and most finished furniture) can be wiped with nontoxic cleaners made for this purpose (the IEP can guide the patient) or may be wiped down after fogging by the IEP. Discarding everything is never the answer. What can be cleaned, what may need to be discarded, and what may be stored in a sealed plastic bin to deal with at a later time is a complex triage situation with several variables. A qualified IEP is the best source for guidance here.

Post-remediation testing

Post-remediation testing is recommended to follow up on levels of mycotoxins, actinomyces, or high spore counts. Periodic physical inspections are also advisable.

Although these measures are the current best practices as recognized by the IEP group at ISEA (the International Society of Environmentally Acquired Illness), there are times when the patient's health may not improve, even after extensive remediation. This may even occur after test results normalize.

> Post-remediation testing is recommended to follow up on levels of mycotoxins, actinomyces, or high spore counts. Periodic physical inspections are also advisable.

We are not always sure why this occurs, but it could be due to undiscovered microbial growth (behind a sealed wall for example) or other unknown factors. How the patient and their family feel in their home is often the best determinate of remediation success.

CHAPTER 11 REFERENCES

1. www.fda.gov/cosmetics/cosmetics-science-research/product-testing-cosmetics, accessed 4/6/2023
2. www.ewg.org/skindeep, accessed 4/6/2023

CHAPTER 12

REDUCE: INFLAMMATION, OXIDATIVE STRESS, AND TOXINS IN THE BODY

Medicine is not only a science; it is also an art. It does not consist of compounding pills and plasters; it deals with the very processes of life, which must be understood before they may be guided.
~ **PARACELSUS**

KEY POINTS

▸ Reducing inflammation, oxidative stress, and toxins/toxicants is a vital step in healing
▸ Reducing inflammation starts with an anti-inflammatory diet
▸ Various medications and supplements can be used to reduce inflammation
▸ Reduction of oxidative stress is usually accomplished with antioxidants from foods or supplements

INFLAMMATION

Inflammation at the appropriate time in the appropriate amount is a good thing. The inflammatory response is initiated by the immune system to respond to infections or damage to tissues. Prolonged (chronic) inflammation over time, however, is damaging to host tissues.

Chronic inflammation has been identified as a causative factor and as a predictor of worse outcomes in many conditions, such as cardiovascular disease, Alzheimer's disease, cancer, bowel diseases, arthritis, cirrhosis, metabolic syndrome, and some pulmonary diseases.[1–4] The cascade of chronic infection begins when blood cells (like monocytes) migrate into tissues, become activated, release inflammatory mediators, and interact with those tissues.[1] In cases of chronic mental or physical illness (including chronic, persistent infections), inflammation can become chronic, which damages normal tissues.[1,3,5] This damage produces damage-associated molecular patterns (DAMPs), which cause further immune activation. Avoiding further immune activation and re-regulating the immune system is vital in PANS and PANDAS.

The role of chronic inflammation in the etiology of cardiovascular disease has become increasingly evident in the last twenty years. Measurement of C-reactive protein (CRP) is commonly used as a marker of increased cardiac risk.[6,7]

There is an ever-increasing body of knowledge demonstrating the fact that inflammation plays a pivotal role in the etiology of various neuropsychiatric disorders, including depression, anxiety, and OCD.[3,5,8–11]

In 2017, Atwells et al. conducted a study using PET scans in patients with OCD and controls.[8] The authors found that the scans indicated that inflammation in the cortico-striato-thalamo-cortical circuit in patients with OCD was significantly higher than in controls. This study confirmed that neuroinflammation secondary to microglial activation is involved in the pathology of OCD. The study also demonstrated that microglial activation in OCD extends *well beyond childhood*, which provides an opportunity for a unique therapeutic target regardless of age.

When microglia are activated, they exhibit what are known as M1 responses, which lead to the release of pro-inflammatory cytokines and reactive oxygen species.[8] Several drugs, including azithromycin and minocycline, have been shown to be able to shift activated microglia from M1 to M2 responses. M2 responses are involved in clearing cellular debris and promoting tissue

> **Inflammation plays a pivotal role in the etiology of various neuropsychiatric disorders, including depression, anxiety, and OCD.**

repair.[12] A study which added minocycline to fluvoxamine in patients with OCD showed significant improvement in symptoms compared to fluvoxamine alone.[13]

An excellent article by Peirce and Alviña describes the central role of neuroinflammation, microglial activation, hypothalamic-pituitary-adrenal (HPA) axis dysfunction, increased intestinal permeability, and the microbiome in the etiology of depression and anxiety.[11] This article should be required reading for all physicians regardless of specialty. A better understanding of the role of neuroinflammation and its link to the intestinal microbiome can transform the diagnosis and treatment of mental illness today. This is the realm in which we practice medicine.

REDUCING INFLAMMATION

The anti-inflammatory diet

The first strategy to combat inflammation involves the adoption of an anti-inflammatory diet (see Chapter 11). This involves eliminating processed foods, refined sugars, gluten, and dairy products. This should never be done in patients with restricted eating behaviors, although more healthy versions of whatever the patients are currently ingesting can be encouraged.

Reducing stress

Stress has been linked to HPA axis dysfunction, which results in immune activation and inflammation. Stress reduction techniques are covered in Chapter 10.

NSAIDS

We are all familiar with the anti-inflammatory uses of various NSAIDS in clinical practice. One clinical trial demonstrated a shortened onset of action of SSRIs in depressed patients when augmented with aspirin.[14] Benefits have also been noted with celecoxib.[15]

A 2017 study in patients with PANS published in the *Journal of Child and Adolescent Psychopharmacology* showed that ibuprofen given within the first thirty days of a flare significantly shortened the flare.[16]

We use ibuprofen in our patients during flares. Some physicians use naproxen sodium, but we have not found this as helpful as ibuprofen in our practice. There are no published studies to show its equivalence or superiority to ibuprofen.

Steroids

We rarely use steroids in the management of PANS and PANDAS as they can only be used short term and, in at least half of our patients, steroids worsen anxiety, irritability, and insomnia.

> Omega 3 fats are neuroprotective and decrease neuroinflammation through interactions with astrocytes and microglia.

Curcumin

Curcumin is a great anti-inflammatory. It is a natural substance that comes from turmeric extracted from the *Curcuma longa* plant. Curcumin exerts its anti-inflammatory effects by various mechanisms. Curcumin reduces neuroinflammation by lowering inflammatory mediators (such as TNF-α, IL-1β, nitric oxide and NFκB gene expression), affecting mitochondrial dynamics, and through epigenetic changes.[17]

In our practice, response to curcumin supplements has been variable. It is available in liquid, capsule, and chewable forms. Curcumin has poor bioavailability unless combined with phospholipids or black pepper extract (piperine).

Omega 3 fats

Omega 3 fats are a type of polyunsaturated fatty acid. Two of the main components are eicosapentaenoic acid (EPA) and docosahexae-noic acid (DHA). Omega 3 fats have strong anti--inflammatory and immune-modulating effects.[18,19] Omega 3 fats are neuroprotective and decrease neuroinflammation through interactions with astrocytes and microglia.[20] No specific studies have been done with omega fats and PANS or PANDAS.

In supplement form, omega 3 fats are usually extracted from fish. Algae sources are used for patients who do not eat fish, although omega content is generally lower per capsule. Other

> **Serrapeptase is an excellent anti-inflammatory without the side effects of NSAIDs.**

foods high in omega 3 fats include flaxseed, chia seeds, and walnuts.

We use omega 3 fats as well as SPMs (specialized pro-resolving mediators) in our patients. SPMs are biosynthesized in the body in response to acute inflammatory responses. They alter expression of pro-inflammatory genes, modulate macrophage function, inhibit microglial activation, and promote resolution of neuroinflammation.[21] SPMs are manufactured in the body through a process called "lipid mediator class switching," which switches pro-inflammatory cytokine synthesis to SPM synthesis.[22]

Serrapeptase

As noted in the discussion of biofilms in Chapter 14, serrapeptase is an excellent anti-inflammatory without the side effects of NSAIDs.

It does not inhibit the production of SPMs, as do some NSAIDS.

Probiotics

Probiotics have immune-modulating properties and can downregulate inflammation.[23] We use probiotics in all of our patients.

Photobiomodulation (red-light therapy)

Photobiomodulation (PBM), specifically red-light therapy, has been shown to reduce inflammation.[24] The science behind red-light therapy is explored in Chapter 17.

OXIDATIVE STRESS

Our body generates reactive oxygen species (ROS) like hydrogen peroxide, superoxide, and peroxynitrite through normal metabolic reactions. These compounds are also known as free radicals. High levels of oxidants can be a result of exposure to environmental pollutants or from cooking fats like vegetable oils at high heats. Charred foods and processed foods are high in oxidants as well.

We have a natural enzymatic system of antioxidants. Foods like fruits and vegetables contain antioxidants. If free radicals exceed the body's capacity to reduce them, oxidative stress occurs. Oxidative stress can lead to inflammation, direct mitochondrial damage, and damage to DNA. It is implicated in cardiovascular disease, cancer, neurodegenerative diseases, and metabolic syndrome.[4,25,26]

Oxidative stress has been implicated in the pathogenesis of several psychiatric disorders (schizophrenia and bipolar disorder); glutathione or its precursors (N-acetylcysteine or NAC) are viable agents to help address oxidative stress[27,28,29] in these conditions. For more information on the role of glutathione and NAC in biotransformation (detoxification), see Chapter 17.

We REDUCE oxidative stress clinically by avoiding processed foods and taking antioxidants like vitamin C, alpha-lipoic acid, vitamin E, vitamin A, and Coenzyme Q10. We also use glutathione, which is considered the body's master antioxidant. Glutathione actually recycles other antioxidants so that they can return to duty in the body. For more information about testing antioxidant levels and glutathione, see Chapter 7.

TOXINS

We are exposed to many toxins in our daily lives. The total of these substances is sometimes referred to as the *exposome*. The exposome may be impacted by toxic foods, mycotoxins from mold exposure, heavy metals, and harmful chemicals found in pesticides and in household cleaners and cosmetics.

We REDUCE these toxins in the body by OPTIMIZING detoxification, which is discussed in detail in Chapter 17.

CHAPTER 12 REFERENCES

1. Libby P. Inflammatory mechanisms: the molecular basis of inflammation and disease. *Nutrition Reviews*. 2007;65(suppl 3):S140–6

2. Holmes C, Cunningham C, Zotova E, et al. Systemic inflammation and disease progression in Alzheimer disease. *Neurology*. 2009;73(10):768–74

3. Halaris A. Inflammation, heart disease, and depression. *Current Psychiatry Reports*. 2013;15(10):1–9

4. Chatterjee S. Oxidative stress, inflammation, and disease. In *Oxidative Stress and Biomaterials*. London, UK. Academic Press. 2016:35–58

5. Gerentes M, Pelissolo A, Rajagopal K, et al. Obsessive-compulsive disorder: autoimmunity and neuroinflammation. *Curr Psychiatry Rep*. 2019;21(8):78:1–10

6. Lagrand WK, Visser CA, Hermens WT, et al. C-reactive protein as a cardiovascular risk factor: more than an epiphenomenon? *Circulation*. 1999;100(1):96–102

7. Ridker PM. High-sensitivity C-reactive protein and cardiovascular risk: rationale for screening and primary prevention. *American Journal of Cardiology*. 2003;92(4):17–22

8. Attwells S, Setiawan E, Wilson AA, et al. Inflammation in the neurocircuitry of obsessive-compulsive disorder. *JAMA Psychiatry*. 2017;74(8):833–40

9. Renna ME, O'Toole MS, Spaeth PE, et al. The association between anxiety, traumatic stress, and obsessive-compulsive disorders and chronic inflammation: a systematic review and meta-analysis. *Depression and Anxiety*. 2018;35(11):1081–94

10. Peirce JM, Alviña K. The role of inflammation and the gut microbiome in depression and anxiety. *Journal of Neuroscience Research*. 2019;97(10):1223–41

11. Amantea D, Bagetta G. Drug repurposing for immune modulation in acute ischemic stroke. *Curr Opin Pharmacol*. 2016;26:124–30

12. Esalatmanesh S, Abrishami Z, Zeinoddini A, Rahiminejad F, Sadeghi M, Najarzadegan MR, Shalbafan MR, Akhondzadeh S. Minocycline combination therapy with fluvoxamine in moderate-to-severe obsessive-compulsive disorder: a placebo-controlled, double-blind, randomized trial. *Psychiatry Clin Neurosci*. 2016;70(11):517–526

13. Turna J, Grosman Kaplan K, Anglin R, et al. The gut microbiome and inflammation in obsessive-compulsive disorder patients compared to age-and sex-matched controls: a pilot study. *Acta Psychiatrica Scandinavica*. 2020;142(4):337–47

14. Mendlewicz J, Kriwin P, Oswald P, et al. Shortened onset of action of antidepressants in major depression using acetylsalicylic acid augmentation: a pilot open-label study. *Int Clin Psychopharmacol*. 2006;21(4):227–31

15. Müller N, Schwarz MJ, Dehning S, et al. The cyclooxygenase-2 inhibitor celecoxib has therapeutic effects in major depression: results of a double-blind, randomized, placebo controlled, add-on pilot study to reboxetine. *Molecular Psychiatry*. 2006;(7):680–684

16. Brown KD, Farmer C, Freeman GM Jr, et al. Effect of early and prophylactic nonsteroidal anti-inflammatory drugs on flare duration in pediatric acute-onset neuropsychiatric syndrome: an observational study of patients followed by an academic community-based pediatric acute-onset neuropsychiatric syndrome clinic. *J Child Adolesc Psychopharmacol*. 2017;27(7):619–628

17. Hatami M, Abdolahi M, Soveyd N, et al. Molecular mechanisms of curcumin in neuroinflammatory disorders: a mini review of current evidence. *Endocrine, Metabolic & Immune Disorders-Drug Targets* (formerly *Current Drug Targets-Immune, Endocrine & Metabolic Disorders*). 2019;19(3):247–58

18. Mori TA, Beilin LJ. Omega-3 fatty acids and inflammation. *Current Atherosclerosis Reports*. 2004;6(6):461–7

19. Simopoulos AP. Omega-3 fatty acids in inflammation and autoimmune diseases. *Journal of the American College of Nutrition*. 2002;21(6):495–505

20. Zendedel A, Habib P, Dang J, et al. Omega-3 polyunsaturated fatty acids ameliorate neuroinflammation and mitigate ischemic stroke damage through interactions with astrocytes and microglia. *Journal of Neuroimmunology*. 2015;278:200–11

21. Ponce J, Ulu A, Hanson C, et al. Role of specialized pro-resolving mediators in reducing neuroinflammation in neurodegenerative disorders. *Frontiers in Aging Neuroscience*. 2022;14:780811:1–11

22. Levy BD, Clish CB, Schmidt B, et al. Lipid mediator class switching during acute inflammation: signals in resolution. *Nat Immunol*. 2001;2(7):612–9

23. Mengheri E. Health, probiotics, and inflammation. *Journal of Clinical Gastroenterology*. 2008;42:S177–8

24. Hamblin MR. Mechanisms and applications of the anti-inflammatory effects of photobiomodulation. *AIMS Biophys*. 2017;4(3):337–361

25. Wu G, Fang YZ, Yang S, et al. Glutathione metabolism and its implications for health. *J Nutr*. 2004;134(3):489–92

26. Ballatori N, Krance SM, Notenboom S, et al. Glutathione dysregulation and the etiology and progression of human diseases. *Biol Chem*. 2009;390(3):191–214

27. Berk M, Ng F, Dean O, et al. Glutathione: a novel treatment target in psychiatry. *Trends Pharmacol Sci*. 2008;29(7):346–51

28. Czarny P, Wigner P, Galecki P, et al. The interplay between inflammation, oxidative stress, DNA damage, DNA repair and mitochondrial dysfunction in depression. *Progress in Neuro-Psychopharmacology and Biological Psychiatry*. 2018;80:309–21

29. Holmay MJ, Terpstra M, Coles LD, et al. N-Acetylcysteine boosts brain and blood glutathione in Gaucher and Parkinson diseases. *Clin Neuropharmacol*. 2013;36(4):103–6

REDUCE: IMMUNE DYSREGULATION

Unconditional love is the most powerful stimulant to the immune system.
~ BERNIE SIEGEL

KEY POINTS

▸ Immune dysregulation is the initial catalyst required for PANS and PANDAS to develop

▸ Low-dose naltrexone is an important agent that helps restore immune regulation

▸ Steroid therapy may be of benefit or may escalate anxiety and aggression

▸ IVIG therapy is only required in about 10% of patients treated with our approach

▸ IVIG should be considered early in the treatment course for children with significant food restriction or who are a danger to themselves or others

▸ IVIG should be used only by experienced physicians and should follow strict protocols to ensure patient safety and to minimize side effects

Typically, PANS and PANDAS are viewed solely as disorders of autoimmunity (overactivity of the immune system with damage to self-tissues). As discussed in Chapter 2, PANS and PANDAS are actually disorders of immune dysregulation.

In addition to demonstrating elements of autoimmunity (for example, Th2 dominance with multiple IgE allergies, elevated ANA, and anti-neuronal antibodies), children with PANS and PANDAS also have a functional immune deficiency.

Many of these children have immunoglobulin deficiencies or a specific antibody deficiency (they don't make antibodies to infections or vaccinations). PANS and PANDAS pathophysiology is initiated by toxin- or stress-induced immune dysregulation. The accompanying immune deficiency allows new or dormant infections to become active and trigger autoimmunity through molecular mimicry, as described in Chapter 2.

Re-regulating the immune system is one of the four vital components of solving the PANS and PANDAS conundrum (along with removing toxins, treating infections, and breaking neurologic loops). If the immune system is not correctly regulated, flares will continue indefinitely. But PANS and PANDAS do not have to be lifelong conditions.

There are three main interventions we employ to directly regulate the immune response and restore it to a state of homeostasis.

Low-Dose Naltrexone (LDN)

The first is low-dose naltrexone (LDN).[1] Naltrexone is a nonselective, pure opioid antagonist. Opiate receptors are present in many parts of the body. Many processes within the body are controlled by the release of natural opiates known as endorphins and enkephalins.

Naltrexone has been approved for the treatment of opiate addiction since 1984[2] in oral doses of 50–100 mg daily.

> Re-regulating the immune system is one of the four vital components of solving the PANS and PANDAS conundrum.

Naltrexone has different actions when used at lower doses. Low-dose naltrexone refers to doses from 1–5 mg daily. It exists as a combination of left (levo-naltrexone) and right (dextro-naltrexone) isomers. The two isomers have different actions.

The dextro-isomer of naltrexone blocks (really antagonizes) toll-like receptor 4 (TLR4), which reduces the production of inflammatory cytokines, thereby reducing the inflammatory response.[1,3] TLR4 receptors are present on microglial cells, mast cells, and macrophages. On microglial cells, activation of TLR4 directly results in production of inflammatory products such as IL-2 and TNF-α.[1,3]

The levo-isomer of naltrexone blocks opiate receptors in the body for a brief period. This increases the natural production of anti-inflammatory (natural) endorphins and upregulates opiate receptors.[1,3] Increased production of endorphins improves neuropsychological health.[4] Increases in met-enkephalin (also known as opioid growth factor or OGF) modulate (improve) the immune response.[5] Increases in OGF have also been shown to decrease the growth of cancerous cells.[6–8]

In addition to improving immune status, LDN also exerts regulatory activity on the immune system, which makes it an ideal agent for auto-immune diseases.[9] Multiple studies have shown that LDN improves symptoms and quality of life in patients with multiple sclerosis.[10–13] In all these studies, the drug was found to be safe and well-tolerated. One of the studies[10] showed increases in the peripheral blood mononuclear cell levels of β-endorphins with LDN administration. Addi-

> In addition to improving immune status, LDN also exerts regulatory activity on the immune system, which makes it an ideal agent for autoimmune diseases.

tional significant improvements have been seen in clinical studies of patients with fibromyalgia,[14–16] IBS,[17] depression,[18] and inflammatory bowel disease (Crohn's disease and ulcerative colitis) in both adults and children.[19–22]

Additional case reports exist showing improvement in patients with complex regional pain syndrome,[23,24] autism,[25] cancer,[26–29] diabetic neuropathy,[30] and Hailey-Hailey disease (a type of chronic familial pemphigus).[31,32] Another case report describes a patient with long-standing postural orthostatic tachycardia syndrome (POTS) and mast cell activation syndrome (MCAS) who achieved significant symptomatic relief with LDN.[33]

A study of autoimmune encephalitis in a mouse model showed that the administration of both OGF and LDN was safe and halted the progression of the disease while reversing neurological deficits and preventing the onset of neurological dysfunction.[34]

While traditional doses of naltrexone for addiction (50–100 mg) are available commercially, low-dose naltrexone must be obtained from a compounding pharmacy. Liquids, capsules, and topical creams are available. We use liquids and capsules in our patients based upon age and weight. The dose must be titrated up over several weeks. It is usually administered at night, as it may induce relaxation. Occasionally, some patients report restless sleep or nightmares. In this case, the medication can be moved to the morning and these symptoms typically completely resolve. Rare headaches may be reported. If headaches are troublesome or if behavior changes for the worse, reducing the daily dose may be helpful.

STEROIDS

Steroid therapy can also be used for immune modulation. This is typically accomplished by using a five-day prednisone burst (1 mg/kg orally for five days). Repeated or prolonged courses are obviously precluded by untoward side effects. Liquid prednisone is very bitter. Pill formulations are typically small and powdery (like a baby aspirin) and can be crushed and placed in foods. They are also quite bitter, so if the pills are to be swallowed intact, ample liquids should be used to take them.

Although steroids are listed as an initial intervention in the original articles by the PANS consortium, we have found that initiating steroids during an acute flare may result in an increase in aggression and anxiety in about half of the treated patients. Later in the course of treatment, we sometimes use a course of steroids in an attempt to avoid IVIG.

INTRAVENOUS IMMUNE GLOBULIN (IVIG)

The final strategy we may use to re-regulate the immune system is IVIG. IVIG is a suspension of immune globulins (antibodies) produced by extracting the serum from thousands of donor plasma samples (1,000–100,000 donors per lot depending on manufacturer). IVIG reflects the immune environment of the donor pool. It typically contains antibodies against multiple infectious agents. Although it is mostly IgG, IVIG also contains small amounts of IgA and IgM.

Traditionally, immune globulin therapy is used for three indications:

1. Replacement therapy for patients with congenital or acquired immune deficiencies (usually hypogammaglobulinemia or agammaglobulinemia)
2. Modulation of autoimmune or inflammatory conditions
3. Treatment or prophylaxis for infections

Replacement therapies for congenital or acquired immune deficiencies (like common variable immune deficiency) are typically administered at a lower dose than the dose used for immune modulation. The immune modulatory dose of IVIG is typically 1–2g/kg IV split over 2–5 days. In PANS and PANDAS, we split the dose (2g/kg) over 2 days.

Evidence for immune modulation and resolution of inflammation

Although some of the mechanisms of the beneficial actions of IVIG are unknown, it has been shown that higher doses of IVIG lead to a reduction of inflammation and lead to immunosuppression.[35,36] IVIG induces anti-inflammatory cytokines and leads to decreased macrophage responses to interferon.[37] It is also cytotoxic to eosinophils and neutrophils, which causes a switch from a proinflammatory to an antinflammatory state.[38] IVIG leads to an expansion of the regulatory (CD4+CD25+) T-cell population.[39] This expansion of the regulatory T-cell population has been shown in mice to prevent the development of experimental autoimmune encephalomyelitis (EAE), which is an accepted animal model for multiple sclerosis (MS).[40,41] IVIG contains natural IgG antibodies to various cytokines, which can neutralize innate inflammatory responses.[42] IVIG therapy in pediatric allergy patients led to reduced levels of IgE.[43,44]

IVIG in patients with PANS and PANDAS

In 1999, a small study was conducted in children with PANDAS.[45] Twenty-nine patients were split into three groups. One group received therapeutic plasma exchange (plasmapheresis). The second group received a placebo. The third group had IVIG. Baseline, one-month, and twelve-month symptom assessment scales were taken. There was no change in the placebo group, even at twelve months (suggesting that PANDAS symptoms don't just go away spontaneously). OCD, anxiety, and overall functioning improved significantly in the plasma exchange and IVIG groups. Over 80% of patients in the IVIG and plasma exchange groups were still very much improved at one year.

Another small study showed that serum antibodies from children with PANDAS bound to specific intercholinergic neurons in the brain of mice in an area of the brain called the striatum, which is implicated in tic disorders.[46] The binding of the antibodies in the children with PANDAS was much higher than in a group of children without PANDAS. After the children with PANDAS received IVIG, the experiment was repeated and the antibody binding in the brains of the mice returned to the normal level seen in the control group of healthy children.

A 2018 Italian study by Pavone et al. involving thirty-four children showed significant improvement in twenty-nine of the thirty-four subjects after three monthly IVIG treatments.[47] In 2021, a study of twenty-one patients who received IVIG for moderate to severe PANS exhibited significant and sustained reductions in OCD scores.[48] Mean baseline measurements for anti-tubulin antibodies and CaM-Kinase II levels were elevated prior to treatment and all patients had previously received antibiotics. A ten-patient, open-label trial in 2022 also showed significant and sustained clinical improvement after monthly IVIG administration for three months.[49]

IVIG is generally well tolerated. It can cause an acute immune reaction (thought to be from excipients and other proteins in the infusion) consisting of fever, chills, and muscle/ joint aches. To avoid this type of reaction, IV decadron or solumedrol, acetaminophen, and diphenhydramine are given just before the infusion. True allergic reactions to IVIG are rare, although patients with low IgA levels are at a higher risk as low IgA may be due to anti-IgA antibodies. In the case of patients with low serum IgA, IgA-poor IVIG preparations are prescribed.

In a minority of cases, IVIG infusions can lead to a delayed onset severe headache with nausea and vomiting (typically 12–24 hours after infusion). This presents very similarly to a post-dural puncture headache and is much worse if patients are (or become) dehydrated. The actual term for this syndrome is "aseptic meningitis," although no CSF testing or therapies for meningitis are needed. We don't usually use this term with parents, as they hear "meningitis" and may become overly concerned. The best way to treat this problem is prevention. We strongly advise parents and patients to aggressively hydrate before, during, and after IVIG.

If these patients develop a severe headache and nausea, the treatment is orally dissolving ondansetron every six hours as needed and prednisone (1 mg/kg daily by mouth for three days). Parents are also advised to increase hydration to treat this once the patient is tolerating oral fluids. If the child is unable to tolerate oral fluids despite medications, evaluation in the emergency department and IV hydration is advisable.

We provide all our patients receiving IVIG with prescriptions for ondansetron and prednisone before the first day of IVIG in case they are needed. In addition, we provide both pre- and post-IVIG intravenous saline as a bolus (150–250 mL) to further reduce the risk of headache. Having a post-IVIG headache after the first infusion does not predict subsequent headaches (mainly because patients and parents are more motivated to aggressively hydrate if they experience this complication).

Side effects (including mild immune reactions and headaches) may also be related to the speed of IVIG infusion. For this reason, IVIG must be administered slowly in a very controlled manner with gradually increasing rates of infusion over several hours. Proper infusion of IVIG with premedications, establishment of a peripheral IV, IV fluids before and after, and immune globulin infusion typically takes 6–8 hours a day for two days. The ordering and administration of IVIG must be approached in a methodical manner to ensure safety and reduce symptoms.

Although some clinicians order initial IVIG infusions at the patients' homes, we prefer to

> **IVIG must be administered slowly in a very controlled manner with gradually increasing rates of infusion over several hours.**

have the child's first infusion done in an infusion center with specially trained personnel, close monitoring, and emergency supplies. If patients do well in this setting with the first infusion, the remaining infusions may be performed in their home if approved by insurance and the family. This tends to be calming for the child.

If there is no change in symptoms after three monthly infusions, we may hold on ordering further IVIG unless the child also has common variable immunodeficiency or some other indication for ongoing IVIG. We do have a few children who experience a sharp uptick in symptoms after discontinuation of IVIG. In these cases, we may reinstitute therapy if the child has previously shown a good response.

Parents often ask about the risk of transmission of infections since IVIG is technically a blood product. Although the absolute infection risk of a

pooled product can never be known with 100% certainty, most sources report that IVIG carries a very low risk of transmission of infections due to the way it is filtered. In a professional article on the mechanisms of action of IVIG,[50] Chaigne and Mouthon state that IVIG processing uses various methods of viral inactivation, pasteurization, and nanofiltration. The authors further state:

> Thus, no transmission of HIV, hepatitis A virus or hepatitis B virus, has been reported. However, before 1995, cases of transmission of hepatitis C virus have been reported following IVIG treatment. Although the risk of transmission of prions is possible, no case of Creutzfeldt-Jakob disease has been reported. To further limit the risk of transmitting any infectious agent, particularly Parvovirus B19 and prions, a nanofiltration process to 35 or 20 nm was added in the manufacturing process of the IVIG.

For these reasons, IVIG is likely safer in many ways than other blood products.

Our own clinical experience has been favorable with IVIG. We typically prescribe 2 g/kg IV, split over two days. Because we address infections, toxins, immune dysregulation, and neural loops in a systematic fashion, only about 10% of our patients end up needing IVIG. Patients for whom we immediately order IVIG at first meeting include children with significantly restricted eating or children with rapid behavioral deterioration (once other neurologic emergencies have been excluded).

As many of our patients with PANS and PANDAS have hypogammaglobulinemia or a specific antibody deficiency, IVIG may be submitted for approval under these diagnoses.

An example of IVIG orders, helpful tips for getting IVIG approved, and a sample appeal letter for IVIG can be found in Appendix E.

CHAPTER 13 REFERENCES

1. www.ldnresearchtrust.org, accessed 3/11/2023
2. Srivastava AB, Gold MS. Naltrexone: a history and future directions. *Cerebrum*. 2018;2018:13–18
3. Toljan K, Vrooman B. Low-dose naltrexone (LDN): review of therapeutic utilization. *Medical Sciences*. 2018;6(4):82:1–18
4. Lutz PE, Kieffer BL. Opioid receptors: distinct roles in mood disorders. *Trends Neurosci*. 2013;36(3):195–206
5. Janković BD, Radulović J. Enkephalins, brain and immunity: modulation of immune responses by methionine-enkephalin injected into the cerebral cavity. *Int J Neurosci*. 1992;67(1–4):241–70
6. Zagon IS, Donahue R, McLaughlin PJ. Targeting the opioid growth factor: opioid growth factor receptor axis for treatment of human ovarian cancer. *Exp Biol Med* (Maywood). 2013;238(5):579–87
7. Rogosnitzky M, Finegold MJ, McLaughlin PJ, et al. Opioid growth factor (OGF) for hepatoblastoma: a novel non-toxic treatment. *Invest New Drugs*. 2013;31(4):1066–70
8. Donahue RN, McLaughlin PJ, Zagon IS. Low-dose naltrexone targets the opioid growth factor-opioid growth factor receptor pathway to inhibit cell proliferation: mechanistic evidence from a tissue culture model. *Exp Biol Med* (Maywood). 2011;236(9):1036–50
9. Li Z, You Y, Griffin N, et al. Low-dose naltrexone (LDN): A promising treatment in immune-related diseases and cancer therapy. *Int Immunopharmacol*. 2018;61:178–184
10. Gironi M, Martinelli-Boneschi F, Sacerdote P, et al. A pilot trial of low-dose naltrexone in primary progressive multiple sclerosis. *Mult Scler*. 2008;14(8):1076–83
11. Turel AP, Oh KH, Zagon IS, et al. Low dose naltrexone for treatment of multiple sclerosis: a retrospective chart review of safety and tolerability. *J Clin Psychopharmacol*. 2015;35(5):609–11
12. Cree BA, Kornyeyeva E, Goodin DS. Pilot trial of low-dose naltrexone and quality of life in multiple sclerosis. *Ann Neurol*. 2010;68(2):145–50
13. Sharafaddinzadeh N, Moghtaderi A, Kashipazha D, et al. The effect of low-dose naltrexone on quality of life of patients with multiple sclerosis: a randomized placebo-controlled trial. *Mult Scler*. 2010;16(8):964–9
14. Younger J, Mackey S. Fibromyalgia symptoms are reduced by low-dose naltrexone: a pilot study. *Pain Med*. 2009;10(4):663–72
15. Younger J, Noor N, McCue R, et al. Low-dose naltrexone for the treatment of fibromyalgia: findings of a small, randomized, double-blind, placebo-controlled, counterbalanced, crossover trial assessing daily pain levels. *Arthritis Rheum*. 2013;65(2):529–38
16. Parkitny L, Younger J. Reduced Pro-Inflammatory Cytokines after Eight Weeks of Low-Dose Naltrexone for Fibromyalgia. *Biomedicines*. 2017;5(2):16:1–10
17. Kariv R, Tiomny E, Grenshpon R, et al. Low-dose naltrexone for the treatment of irritable bowel syndrome: a pilot study. *Dig Dis Sci*. 2006;51(12):2128–33

18. Mischoulon D, Hylek L, Yeung AS, et al. Randomized, proof-of-concept trial of low dose naltrexone for patients with breakthrough symptoms of major depressive disorder on antidepressants. *J Affect Disord.* 2017;208:6–14

19. Parker CE, Nguyen TM, Segal D, et al. Low dose naltrexone for induction of remission in Crohn's disease. *Cochrane Database Syst Rev.* 2018;4(4):CD010410:1–27

20. Smith JP, Stock H, Bingaman S, et al. Low-dose naltrexone therapy improves active Crohn's disease. *Am J Gastroenterol.* 2007;102(4):820–8

21. Lie MRKL, van der Giessen J, Fuhler GM, et al. Low dose Naltrexone for induction of remission in inflammatory bowel disease patients. *J Transl Med.* 2018;16(1):55:1–20

22. Raknes G, Simonsen P, Småbrekke L. The effect of low-dose naltrexone on medication in inflammatory bowel disease: a quasi experimental before-and-after prescription database study. *J Crohns Colitis.* 2018;12(6):677–686

23. Chopra P, Cooper MS. Treatment of complex regional pain syndrome (CRPS) using low dose naltrexone (LDN). *J Neuroimmune Pharmacol.* 2013;8(3):470–6

24. Weinstock LB, Myers TL, Walters AS, et al. Identification and treatment of new inflammatory triggers for complex regional pain syndrome: small intestinal bacterial overgrowth and obstructive sleep apnea. *A A Case Rep.* 2016;6(9):272–6

25. Bouvard MP, Leboyer M, Launay JM, et al. Low-dose naltrexone effects on plasma chemistries and clinical symptoms in autism: a double-blind, placebo-controlled study. *Psychiatry Res.* 1995;58(3):191–201

26. Berkson BM, Rubin DM, Berkson AJ. The long-term survival of a patient with pancreatic cancer with metastases to the liver after treatment with the intravenous alpha-lipoic acid/low-dose naltrexone protocol. *Integr Cancer Ther.* 2006;5(1):83–9

27. Berkson BM, Rubin DM, Berkson AJ. Revisiting the ALA/N (alpha-lipoic acid/low-dose naltrexone) protocol for people with metastatic and nonmetastatic pancreatic cancer: a report of 3 new cases. *Integr Cancer Ther.* 2009;8(4):416–22

28. Berkson BM, Rubin DM, Berkson AJ. Reversal of signs and symptoms of a B-cell lymphoma in a patient using only low-dose naltrexone. *Integr Cancer Ther.* 2007;6(3):293–6

29. Rogosnitzky M, Finegold MJ, McLaughlin PJ, Zagon IS. Opioid growth factor (OGF) for hepatoblastoma: a novel non-toxic treatment. *Invest New Drugs.* 2013;31(4):1066–70

30. Hota D, Srinivasan A, Dutta P, et al. Off-label, low-dose naltrexone for refractory painful diabetic neuropathy. *Pain Med.* 2016;17(4):790–1

31. Campbell V, McGrath C, Corry A. Low-dose naltrexone: a novel treatment for Hailey-Hailey disease. *Br J Dermatol.* 2018;178(5):1196–1198

32. Ibrahim O, Hogan SR, Vij A, et al. Low-dose naltrexone treatment of familial benign pemphigus (Hailey-Hailey disease). *JAMA Dermatol.* 2017;153(10):1015–1017

33. Weinstock LB, Brook JB, Myers TL, et al. Successful treatment of postural orthostatic tachycardia and mast cell activation syndromes using naltrexone, immunoglobulin and antibiotic treatment. *BMJ Case Rep.* 2018;2018:bcr2017221405:1–6

34. Rahn KA, McLaughlin PJ, Zagon IS. Prevention and diminished expression of experimental autoimmune encephalomyelitis by low dose naltrexone (LDN) or opioid growth factor (OGF) for an extended period: therapeutic implications for multiple sclerosis. *Brain Res.* 2011;1381:243–53

35. Nimmerjahn F, Ravetch JV. Anti-inflammatory actions of intravenous immunoglobulin. *Annu Rev Immunol.* 2008;26:513–33

36. Schwab I, Nimmerjahn F. Intravenous immunoglobulin therapy: how does IgG modulate the immune system? *Nat Rev Immunol.* 2013;13(3):176–89

37. Park-Min KH, Serbina NV, Yang W, et al. FcgammaRIII-dependent inhibition of interferon-gamma responses mediates suppressive effects of intravenous immune globulin. *Immunity.* 2007;26(1):67–78

38. Casulli S, Topçu S, Fattoum L, et al. A differential concentration-dependent effect of IVIg on neutrophil functions: relevance for anti-microbial and anti-inflammatory mechanisms. *PLoS One.* 2011;6(10):e26469:1–14

39. Massoud AH, Guay J, Shalaby KH, et al. Intravenous immunoglobulin attenuates airway inflammation through induction of forkhead box protein 3-positive regulatory T cells. *J Allergy Clin Immunol.* 2012;129(6):1656–65

40. Ephrem A, Chamat S, Miquel C, et al. Expansion of CD4+CD25+ regulatory T cells by intravenous immunoglobulin: a critical factor in controlling experimental autoimmune encephalomyelitis. *Blood.* 2008;111(2):715–22

41. Galeotti C, Kaveri SV, Bayry J. IVIG-mediated effector functions in autoimmune and inflammatory diseases. *International Immunology.* 2017;29(11):491–8

42. Svenson M, Hansen MB, Bendtzen K. Binding of cytokines to pharmaceutically prepared human immunoglobulin. *J. Clin. Invest.* 1993;92:2533:1–7

43. Mazer BD, Gelfand EW. An open-label study of high-dose intravenous immunoglobulin in severe childhood asthma. *J Allergy Clin Immunol.* 1991;87(5):976–83

44. Zhuang Q, Mazer B. Inhibition of IgE production in vitro by intact and fragmented intravenous immunoglobulin. *J Allergy Clin Immunol.* 2001;108(2):229–34

45. Perlmutter S, Leitman SF, Garvey MA, et al. Therapeutic plasma exchange and intravenous immunoglobulin for obsessive-compulsive disorder and tic disorders in childhood. *Lancet.* 1999;354(9185):1153–1158

46. Frick LR, Rapanelli M, Jindachomthong K, et al. Differential binding of antibodies in PANDAS patients to cholinergic interneurons in the striatum. *Brain, Behavior, and Immunity.* 2018;69:304–311

47. Pavone P, Falsaperla R, Cacciaguerra G, et al. PANS/PANDAS: clinical experience in IVIG treatment and state of the art in rehabilitation approaches. *NeuroSci.* 2020;1(2):75–84

48. Melamed I, Kobayashi RH, O'Connor M, Kobayashi AL, Schechterman A, Heffron M, Canterberry S, Miranda H, Rashid N. Evaluation of intravenous immunoglobulin in pediatric acute-onset neuropsychiatric syndrome. *J Child Adolesc Psychopharmacol.* 2021 Mar;31(2):118–128

49. Hajjari P, Oldmark MH, Fernell E, et al. Paediatric acute-onset neuropsychiatric syndrome (PANS) and intravenous immunoglobulin (IVIG): comprehensive open-label trial in ten children. *BMC Psychiatry.* 2022;22:535:1–13

50. Chaigne B, Mouthon L. Mechanisms of action of intravenous immunoglobulin. *Transfus Apher Sci.* 2017;56(1):45–49

CHAPTER 14

CONSIDERATIONS FOR ANTIMICROBIAL THERAPY, BIOFILMS, AND INITIAL ANTIBIOTIC CHOICES

Medicine is a science of uncertainty and an art of probability.
~ SIR WILLIAM OSLER

KEY POINTS

▸ Like many serious infections, PANS and PANDAS may require a longer course of therapy than other, less serious infections
▸ Steps should be taken to prevent yeast overgrowth and to protect the microbiome
▸ Biofilms are common in many bacterial infections and act as a source of resistance to antimicrobials and host immune defenses
▸ Biofilms can be reliably eradicated with certain enzyme therapies
▸ The PANS Initial Antibiotic Decision Scale is useful to guide the initial choice of antimicrobials at the first visit or in response to a flare at any stage of treatment

In this chapter and the two that follow, we will discuss antimicrobial therapies to REDUCE infections that are part of the pathophysiology of PANS and PANDAS. We emphasize that infections are merely part of the process, as immune dysregulation, toxins, inflammation, and neural loops (habitual rituals, beliefs, and behaviors) are also part of the process when flares occur.

At times, treating infections produces rapid, dramatic improvements in the status of the patient. Although antibiotic therapy is often the mainstay of this treatment, the addition of single herbal products and herbal combinations will be discussed where applicable.

> **Biofilms prevent host immune defenses from clearing infections and shield the pathogens from antimicrobials.**

The treatment of children with PANS and PANDAS is complex and must be dynamic. You must institute therapy, see how the child responds, and potentially adjust course. For this reason, there are no hard-and-fast protocols for treatment. Also, for this reason, there are few if any peer-reviewed references available regarding specific treatments. Much of what is included in the REDUCE chapters is based upon what we have found to be clinically successful.

This chapter includes an introduction that will address common questions we get regarding duration of antibiotics, risks, benefits, and some adjunctive therapies. It also contains information on biofilms, a relatively new but extremely important topic when treating infections. Finally, we will present a chart we have developed to help guide our initial antibiotic choice if we are initiating antimicrobial treatment before the results of tests for specific infections are available.

ANTIBIOTIC STEWARDSHIP

Antibiotic resistance is a growing problem all over the world.[1] The development of new and improved antibiotics to battle resistance and cover serious infections continues. In the mid-1990s, it seemed like a new cephalosporin was coming out every week.

In our patients with PANS and PANDAS, we typically use antibiotics for longer courses than would be prescribed for common infections like *Strep* throat. This reflects the fact that PANDAS is similar to the sequelae of rheumatic fever (Sydenham chorea) as discussed in Chapter 2. The current AHA recommendations for treatment and prophylaxis of rheumatic fever are to continue prophylactic antibiotics for five years or until age twenty-one (whichever is longer).[2] We don't treat with antibiotics for that duration since we usually see a resolution of symptoms well before that point.

Another reason for prolonged courses of antibiotics in PANS and PANDAS is that tick-borne infections are commonly seen in these disorders and experienced physicians have discovered that traditional 14–21 day courses of antibiotics are insufficient to eradicate these infections.

Finally, *Strep*, *Mycoplasma*, and some tick-borne infections exist in a biofilm (discussed later in this chapter). Biofilms prevent host immune defenses from clearing infections and shield the pathogens from antimicrobials.

We often see patients who have received a 7–10 day course of antibiotics from another clinician in an attempt to treat PANDAS, only to have a more severe flare when the antibiotic course is over. In our clinical experience, antibiotics may be required for 2–6 months, although we sometimes give breaks from therapy depending upon the clinical course and parental preference.

As much as we want to avoid contributing to antibiotic resistance, PANS and PANDAS should be recognized to be the emergencies that they are. In addition to rheumatic fever, patients with tuberculosis and vesicoureteral reflux are often prescribed prolonged courses of antibiotics.

Ultimately, if prescribers stopped writing prescriptions for amoxicillin and azithromycin for patients with clear cases of viral illness, we would strike a far more decisive blow against antibiotic resistance. Careful use of antibiotics for upper respiratory infections may not result in optimal Press Ganey scores, but just may save us all from resistant infections. Using natural compounds rather than antibiotics in animal feed could also be a protective measure against antibiotic resistance.[1]

PROTECTING THE GUT

In integrative medicine, we spend a lot more time talking about gut health than other physicians do. In many of the training courses in integrative medicine, antibiotics are demonized because they can disrupt the healthy microbiome and lead to overgrowth of pathogenic bacteria like *C. difficile*. Antibiotic use has also been shown to increase intestinal permeability.[3] Although these are valid concerns, careful attention to gut preservation while on antibiotics and gut recovery after treatment can help patients recover microbiome diversity.

Unless there is food restrictive behavior, we have patients REDUCE (or better, remove) foods that can contribute to increased intestinal permeability, like processed foods, sugars, gluten, and dairy, as discussed in Chapter 11.

> Careful attention to gut preservation while on antibiotics and gut recovery after treatment can help patients recover microbiome diversity.

When we prescribe antibiotics, we supplement with butyrate. Butyrate is a short-chain fatty acid that feeds the colonic epithelial cells. It also contributes to the release of natural antimicrobial substances in the gut to keep pathogens in check,[4] induces host defensin production,[1] and activates the innate and adaptive immune responses.[1] Animal studies demonstrate that butyrate reduces inflammatory markers, reduces bacterial translocation in the gut, and repairs the intestinal barrier.[1,5]

Butyrate is produced by anaerobic bacterial fermentation of indigestible dietary fiber. We typically use butyrate supplements instead of just relying on natural production from dietary fiber, since dietary modification in these children is difficult and the addition of more fiber just adds stress to the parents. There are no palatable liquid butyrate supplements, so children must be able to swallow pills to take it.

We add multi-strain probiotics and *Saccharomyces boulardii* to help preserve some of the healthy gut microbiome. Probiotics have been shown in several meta-analyses to reduce the risk of antibiotic-associated diarrhea and are an effective treatment adjunct for *C. diff* infection.[6,7]

Saccharomyces boulardii is actually a type of "friendly" yeast which acts similarly to a probiotic. It has been shown to prevent antibiotic-associated diarrhea in adults and children.[8–10] Probiotics and *S. boulardii* are both available in capsule and powdered form. They may be given together, but both should be given at least two hours from antibiotics. Probiotics and *S. boulardii* should not be used in children or adults who are severely immunocompromised (like hospitalized patients with neutropenia).

Fortunately, we have not seen any significant acute or chronic sequelae of antibiotic use in our practice. The most common side effects of antibiotic use we have seen are nausea, abdominal pain, and mild diarrhea. We have not seen side effects with butyrate, probiotics, or *Saccharomyces boulardii*.

PREVENTING YEAST OVERGROWTH

Traditionally, thrush or vaginal yeast infections from antibiotic use are only treated once they have occurred. Instead, we prefer to prophylactically use an oral antifungal (nystatin) as soon as patients are placed on antibiotics. Nystatin is a good choice because it is not absorbed systemically[11] and it does not react with other medications such as SSRIs. Probiotics (especially *Saccharomyces*) should be taken at least two hours from nystatin, as the drug is fungicidal to *Saccharomyces*.[12] Pill forms and an oral suspension of nystatin are available.

CAN YOU JUST USE HERBAL ANTIMICROBIALS INSTEAD OF PRESCRIPTION ANTIBIOTICS?

The simple answer is no, but we would if we could. In our practice, we often use herbals as an adjunct to antibiotics and sometimes even as a sole agent to treat more minor infections. However, for children in crisis with severe neuro-

> **Probiotics have been shown in several meta-analyses to reduce the risk of antibiotic-associated diarrhea and are an effective treatment adjunct for *C. diff* infection.**

psychiatric symptoms, antibiotics are clearly indicated. In the next two chapters we discuss some of the herbal options to consider.

"HERX" REACTIONS

The Jarisch-Herxheimer reaction[13] (JHR) was first described in the late nineteenth century. It is a reaction which can occur when a patient with a spirochetal disease receives antibiotics. It typically consists of fever, chills, joint pain, headache, malaise, and may also worsen the skin rashes seen with syphilis. It was originally described with syphilis but has been seen in other spirochetal diseases like Lyme disease, relapsing fever (louse borne and tick-borne), and leptospirosis.

The reaction usually occurs within two hours of antibiotic administration and usually subsides within 8–12 hours. In Lyme disease, the reaction is usually mild to moderate in severity. In leptospirosis, and occasionally in relapsing fever, reactions can be more severe, including hypotension, altered mental status, nuchal rigidity, ARDS, and kidney impairment. Deaths have been reported but are very rare. The JHR has been seen after administration of penicillin, ceftriaxone, macrolides, meropenem, and fluoroquinolones.[13]

The JHR can be differentiated from a simple drug reaction as drug reactions are typically skin rashes or anaphylactic in nature, while JHR comes with a host of constitutional symptoms. The exact etiology of the JHR is unknown at this time, though it has been proposed that it may be from release of spirochetal endotoxin, innate immune system activation, or host phagocytosis with intracellular spirochetal uptake.

We have not seen any *true* JHR in clinical practice even though we have treated many pediatric and adult patients with Lyme disease and *Borrelia miyamotoi*.

Many lay people and online sources describe any adverse reaction during antibiotic, antiviral, or herbal treatments as a JHR or, in nonscientific circles, a "herx reaction." This term has been used for a wide variety of reactions including headaches, joint pain, nausea, or brain fog. It is very unlikely that any of these reactions are from a true JHR. The term is also used by the same sources when these symptoms are seen when non-spirochetal infections are treated with natural or prescription antimicrobials.

We do sometimes see worsened behavioral flares in children when antibiotics are instituted for various infections in PANS and PANDAS. These reactions are not true JHR, as they may last for several days while on therapy and never cause fever. They may be due to the human immune system reaction to bacterial, viral, or spirochetal removal. We prefer to refer to these symptoms as "the healing response." Binders like activated charcoal, chlorella, citrus pectin, and clay may be used to help alleviate these symptoms. If significant behavioral changes are seen,

> Biofilms can protect organisms from antibiotics and facilitate immune evasion by preventing host phagocytosis and host immune cell modulation.

antibiotic, antiviral, or herbal therapies may be held for a few days and reinstituted slowly, then gradually tapered up to the full dose.

REDUCING BIOFILMS

In the natural environment or in animal hosts, microbes can exist as free-floating organisms (called planktonic growth) or can become adherent (or sessile) by attaching to surfaces or host cells. Once attached, microorganisms most often exist in biofilms.

Biofilms are highly organized, three-dimensional matrices of extracellular polymeric substances (EPS). They are produced by microbes themselves and closely regulate the hydration, oxygen tension, and pH of the environment.[14] Biofilms can protect organisms from antibiotics and facilitate immune evasion by preventing host phagocytosis and host immune cell modulation.[15] Within the biofilm, cell-to-cell communication occurs through a chemical process called *quorum sensing*.[14–16]

Due to the compartmentalization of different portions of the matrix, organisms within the biofilm may be a single species or multiple, phylogenetically unrelated species.[15] Enzymes produced in the biofilm can remove components of the matrix and can act as virulence factors.[14] Different species may also horizontally transfer genetic material between biofilm cells and may exchange bacterial resistance mechanisms.[15] For these reasons, some consider biofilms the most successful form of life on earth.[14]

It is estimated that 99% of the microorganisms on earth live in biofilms.[17] The National Institutes of Health has stated that biofilms account for 80% of microbial infections in the human body.[18] Over 60% of hospital-acquired infections are caused by biofilm colonization of medical devices such as catheters, contact lenses, mechanical cardiac valves, and endotracheal tubes.[17]

Although we may first think of implanted device colonization when we hear the term *biofilm*, adherent biofilms on various host tissues are far more common.[15] Unfortunately, the role of biofilms in serious infections is not emphasized in modern medicine, even in the field of infectious disease. Most current medical textbooks contain minimal information on biofilms and nothing about measures to eradicate them in chronic disease.

Although viruses, fungi, and parasites can also exist in biofilms, most of the discussion of this topic within the field of medicine (and within this textbook) deals with bacterial infections, in which biofilms play a pivotal role in propagation of illness.

Biofilms present two significant obstacles when diagnosing and caring for patients with bacterial infections. First, unlike acute illness, cultures may not be reliable in detecting bacteria in biofilms due to inadequate sampling or inadequate media in which to grow the organisms.[16] Second, and perhaps more importantly, biofilms can select out "persister" organisms that may reform the biofilm, shed new planktonic cells after antibiotic therapy has been discontinued, and cause a relapse of the infection.[15,19] The development of persister organisms within the biofilm matrix may necessitate prolonged courses of antimicrobial treatments[15,19] and novel strategies to disrupt biofilms, as noted below.

In terms of the organisms which are associated with or triggers for PANS and PANDAS, biofilms have been associated with *Streptococcus pyogenes*,[16,20] *Mycoplasma pneumoniae*,[21] *Borrelia burgdorferi*,[22,23] *Bartonella*,[24] and *Candida*.[19] *Staphylococcus aureus* is also a notorious biofilm producer which accounts for a significant proportion of nosocomial and implanted device related infections.[14–17,25,26] In addition to *Candida*, molds such as *Aspergillus* produce well-defined biofilms very similar to the extracellular matrix of bacteria.[27]

Since biofilms may prevent penetration of antibiotics or promote antibiotic resistance, strategies for removing or dissolving biofilms are

> **Biofilms account for 80% of microbial infections in the human body.**

needed. In the last several years, various biofilm disruption strategies have been investigated.

One of the most promising anti-biofilm therapies that we have found is the use of various types of digestive and fibrinolytic enzymes. Currently, antibacterial and anti-biofilm liquid enzymes are used as surface-cleaning materials in commercial applications.

Impregnating proteolytic enzymes such as lysostaphin into creams and bandages has been shown experimentally in animal models to be effective at reducing and clearing MRSA. Dairy cows who were genetically engineered to secrete lysostaphin in their milk had a lower incidence of mastitis from *Staph*.[17]

Amylase and lysozyme are polysaccharide-degrading enzymes which are used in the food and medical industry for their antibacterial properties.[17] Disruption of biofilms is best accomplished by a combination of proteases and polysaccharide-degrading enzymes.[17]

There are several commercially available over-the-counter enzyme supplements. One group which has been studied is fibrinolytics. This group contains lumbrokinase, nattokinase, and serrapeptase (also known as serratiopeptase). Studies have been done which have demonstrated the effectiveness of fibrinolytic enzymes against *Staph aureus* biofilms, including MRSA in vitro and in vivo in animal models.[25,26,28] These studies were done both with and without anti-staphylococcal antibiotics. These fibrinolytic enzymes did not affect the immune response and were not found to be cytotoxic to host cells.[25] Of the fibrinolytic agents, serrapeptase has been studied most extensively.

The review article authored by Jadhav et al. outlines the properties and therapeutic potential of serrapeptase.[29] Serrapeptase has been used therapeutically for decades in Europe and Japan for a variety of indications. It has been shown to modify the virulent phenotype of the bacteria in biofilms (including mature biofilms) and it enhances the bactericidal effect of antibiotics. The enzyme disrupts the biofilm by acting as a "nano-drill" to disrupt the biofilm membrane. In a rat model of Alzheimer's disease, serrapeptase reduced amyloid more effectively than nattokinase and reduced transforming growth factor-β and IL-6. In an animal model of ulcerative colitis, serrapeptase reduced disease activity, C-reactive protein, glutathione depletion, myeloperoxidase, and lipid peroxidation. These findings indicate less inflammation and oxidative stress. Serrapeptase is considered safe with very rare side effects.

In addition to its role as a biofilm disruptor, serrapeptase is an outstanding anti-inflammatory drug. A comprehensive review by Manju Tiwari outlines the anti-inflammatory effects of serrapeptase.[30] It provides at least equal, if not superior resolution of inflammation and pain control as NSAIDS. In addition, as Tiwari points out, lipid mediators derived from polyunsaturated fatty acids are required for resolution of inflammation. These mediators

> In addition to its role as a biofilm disruptor, serrapeptase is an outstanding anti-inflammatory drug.

are known as specialized pro-resolving mediators (SPMs). Some NSAIDS inhibit lipoxygenase (LOX) enzymes, which are required to produce SPMs. This could theoretically slow resolution of inflammation. Serrapeptase does not inhibit LOX pathways. Another article by Nair and Devi further outlines the anti-inflammatory efficacy of serrapeptase.[31]

Amylase is an enzyme that breaks down starches into simple sugars through hydrolysis. In humans it is present in saliva and pancreatic fluid. Supplements containing amylase are commercially available. Studies have shown that commercially available α-amylase compounds can break down *Staph aureus* biofilms in vitro.[32]

Papain is a mixture of proteolytic enzymes and peroxidases found in papaya. It has been used since the early 1980s in some regions of the world to accelerate wound healing.[33] It is believed that it works by breaking down and removing damaged tissue and by disrupting bacterial biofilms. In vitro studies have shown that papain has antibacterial properties, that it breaks down mature biofilms, and that it prevents biofilm formation of methicillin-resistant *Staphylococcus epidermidis* and methicillin-resistant *Staphylococcus haemolyticus*. In vitro studies have also demonstrated that papain reduces and inhibits biofilms of *Klebsiella pneumoniae*.[34]

Bromelain is a group of proteolytic enzymes found in the fruit and stems of the pineapple plant. A review by Jančič and Gorgieva details several benefits of bromelain.[35] This group of enzymes has been shown to have antimicrobial activity against both gram positive and gram-negative bacteria. Bromelain inhibits the growth of fungal pathogens and increases the effectiveness of antibiotics by potentiating their absorption. It is also strongly anti-inflammatory and has some fibrinolytic activity.

Bromelain inhibits bacterial cell adhesion. It is safe and well-tolerated in humans, even at high doses. Topical preparations speed wound and burn healing, removing necrotic tissue while sparing healthy tissues. An in vitro study by Carter et al. showed that bromelain dissolved 80% of biofilms produced by *Pseudomonas aeruginosa* on hernia mesh.[36] In the study, this effect was potentiated by a combined product containing bromelain and N-acetyl cysteine.

> **Bromelain inhibits bacterial cell adhesion.**

In our practice, we use a combination of enzymes along with serrapeptase.

Master herbalist and physician Dr. Stephen Buhner has written that the herbs *Andrographis paniculata*, *Houttuynia cordata*, *Polygonum cuspidatum*, *Rhodiola spp*, and *Scutellaria baicalensis* can help break up biofilms.[37] Although we use some herbal products as natural antimicrobials, we don't use any herbs solely as anti-biofilm agents.

Disruption of nasal biofilms can be accomplished with xylitol and grapefruit seed extract. Xylitol is a sugar alcohol. It has been shown in vitro to significantly reduce biofilm biomass (*S. epidermidis*), inhibit biofilm formation (*S. aureus and P. aeruginosa*), and reduce growth of planktonic bacteria (*S. epidermidis, S. aureus,* and *P. aeruginosa*) in chronic rhinosinusitis patients.[38] Grapefruit seed extract (GSE) has been shown in vitro to degrade biofilms from *Staph aureus* and *E. coli*.[39] GSE also inhibits growth and decreases biofilm formation of clinical isolates of *K. pneumoniae* (including drug-resistant strains).[40] It has also been shown to have a persistent inhibitory effect on biofilm development for *C. albicans* on denture-based resin.[41]

We recommend X-lear nasal spray (www. xlear.com/xlear-sinus-care) to our patients with chronic sinus issues to break up nasal biofilms from bacterial or fungal pathogens, as it contains xylitol, GSE, and saline.

Nasal irrigation with distilled water and NeilMed premixed packets (www.neilmed.com/ usa) containing sodium chloride and sodium bicarbonate is also effective for clearing mucus from the sinus passages. Only distilled water should be used for nasal irrigation to prevent the rare but serious parasitic brain infections which may occur after using tap water. It is unknown whether the plain NeilMed packets disrupt biofilms, but the company also makes a variety with xylitol.

Inhibiting quorum-sensing in biofilms could potentially inhibit the development of resistance to antimicrobials and decrease pathogen virulence.[42] Anti-quorum-sensing enzymes, polyphenols, and herbs may be useful agents to battle biofilm-producing organisms in the future as this would help decrease bacterial virulence. One article on anti-quorum-sensing plant extracts found experimental evidence of anti-quorum-sensing activity for baicalein (from Chinese skullcap), quercetin, caffeine, oregano oil, manuka honey, ginger, and garlic extract, among others.[43] Anti-quorum-sensing properties have also been noted in vanilla extract.[44]

No controlled trials have been done on enzymes or anti-quorum-sensing compounds in PANS and PANDAS, tick-borne illness, or other infections in vivo, but the basic science is compelling, which makes these agents a logical (and safe) choice for our patients.

INITIAL ANTIBIOTIC CHOICE IN PANS AND PANDAS

If patients present to our office for the initial appointment and are not in an extreme flare, we prefer to wait for some test results before beginning an antibiotic or herbal regimen. Unfortunately, this is not usually the case. As a Center of Excellence for PANS and PANDAS, we typically see patients who are particularly severe or have failed treatment with antibiotics or IVIG previously.

In these cases, after a discussion with parents, we start an antibiotic empirically while waiting for test results and cultures. Once results are available, the antibiotic or herbal coverage can be changed or narrowed. In the original literature from the PANS consortium[45] and in algorithms on the PANDAS Physicians Network website,[46] initial empiric antibiotics are suggested.

In cases of PANS, we are dealing with many different pathogens, not just *Strep*. For this reason, β-lactams and cephalosporins are not always the best initial choice. Some physicians treating patients with PANS and PANDAS use azithromycin initially in all cases since it should provide coverage for *Strep*, tick-borne illnesses, and *Mycoplasma*. We prefer not to do this since macrolide resistance (particularly in *Strep* and *Mycoplasma*) is increasing at an alarming rate, and we don't want to contribute to this phenomenon.

Since choosing between providing coverage for *Strep* versus tick-borne illnesses and *Mycoplasma* can be challenging, we have developed the PANS Initial Antibiotic Decision Scale (PIADS). The scale basically helps choose between two main groups of antibiotics: β-lactams/cephalosporins or macrolides/tetracycline derivatives for empiric treatment. Obviously, if patients are allergic to a certain antibiotic or class, are on a medication which will react with a certain antibiotic, or cannot take a particular antibiotic for some other reason, an alternative agent should be chosen.

THE PANS INITIAL ANTIBIOTIC DECISION SCALE

Score Column A and Column B (the highest score can be used to guide initial treatment)

Column A		Column B	
Previous improvement in behavior, anxiety, or OCD with β-lactam or cephalosporin	+5	Behavioral flares better with macrolide or tetracycline compound	+2
History of elevated ASO and/or Anti-DNase titers	+2	History of elevated *Mycoplasma* antibody titers	+2
Any history of prior behavioral flares with positive *Strep* culture or antigen	+3	Restrictive eating (current symptoms)	+5
Positive *Strep* culture or antigen within 60 days of initial appointment	+2	Restrictive eating (past history, now gone)	+3
Frequent tics, particularly head and neck	+2	Asthma (new onset within 90 days of initial flare)	+2
Scarlatina diagnosis or peri-anal *Strep* diagnosis within 60 days of initial appointment	+2	History of asthma remote onset (>90 days before first flare)	+1
History of peri-anal *Strep*	+1	Joint or muscle pain	+2
Sore throat more than 3 times per year (without testing)	+1	Known tick exposure	+2
Enlarged anterior cervical nodes or enlarged tonsils on exam	+2	Rage or extreme irritability is worse than anxiety	+1
TOTAL:		**TOTAL:**	

If the total for Column A is higher, we choose a β-lactam or cephalosporin antibiotic. If the total for Column B is higher, we choose a macrolide or a tetracycline derivative. If the totals are equal, we choose to begin therapy with a macrolide or a tetracycline derivative. See Appendix B for information on the dosages we commonly use.

When using antibiotics, we use regular probiotics plus saccharomyces to protect the gut. We also add oral nystatin to prevent yeast overgrowth and add enzymes to help break down biofilms. Dosage information can be found in Appendix B.

CHAPTER 14 REFERENCES

1. Du K, Bereswill S, Heimesaat MM. A literature survey on antimicrobial and immune-modulatory effects of butyrate revealing non-antibiotic approaches to tackle bacterial infections. *European Journal of Microbiology and Immunology*. 2021;11(1):1–9

2. Kumar RK, Antunes MJ, Beaton A, et al. American Heart Association Council on Lifelong Congenital Heart Disease and Heart Health in the Young; Council on Cardiovascular and Stroke Nursing; and Council on Clinical Cardiology. Contemporary diagnosis and management of rheumatic heart disease: implications for closing the gap: a scientific statement from the American Heart Association. *Circulation*. 2020;142(20):e337–e357

3. Spiller RC. Hidden dangers of antibiotic use: increased gut permeability mediated by increased pancreatic proteases reaching the colon. *Cellular and Molecular Gastroenterology and Hepatology*. 2018;6(3):347–349

4. Raqib R, Sarker P, Bergman P, et al. Improved outcome in shigellosis associated with butyrate induction of an endogenous peptide antibiotic. *Proceedings of the National Academy of Sciences*. 2006;103(24):9178–83

5. Li C, Chen X, Zhang B, et al. Sodium butyrate improved intestinal barrier in rabbits. *Italian Journal of Animal Science*. 2020;19(1):1482–92

6. Videlock EJ, Cremonini F. Meta-analysis: probiotics in antibiotic-associated diarrhoea. *Alimentary pharmacology & therapeutics*. 2012;35(12):1355–69

7. McFarland LV. Evidence-based review of probiotics for antibiotic-associated diarrhea and Clostridium difficile infections. *Anaerobe*. 2009;15(6):274–80

8. Szajewska H, Kołodziej M. Systematic review with meta-analysis: Saccharomyces boulardii in the prevention of antibiotic-associated diarrhoea. *Alimentary Pharmacology & Therapeutics*. 2015;42(7):793–801

9. Surawicz CM, Elmer GW, Speelman P, McFarland LV, Chinn J, Van Belle G. Prevention of antibiotic-associated diarrhea by *Saccharomyces boulardii*: a prospective study. *Gastroenterology*. 1989;96(4):981–8

10. Kotowska M, Albrecht P, Szajewska H. *Saccharomyces boulardii* in the prevention of antibiotic-associated diarrhoea in children: a randomized double-blind placebo-controlled trial. *Aliment Pharmacol Ther*. 2005;21(5):583–90

11. www.pdr.net/drug-summary/Nystatin-Tablets-nystatin-1531.302, accessed 2/8/2023

12. Venables P, Russell AD. Nystatin-induced changes in *Saccharomyces cerevisiae*. *Antimicrob Agents Chemother*. 1975;7(2):121–7

13. Butler T. The Jarisch-Herxheimer reaction after antibiotic treatment of spirochetal infections: a review of recent cases and our understanding of pathogenesis. *Am J Trop Med Hyg*. 2017;96(1):46–52

14. Flemming HC, Wingender J. The biofilm matrix. *Nature Reviews Microbiology*. 2010;8(9):623–33

15. Schulze A, Mitterer F, Pombo JP, Schild S. Biofilms by bacterial human pathogens: Clinical relevance: development, composition and regulation: therapeutical strategies. *Microb Cell*. 2021;8(2):28–56

16. Hall-Stoodley L, Stoodley P. Evolving concepts in biofilm infections. *Cell Microbiol*. 2009;11(7):1034–43

17. Thallinger B, Prasetyo EN, Nyanhongo GS, et al. Antimicrobial enzymes: an emerging strategy to fight microbes and microbial biofilms. *Biotechnology Journal.* 2013;8(1):97–109

18. National Institutes of Health. *SBIR/STTR Study and Control of Microbial Biofilms (PA-99-084).* http://grants.nih.gov/grants/guide/pa-files/PA-99-084.html. Published April 21, 1999. Accessed 2/28/2023

19. Lewis KI. Riddle of biofilm resistance. *Antimicrobial agents and chemotherapy.* 2001;45(4):999–1007

20. Young C, Holder RC, Dubois L, D. S Reid. *Streptococcus pyogenes* biofilm. 2022 Aug 21 [updated 2022 Oct 4]. In Ferretti JJ, Stevens DL, Fischetti VA, editors. *Streptococcus pyogenes: Basic Biology to Clinical Manifestations* [Internet]. 2nd ed. Oklahoma City (OK): University of Oklahoma Health Sciences Center; 2022. Chapter 15

21. Feng M, Schaff AC, Balish MF. *Mycoplasma pneumoniae* biofilms grown in vitro: traits associated with persistence and cytotoxicity. *Microbiology* (Reading). 2020;166(7):629–640

22. Di Domenico EG, Cavallo I, Bordignon V, et al. The emerging role of microbial biofilm in Lyme neuroborreliosis. *Front Neurol.* 2018;9:1048

23. Sapi E, Bastian SL, Mpoy CM, et al. Characterization of biofilm formation by *Borrelia burgdorferi* in vitro. *PLoS One.* 2012;7(10):e48277:1–11

24. Zheng X, Ma X, Li T, et al. Effect of different drugs and drug combinations on killing stationary phase and biofilms recovered cells of *Bartonella henselae* in vitro. *BMC Microbiol.* 2020;20(1):87:1–9

25. Hogan S, O'Gara JP, O'Neill E. Novel treatment of *Staphylococcus aureus* device-related infections using fibrinolytic agents. *Antimicrob Agents Chemother.* 2018;62(2):e02008–17

26. Hogan S, Zapotoczna M, Stevens NT, et al. Potential use of targeted enzymatic agents in the treatment of *Staphylococcus aureus* biofilm-related infections. *J Hosp Infect.* 2017;96(2):177–182

27. Morelli KA, Kerkaert JD, Cramer RA. *Aspergillus fumigatus* biofilms: toward understanding how growth as a multicellular network increases antifungal resistance and disease progression. *PLoS Pathog.* 2021;17(8):e1009794:1–23

28. Katsipis G, Pantazaki AA. Serrapeptase impairs biofilm, wall, and phospho-homeostasis of resistant and susceptible *Staphylococcus aureus. Appl Microbiol Biotechnol.* 2023;107(4):1373–1389

29. Jadhav SB, Shah N, Rathi A, et al. Serratiopeptidase: insights into the therapeutic applications. *Biotechnol Rep* (Amst). 2020;28:e00544:1–9

30. Tiwari M. The role of serratiopeptidase in the resolution of inflammation. *Asian J Pharm Sci.* 2017;12(3):209–215

31. Nair SR, Devi S. Serratiopeptidase: an integrated view of multifaceted therapeutic enzyme. *Biomolecules.* 2022;12(10):1468:1–12

32. Craigen B, Dashiff A, Kadouri DE. The use of commercially available alpha-amylase compounds to inhibit and remove Staphylococcus aureus biofilms. *The Open Microbiology Journal.* 2011;5:21:1–11

33. Oliveira HL, Fleming ME, Silva PV, et al. Influence of papain in biofilm formed by methicillin-resistant *Staphylococcus epidermidis* and methicillin-resistant *Staphylococcus haemolyticus* isolates. *Brazilian Journal of Pharmaceutical Sciences.* 2014;50:261–7

34. Mohamed SH, Mohamed MS, Khalil MS, et al. Antibiofilm activity of papain enzyme against pathogenic Klebsiella pneumoniae. *Journal of Applied Pharmaceutical Science.* 2018;8(6):163–8

35. Jančič U, Gorgieva S. Bromelain and nisin: The natural antimicrobials with high potential in biomedicine. *Pharmaceutics.* 2021;14(1):76

36. Carter CJ, Pillai K, Badar S, et al. Dissolution of biofilm secreted by three different strains of *Pseudomonas aeruginosa* with bromelain, N-acetylcysteine, and their combinations. *Applied Sciences*. 2021;11(23):11388:1–13

37. Buhner SH. *Healing Lyme: Natural Healing of Lyme Borreliosis and the Coinfections Chlamydia and Spotted Fever Rickettsioses*. Raven Press, Boulder, CO; 2015:236–237

38. Jain R, Lee T, Hardcastle T, et al. The in vitro effect of xylitol on chronic rhinosinusitis biofilms. *Rhinology*. 2016;54(4):323–328

39. Song YJ, Yu HH, Kim YJ, et al. Anti-biofilm activity of grapefruit seed extract against *Staphylococcus aureus* and *Escherichia coli*. *Journal of Microbiology and Biotechnology*. 2019;29(8):1177–1183

40. Barawi S, Hamzah H, Hamasalih R, et al. Antibacterial mode of action of grapefruit seed extract against local isolates of beta-lactamases-resistant *Klebsiella pneumoniae* and its potential application. *International Journal of Agriculture and Biology*. 2021;26:499–508

41. Tsutsumi-Arai C, Takakusaki K, Arai Y, et al. Grapefruit seed extract effectively inhibits the Candida albicans biofilms development on polymethyl methacrylate denture-base resin. *PLoS One*. 2019;14(5):e0217496

42. Abraham WR. Going beyond the control of quorum-sensing to combat biofilm infections. *Antibiotics* (Basel). 2016;5(1):3:1–16

43. Asfour HZ. Anti-quorum sensing natural compounds. *J Microsc Ultrastruct*. 2018;6(1):1–10

44. Choo JH, Rukayadi Y, Hwang JK. Inhibition of bacterial quorum sensing by vanilla extract. *Lett Appl Microbiol*. 2006;42(6):637–41

45. Cooperstock MS, Swedo SE, Pasternack MS, et al. Clinical management of pediatric acute-onset neuropsychiatric syndrome: part III: treatment and prevention of infections. *J Child Adolesc Psychopharmacol*. 2017;27(7):594–606

46. www.pandasppn.org/severe, accessed 3/10/2023

CHAPTER 15

TREATING *STREP*, *MYCOPLASMA*, AND OTHER BACTERIAL, PARASITIC, AND VIRAL INFECTIONS

There really is no such thing as a sick child;
there are children who happen to be sick.
~ PAUL NEWMAN

KEY POINTS

▸ *Strep* infections can be effectively treated with either β-lactam or cephalosporin antibiotics and biofilm-disrupting agents

▸ Clinical studies do not conclusively show a reduction in *Strep* infections or PANDAS symptoms after tonsillectomy

▸ *Mycoplasma* infections are best treated with a combination of tetracycline or macrolide antibiotics, herbal preparations, and biofilm-disrupting agents

▸ EBV infections are best treated with herbal agents in children

▸ Pathogens in the GI tract should be treated only when found on testing

In this chapter we begin with two of the major players as far as infections in PANS and PANDAS: *Strep* and *Mycoplasma*. We also discuss other bacteria, viruses, and gut pathogens. (See Chapter 16 for an in-depth discussion of the treatment of Lyme disease and other tick-borne infections.)

GROUP A β-HEMOLYTIC STREP

When the initial case definition of PANDAS came to light in 1997,[1] the focus was on antibiotics targeted at *Streptococcus pyogenes* (group A β-hemolytic *Strep* or "GABHS"). Since there is still no known in vitro resistance of *Strep* bacteria to β-lactam antibiotics, penicillin or amoxicillin are typically recommended as first-line treatments.

In clinical practice, however, some patients who have documented *Strep* pharyngitis fail to improve with these agents. Studies have shown that oral and injectable penicillin fail to eradicate GABHS in about 35% of cases.[2] In these cases, it is not a case of traditional antibiotic resistance since GABHS does not make β-lactamase; it is more appropriately referred to as "antibiotic failure."

There are five main contributors to β-lactam antibiotic failure in GABHS infections:

1. GABHS can enter the epithelial cells (a process called internalization) to escape antibiotics.[3] Penicillin does not penetrate the walls of epithelial cells well.[4] Strains recovered from patients with GABHS eradication failure have increased intracellular survival. Cephalosporins and clindamycin are more effective at killing intracellular GABHS and maintain a higher concentration in the tonsillar surface fluid for a longer duration than penicillin.[5]

2. Treatment with penicillin can result (over time) in increased selection of β-lactamase-producing species such as *Haemophilus* species, *Staphylococcus aureus* (including MRSA), *M.*

catarrhalis, *Prevotella*, and *Fusobacterium spp*. These species are typically recovered after treatment with β-lactam antibiotics and are seen in 85% of tonsillar tissue removed from patients with recurrent GABHS infections.[5] Cephalosporins, clindamycin, and amoxicillin-clavulanate are effective at eradicating GABHS in patients with increased β-lactamase activity.[5]

3. The organism *M. catarrhalis* increases GABHS adherence to human epithelial cells. The two bacteria have a symbiotic relationship.[5] *H. influenzae* also shares a symbiotic relationship with GABHS. Both *M. catarrhalis* and *H. influenzae* also produce β-lactamase. Second-generation, extended-spectrum, and third-generation cephalosporins and amoxicillin-clavulanate all have activity against these two pathogens.[5]

4. Biofilms are aggregates of bacteria hidden within an extracellular matrix which allows the bacteria to resist the human immune system as well as antibiotics.[6] Biofilms and solutions to help reduce them are discussed in Chapter 14.

5. The normal healthy oropharyngeal microbiome contains aerobic and anaerobic organisms which interfere with or inhibit growth of pathogenic bacteria like GABHS.[7,8] Some of these bacterial species include α- and γ-hemolytic *Strep*, *Peptostreptococcus*, and *Prevotella*. These helpful species may compete for nutrients or may produce antibiotic-like substances called bacteriocins to kill other bacteria.[7] Only one-third of patients with recurrent *Strep* pharyngitis are colonized with these interfering

bacteria, while GABHS-free patients harbor these bacteria 85% of the time. Lack of these interfering bacteria can lead to frequent recurrence of *Strep* infection.

Several studies have shown that therapeutic colonization of the oropharynx with α-hemolytic *Strep* (*Strep salivarius* K12) lozenges or nasal sprays is safe and can reduce recurrence of *Strep* pharyngitis and upper respiratory tract infections, especially in children.[9–12] This bacterium, in oral probiotic form (dissolvable, chewable, or liquid), has been shown to decrease inflammation.[13] It also inhibits immune activation in periodontal disease.[14] Limiting immune activation in PANS and PANDAS is an especially attractive property of this agent.

One preliminary study showed that *Strep salivarius* K12 probiotics were effective in improving laboratory parameters of illness and increasing survival in hospitalized patients with COVID-19.[15] *Strep salivarius* K12 has also been shown to disrupt biofilms.[14] We use a lozenge form of this oral probiotic from BLIS (blis.co.nz) for our patients with PANS and PANDAS.

Although amoxicillin-clavulanate is more effective against *Strep* than penicillin or plain amoxicillin, it also has strong activity against these beneficial interfering bacteria and thus can potentially lead to higher risk of GABHS recurrence.[5] One study which compared amoxicillin-clavulanate to cefdinir showed that at the end of the treatment course, patients treated with amoxicillin-clavulanate had more depletion of aerobic and anaerobic interfering bacteria than the cefdinir group.[16] This depletion persisted for at least two months and led to quicker reacquisition of infection in the amoxicillin-clavulanate group.

Until recently, macrolides (azithromycin, clarithromycin, and erythromycin) have been an attractive option to treat GABHS as they are resistant to β-lactamase, have activity against *H. influenzae* and *M. catarrhalis*, and produce high intracellular levels of antibiotic which can battle internalization of microbes.[5]

The problem we are now facing is that GABHS is developing true resistance to macrolides at an alarming rate. In the period from 2010 to 2017, erythromycin resistance nearly tripled from 8% to 23%.[17] In the same time period, clindamycin resistance has risen to 22%.[17]

Tetracycline is not used due to *Strep* resistance. Doxycycline and minocycline may be used but are not first-line therapies for isolated *Strep* infections.

Currently, amoxicillin-clavulanate, cephalexin, and cefdinir appear to be good therapeutic choices for GABHS.

Clavulanate as a compound has excellent penetration of the blood-brain barrier. It has also been shown in animal models to increase dopamine levels, decrease anxiety, and act as a neuroprotective agent in chemically induced models of neurodegenerative disease.[18–20]

Patients who have a penicillin allergy may have a cross reactivity to cephalosporins in about 10% of cases. In patients with true allergies, we prescribe clindamycin or a macrolide.

There are no randomized studies which address the question of the optimal length of GABHS antibiotic prophylaxis in children with PANDAS, but recommendations from the PANS consortium group and our own clinical experience suggest that antibiotic treatment for one year is reasonable.[21] Some experts believe that children with the most severe cases may require prophylactic antibiotics until age eighteen, as in rheumatic fever.[21]

There are no specific herbal treatments for GABHS.

As noted in the last chapter, we commonly use digestive enzymes and serrapeptase to help with biofilm disruption.

WHAT ABOUT TONSILLECTOMY?

Since GABHS is the causative agent in PANDAS, it would seem that tonsillectomy might be a good option to help remove a reservoir for *Strep* and thus help reduce recurrence of PANDAS symptoms. In fact, some physicians will not see patients with PANS or PANDAS unless their parents agree to have the child get a tonsillectomy.

But what does the literature say?

There are basically four questions which must be answered:

1. Does tonsillectomy reduce the incidence of *Strep* recurrence in children?

The updated clinical practice guidelines for tonsillectomy by the American Academy of Otolaryngology–Head and Neck Surgery, lists indications for tonsillectomy as the occurrence of seven or more episodes of throat infection in one year or five episodes a year for two consecutive years, or three episodes per year for three consecutive years.[22]

The guidelines state that to qualify, the throat infection should have *at least one* of the following additional criteria: temperature >101°F, cervical adenopathy, tonsillar exudate, or a positive test for GABHS. Since many viral infections cause fever, adenopathy, and exudate, it is unclear whether the procedures are actually being done in patients with infections caused by *Strep* exclusively.

This guideline also states that, although infections and missed school days may decrease immediately after the procedure, this benefit is not sustained long term.[22] A systematic review of the literature in the journal *Pediatrics* confirmed that short-term benefits (moderate strength of evidence) for decreased infections and missed school do not persist over time.[23]

For these reasons, it has not been conclusively demonstrated that tonsillectomy will reli-

> It has not been conclusively demonstrated that tonsillectomy will reliably reduce infections from GABHS long term.

ably reduce infections from GABHS long term. Research has documented that patients who have had a tonsillectomy still get *Strep* throat infections.[24] We also see *Strep* cellulitis and recurrent peri-anal *Strep*, which are unaffected by tonsillectomy.

2. Does tonsillectomy reduce the frequency or intensity of PANDAS flares?

Although some small case reports of children with PANDAS who improved after tonsillectomy exist, larger prospective studies have not demonstrated the benefits of tonsillectomy in this population.[25] In a well-done study by Pavone et al., 120 children who met strict criteria for PANDAS were split into a surgical group that underwent tonsillectomy (or adenotonsillectomy) and a control group that did not.[26] After two years of follow-up every two months post-surgery, no improvements were seen in symptom progression, *Streptococcal* or anti--neuronal antibodies, or the clinical severity of neuropsychiatric symptoms in the surgical group as compared to the control group.

Additional case study reviews have found that there is no conclusive proof that tonsillectomy improves the clinical course of PANDAS or prevents recurrences of flares.[27,28] Although a survey of parents of children with PANDAS who had a tonsillectomy reported high parental satisfaction with the procedure, the results were subjective and based upon questionnaires filled out by only the parents who could be reached.[29] The PANS consortium also maintains that there is insufficient evidence that tonsillectomy reliably improves symptoms in PANDAS patients.[21]

3. What is the role of the tonsils in protective immunity?

The tonsils are part of Waldeyer's ring of lymphoid tissue. They are an important part of the nasopharyngeal and respiratory immune system. The tonsils and adenoids help with clonal B-cell expansion, B-cell receptor maturation, and differentiation of B memory cells and plasma cells.[30-31] The authors of a comprehensive review of the immunology of the tonsils and adenoids in the *International Journal of Pediatric Otorhinolaryngology* suggest that, due to the vital role of the tonsils and adenoids, a conservative attitude toward adenotonsillectomy, especially in younger children, is warranted.[30]

4. What are the immediate risks and long-term sequelae of tonsillectomy?

The short-term risks of adenotonsillectomy include anesthesia risks, infection, intraoperative surgical complications, and post-tonsillectomy bleeding and pain. Post-surgical pain is especially concerning in children who already have food restriction or OCD-related globus symptoms.

> **Due to the vital role of the tonsils and adenoids, a conservative attitude toward adenotonsillectomy, especially in younger children, is warranted.**

In terms of long-term risks, there is one large study which demonstrated that patients who have had a tonsillectomy may have some long-term immune issues. The study was performed in Denmark and followed over one million children longitudinally for 10–30 years. The authors found that patients who had had tonsillectomy had increased long-term risks of respiratory, infectious, and allergic diseases as compared to controls who had not had surgery.[32] This was an observational study and may not prove causation.[33] Nevertheless, patients and/or their parents should be counseled about potential long-term risks from adenotonsillectomy.

We do not currently recommend tonsillectomy unless the procedure is recommended by a specialist due to sleep-disordered breathing.

MYCOPLASMA PNEUMONIAE

Mycoplasma pneumoniae is a common cause of atypical pneumonia and bronchitis. Studies have demonstrated a link between *Mycoplasma pneumoniae* in children and tics, OCD, and Tourette syndrome.[34–36] In our practice, we have found a direct link between children with PANS who have food restriction and avoidance and *Mycoplasma* infection.

An excellent review by Garth Nicolson, PhD, outlines the following methods by which pathogenic *Mycoplasma* infections can evade host immune mechanisms.[37] The organism has variable and changing surface membrane antigens and can scavenge host structures and apply them to their own surface glycolipids to avoid detection.

Mycoplasma can also suppress host immune cells and trigger the host to release inflammatory cytokines such as IL-2, IL-6, and TNF-α. The release of inflammatory cytokines is predictive

> **Anti-neuronal antibodies have been identified in 100% of patients with CNS involvement.**

of refractory infections in children. *Mycoplasma* can also induce apoptosis in host immune cells. These immune evading strategies are important for the survival of *Mycoplasma* since it is slow growing.

The fact that the adhesin molecules and glycolipids of the *Mycoplasma* cell membrane share homology with mammalian tissues, coupled with the fact that these organisms scavenge and use host cell membranes as camouflage, has

been shown to trigger autoimmunity in multiple organ systems through the process of molecular mimicry.[37,38,39] Specific diseases associated with molecular mimicry are rheumatoid (and other types of) arthritis, asthma, MS, and some neurodegenerative diseases.[37]

Central nervous system complications, including encephalitis, diplopia, mental confusion, and acute psychosis are the most common extrapulmonary manifestations of *Mycoplasma*. Anti-neuronal antibodies have been identified in 100% of patients with CNS involvement.[40]

Antibiotic treatment[40,41]

Since *Mycoplasma* lacks a cell wall, traditional β-lactam antibiotics such as penicillin and amoxicillin are ineffective. Macrolides and tetracyclines are effective. Azithromycin tends to have lower MICs than other macrolides. Since patients with PANS and PANDAS often have persistent infection due to immune dysregulation and/or hypogammaglobulinemia, a five-day course of azithromycin or a ten-day course of clarithromycin are seldom sufficient to clear the infection. Longer courses (30–60 days) are generally needed. Azithromycin and clarithromycin are better tolerated by patients than erythromycin and doxycycline, which tend to cause more nausea and abdominal pain.

Erythromycin and clarithromycin are strong inhibitors of CYP3A4 enzymes in the liver which can affect the metabolism of other medications.[42] In contrast, azithromycin is a weak substrate for the enzyme and does not inhibit or induce the enzyme.[42] This means that azithromycin is less likely to interact with the metabolism of other medications.

One concern when using macrolides is prolongation of the QT interval and subsequent risk of dangerous or fatal cardiac arrhythmias. This concern was brought to light by an article in the *New England Journal of Medicine* by Ray et al. from 2012.[43] This paper describes a retrospective correlational study of Medicaid data from Tennessee.

It compared patients getting various outpatient antibiotics (including azithromycin) to patients not receiving antibiotics. A large group of patients with prescriptions for azithromycin, amoxicillin, levofloxacin, ciprofloxacin, and controls were considered in the study. Increased risk of death at day four of therapy was suggested in patients receiving azithromycin as compared to amoxicillin or no antibiotic. In addition to being a retrospective cohort study (which suggests correlation but does not prove causation), the patients in the study who received azithromycin were more likely to be treated for pneumonia or COPD, which would place them at higher risk of death in general. Nevertheless, this study resulted in an FDA warning to prescribers that implicated azithromycin as an increased risk factor for cardiovascular death due to QT interval prolongation.

A subsequent, very large Danish study by Svanström et al. in the *New England Journal of Medicine* found no increased risk of death from azithromycin as compared to penicillin.[44] A 2014 meta-analysis of twelve randomized controlled studies (15,588 patients) by Almalki—which compared azithromycin to placebo in patients with COPD, severe sepsis, and cardiovascular disease—showed a trend toward decreased mortality in the azithromycin group.[45]

> Macrolides have anti-inflammatory and immunomodulating properties.

Prolongation of the QT interval, which may rarely result in serious ventricular dysrhythmias, has been demonstrated with both erythromycin and clarithromycin.[46] This QTc prolongation is associated with inhibition of the hERG potassium channel by both of these drugs. Azithromycin, however, has a very low affinity for the hERG receptor, even at high concentrations.[46] In the presence of low extracellular potassium, both erythromycin and clarithromycin (but not azithromycin) have been shown to induce torsade de pointes[46] by delaying cardiac repolarization.

In contrast, although azithromycin prolongs the QTc, it does so by prolonging the action potential itself rather than delaying cardiac repolarization.[47] In a study in dogs, this QTc prolongation was mild and did not induce torsade de pointes.[47] This prolongation of the action potential by azithromycin could actually give this agent *antiarrhythmic* properties.[48]

Although the evidence in the preceding paragraphs calls into question the connection between azithromycin-induced QTc prolongation and increased cardiovascular events, most drug interaction programs (like www.epocrates.com) and the package insert[49] for azithromycin list QTc prolongation as an adverse reaction and recommend avoiding coadministration of this antibiotic with other medication which may prolong the QT interval. For this reason, we avoid using azithromycin in patients taking SSRIs and antipsychotics (which have both been shown to increase the QT interval independently) if possible. If azithromycin is necessary in patients on these medications, we may taper and discontinue the psychiatric medications before starting the azithromycin.

One interesting fact about macrolides is that they have been shown to have anti-inflammatory and immunomodulating properties.[50] For this reason, azithromycin remains an attractive initial choice for patients with PANS in whom *Strep* is not considered the primary driver of the syndrome.

As with *Strep* bacteria, though, macrolide resistance in *Mycoplasma pneumoniae* is rising in the United States. According to a multi-site study conducted between 2012 and 2014, resistance rates to macrolides were as high as 13.2%.[51] A global meta-analysis from 2022 shows that resistance in some areas of Asia can be as high as 53.4% in some strains.[52] While we don't recommend macrolide use if *Strep* infection is the primary concern, it is an appropriate choice for *Mycoplasma* infections and tick-borne infections.

> Studies have shown no teeth staining in children younger than age eight who were treated with doxycycline compared to controls.

Tetracyclines

Tetracyclines are effective against *Mycoplasma pneumoniae* (and other intracellular) infections. There are two oral tetracycline derivatives used in clinical practice today: doxycycline and minocycline. There is also evidence that doxycycline is effective against macrolide-resistant *Mycoplasma pneumoniae*.[53–55]

Both doxycycline and minocycline are available in capsules but are not widely available in liquid form. The capsules cannot be opened and added to foods, as the powder is very irritating. Even in capsule form, these medications can irritate the esophagus and stomach and must be taken with at least 8 ounces of water. In our experience, the monohydrate formulation of doxycycline is preferable, as it is associated with fewer gastrointestinal side effects.

Patients on any of the tetracyclines may experience a photosensitivity reaction when exposed to bright sunlight outdoors. This can range from mild skin irritation (like a first-degree sunburn) to more severe reactions with blistering. We advise patients that routine periods outside may be fine (with sunscreen), but sunbathing or extended time at the beach is not advisable while on these meds.[55]

Minocycline occasionally causes dizziness or vertigo.[56] This may be because it is more lipophilic and achieves higher CNS concentrations.[57] We have not found minocycline to be any more efficacious than doxycycline in our patients with PANS. Doxycycline has fewer reported adverse effects than minocycline.[57]

Since permanent staining and enamel hypoplasia of secondary teeth has been a rare but reported side effect seen with tetracyclines, they are usually recommended only for patients over the age of eight.[56,57] Careful review of the literature, however, shows that this staining is seen with minocycline and tetracycline, but has not conclusively been demonstrated with doxycycline.

In fact, several studies have shown no teeth staining in children younger than age eight who were treated with doxycycline compared to controls.[58–60] At least one of these studies included children who took doxycycline for as long as twenty-eight days. There is one article which describes four patients who developed some temporary yellow staining of the teeth with doxycycline, which was resolved with dental cleaning.[61]

Tetracyclines, including doxycycline and minocycline, are all labeled class D in pregnancy due to concerns for developmental bone issues, teeth staining, and teratogenicity.[57,62] These effects have not been shown with doxycycline in two review articles which succinctly summarize the current state of the literature on the matter.[57,62] Neither article advocates for use in pregnant women but rather calls for a reappraisal of the evidence and softening of the current restrictions. We still advise our patients of childbearing age to avoid any chance of pregnancy while on minocycline or doxycycline.

Nonantimicrobial effects of the tetracyclines[63,64]

Like macrolides, tetracyclines (especially minocycline and doxycycline) have been shown to have anti-inflammatory and immune-modulating effects. These drugs modify inflammation and immune hyperactivity and have been shown to provide clinical improvement in symptoms in patients with treatment-resistant rheumatoid arthritis.[65–67]

Doxycycline can inhibit matrix metalloproteinases which break down tissue matrices.[68,69] Minocycline has been shown to decrease excitotoxicity in microglial cells and has been studied in experimental models of autoimmune encephalitis.[70,71] The use of minocycline in patients with active relapsing remitting multiple sclerosis was associated with reduced gadolinium activity on MRI, greatly reduced relapse rates over the monitoring period, and decreased matrix metalloproteinase 9 (MMP-9) levels.[72]

Doxycycline has been shown to reduce

> Doxycycline has been shown to reduce microglial activation through the inhibition of NFκB nuclear translocation.

microglial activation through the inhibition of NFκB nuclear translocation.[73] It also reduces the production of reactive oxygen species and reduces proinflammatory cytokines (TNF-α and IL-1β).[74] In animal models, doxycycline can reduce the progression and severity in neurodegenerative diseases such as Parkinson's disease and Alzheimer's.[74,75]

Herbals

The work of Dr. Stephen Buhner contains a wealth of knowledge about effective herbs for *Mycoplasma* and other infectious diseases, and contains much of the basic science about cytokines and immune alteration from *Mycoplasma*.[76]

Based upon this work, as well as other independent research, we use several herbal products to help eradicate *Mycoplasma*. Antibiotics seldom affect antibody levels. Clinical improvement is enhanced by adding herbals to traditional antimicrobials.

We use a combination product which contains *Isatis*, *Cordyceps*, *Houttuynia*, *Scutteraria*, cat's claw, *Sida acuta*, *Uva-ursi*, and *Stillingia*. It is made by by Researched Nutritionals, and it does have a strong taste. If children are more sensitive to taste, herbal products from Beyond Balance such as ENL-MC are preferable.

IVIG

In addition to its immunomodulatory effects, IVIG also has antibacterial and antiviral properties. One in vitro study demonstrated that five commercial IVIG preparations had high levels of antibody activity against *Mycoplasma*.[38,77] An example of IVIG orders, helpful tips for getting IVIG approved, and a sample appeal letter for IVIG can be found in Appendix E.

CHLAMYDIA PNEUMONIAE

Treatment approaches targeted at *Mycoplasma* species (antibiotics and herbals) are also effective against *Chlamydia pneumoniae*. Some research has demonstrated links between *Chlamydia pneumoniae* and dementia.[78] This organism also causes neuroinflammation. Commercial preparations of IVIG have also been shown to have high activity against *C. pneumoniae*.[77]

TOXOPLASMOSIS

In Chapter 8, we presented the evidence for toxoplasmosis as a trigger for neuropsychiatric syndromes. There are two case reports of children who had presentations of sudden onset OCD in the setting of positive titers for *Toxoplasma gondii*.[79] Both children in this report improved with antimicrobial treatment with trimethoprim/sulfamethoxazole.

Cases of acute, severe toxoplasmosis may be referred to infectious disease. Patients with positive titers who have PANS may respond to antimicrobial herbs.

EPSTEIN-BARR VIRUS (EBV)

We typically use a product called IMN-VII from Beyond Balance to treat EBV. Alternatively, if the child can swallow capsules, we may use a combination herbal product containing monolaurin, lysine, olive leaf extract, cinnamon, and bee propolis (see Appendix B).

REDUCING ABNORMAL BACTERIAL PATHOGENS, PARASITES, AND YEAST IN THE GI TRACT

Careful balance of the different species of bacteria in the gut microbiome is essential, as noted in Chapter 7. *Bacterial dysbiosis* is the term which refers to microbial imbalances in the gut. Pathologic bacteria (sometimes referred to as dysbiotic bacteria) can overgrow, lead to inflammation in the gut, and can contribute to immune dysfunction.

As mentioned in Chapter 7, we use a three-day stool test to quantify and speciate stool bacteria. One of the things that this test does is identifies pathologic bacterial overgrowth. If overgrowth of pathogens is found, the test also provides culture and sensitivity results for both antibiotics and for natural substances such as caprylic acid and *Uva ursi*.

We do not use prescription antibiotics in these cases unless something like *C. difficile* is found and the patient is very symptomatic. In most cases, we will use an herbal like ginger, sodium caprylate, oregano, or a combination product. For younger children who do not swallow pills and do not care for the powders mixed in foods (the taste can still be strong), we use products from Beyond Balance such as Pro-Myco.

If we find yeast overgrowth on stool testing or elevated yeast markers on the Metabolomix test from Genova Diagnostics, we treat it with nystatin or herbs (depending on what the sensitivity says on the stool test). We also use Pro-Myco from Beyond Balance in these cases for children unable to swallow pills.

In recent years, many in the online health and wellness space have begun to discuss parasites as a cause of chronic illness. Unfortunately, many of the proponents of this theory do not base their diagnosis on any actual testing. Instead, they tell their clients that if they have any symptoms on a long laundry list (such as grinding their teeth at night), they must have parasites. These practitioners (most without medical training) commonly recommend over-the-counter parasite cleanses.

In contrast, we only treat parasites we find on stool testing. Once we have identified the type of parasite (*Giardia* vs. *Blastocystis*, etc.), we can then decide upon treatment. Prescription treatment ranges from metronidazole to nitazoxanide. We have found Parazomin drops by Beyond Balance particularly helpful for parasites.

CHAPTER 15 REFERENCES

1. Swedo SE, Leonard HL, Mittleman BB, et al. Identification of children with pediatric autoimmune neuropsychiatric disorders associated with streptococcal infections by a marker associated with rheumatic fever. *American Journal of Psychiatry*. 1997;154(1):110–112

2. Kaplan EL, Chhatwal GS, Rohde M. Reduced ability of penicillin to eradicate ingested group A streptococci from epithelial cells: clinical and pathogenetic implications. *Clin Infect Dis*. 2006;43(11):1398–1406

3. Hagman MM, Dale JB, Stevens DL. Comparison of adherence to and penetration of a human laryngeal epithelial cell line by group A streptococci of various M protein types. *FEMS Immunol Med Microbiol*. 1999;23:195–204

4. Stjernquist-Desatnik A, Samuelsson P, Walder M. Penetration of penicillin V to tonsillar surface fluid in healthy individuals and in patients with acute tonsillitis. *J Laryngol Otol*. 1993;107(4):309–312

5. Brook I. Treatment challenges of group A beta-hemolytic streptococcal pharyngo-tonsillitis. *International Archives of Otorhinolaryngology*. 2017;21:286–96

6. Johnson AF, LaRock CN. Antibiotic treatment, mechanisms for failure, and adjunctive therapies for infections by group A *Streptococcus*. *Front Microbiol*. 2021;12:760255:1–9

7. Brook I, Gober AE. Interference by aerobic and anaerobic bacteria in children with recurrent group A beta-hemolytic streptococcal tonsillitis. *Arch Otolaryngol Head Neck Surg*. 1999;125(5): 552–554

8. Brook I. Penicillin failure in the treatment of streptococcal pharyngo-tonsillitis. *Curr Infect Dis Rep*. 2013;15:232–235

9. Di Pierro F, Donato G, Fomia F, et al. Preliminary pediatric clinical evaluation of the oral probiotic *Streptococcus salivarius* K12 in preventing recurrent pharyngitis and/or tonsillitis caused by *Streptococcus pyogenes* and recurrent acute otitis media. *Int J Gen Med*. 2012;5:991–7

10. Di Pierro F, Colombo M, Giuliani MG, et al. Effect of administration of *Streptococcus salivarius* K12 on the occurrence of streptococcal pharyngo-tonsillitis, scarlet fever and acute otitis media in 3 years old children. *Eur Rev Med Pharmacol Sci*. 2016;20(21):4601–4606

11. Burton JP, Wescombe PA, Moore CJ, Chilcott CN, Tagg JR. Safety assessment of the oral cavity probiotic *Streptococcus salivarius* K12. *Appl Environ Microbiol*. 2006;72(4):3050–3

12. Bidossi A, De Grandi R, Toscano M, Bottagisio M, De Vecchi E, Gelardi M, Drago L. Probiotics *Streptococcus salivarius* 24SMB and *Streptococcus oralis* 89a interfere with biofilm formation of pathogens of the upper respiratory tract. *BMC Infect Dis*. 2018;18(1):653:1–19

13. Kaci G, Goudercourt D, Dennin V, et al. Anti-inflammatory properties of Streptococcus salivarius, a commensal bacterium of the oral cavity and digestive tract. *Appl Environ Microbiol*. 2014;80(3):928–34

14. MacDonald KW, Chanyi RM, Macklaim JM, et al. *Streptococcus salivarius* inhibits immune activation by periodontal disease pathogens. *BMC Oral Health*. 2021;21(1):245:1–22

15. Di Pierro F, Iqtadar S, Mumtaz SU, et al. Clinical effects of *Streptococcus salivarius* K12 in hospitalized COVID-19 patients: results of a preliminary study. *Microorganisms*. 2022;10(10):1926:1–13

16. Brook I, Gober AE. Long-term effects on the nasopharyngeal flora of children following antimicrobial therapy of acute otitis media with cefdinir or amoxicillin-clavulanate. *J Med Microbiol*. 2005;54(Pt 6):553–556

17. www.cdc.gov/drugresistance/pdf/threats-report/gas-508.pdf, accessed 2/11/2023

18. Kost GC, Selvaraj S, Lee YB, et al. Clavulanic acid increases dopamine release in neuronal cells through a mechanism involving enhanced vesicle trafficking. *Neurosci Lett*. 2011;504(2):170–175

19. Anoush M, Pourmansouri Z, Javadi R, et al. Clavulanic acid: a novel potential agent in prevention and treatment of scopolamine-induced Alzheimer's disease. *ACS Omega*. 2022;7(16):13861–13869

20. Huh Y, Ju MS, Park H, et al. Clavulanic acid protects neurons in pharmacological models of neurodegenerative diseases. *Drug Development Research*. 2010;71(6):351–7

21. Cooperstock MS, Swedo SE, Pasternack MS, et al. Clinical management of pediatric acute-onset neuropsychiatric syndrome: part III: treatment and prevention of infections. *J Child Adolesc Psychopharmacol*. 2017;27(7):594–606

22. Mitchell RB, Archer SM, Ishman SL, et al. Clinical practice guideline: tonsillectomy in children (update): executive summary. *Otolaryngol Head Neck Surg*. 2019;160(2):187–205

23. Morad A, Sathe NA, Francis DO, et al. Tonsillectomy versus watchful waiting for recurrent throat infection: a systematic review. *Pediatrics*. 2017;139(2):e20163490:1–11

24. Orvidas LJ, St Sauver JL, Weaver AL. Efficacy of tonsillectomy in treatment of recurrent group A beta-hemolytic streptococcal pharyngitis. *Laryngoscope*. 2006;116(11):1946–50

25. Demesh D, Virbalas JM, Bent JP. The role of tonsillectomy in the treatment of pediatric autoimmune neuropsychiatric disorders associated with streptococcal infections (PANDAS). *JAMA Otolaryngology: Head & Neck Surgery*. 2015;141(3):272–5

26. Pavone P, Rapisarda V, Serra A, et al. Pediatric autoimmune neuropsychiatric disorder associated with group a streptococcal infection: the role of surgical treatment. *Int J Immunopathol Pharmacol*. 2014;27(3):371–8

27. Windfuhr JP. Tonsillectomy remains a questionable option for pediatric autoimmune neuropsychiatric disorders associated with streptococcal infections (PANDAS). *GMS Curr Top Otorhinolaryngol Head Neck Surg.* 2016 Dec 15;15:Doc07:1–10

28. Rajgor AD, Hakim NA, Ali S, et al. Paediatric autoimmune neuropsychiatric disorder associated with group a beta-haemolytic streptococcal infection: an indication for tonsillectomy? A review of the literature. *Int J Otolaryngol.* 2018;2018:2681304:1–11

29. Prasad N, Johng S, Powell D, et al. Role of tonsillectomy and adenoidectomy in parental satisfaction of treatments for PANDAS. *American Journal of Otolaryngology.* 2021;42(4):102963:1–7

30. Brandtzaeg P. Immunology of tonsils and adenoids: everything the ENT surgeon needs to know. *Int J Pediatr Otorhinolaryngol.* 2003;67 Suppl 1:S69–76

31. Kato A, Hulse KE, Tan BK, Schleimer RP. B-lymphocyte lineage cells and the respiratory system. *J Allergy Clin Immunol.* 2013;131(4):933–57

32. Byars SG, Stearns SC, Boomsma JJ. Association of long-term risk of respiratory, allergic, and infectious diseases with removal of adenoids and tonsils in childhood. *JAMA Otolaryngol Head Neck Surg.* 2018;144(7):594–603

33. Rosenfeld RM. Old Barbers, Young Doctors, and Tonsillectomy. *JAMA Otolaryngol Head Neck Surg.* 2018;144(7):603–604

34. Muller N, Riedel M, Forderreuther S, Blendinger C, AbeleHorn M. Tourette's syndrome and *Mycoplasma pneumoniae* infection [letter]. *American Journal of Psychiatry.* 2000;157:481–482

35. Müller N, Riedel M, Blendinger C, et al. *Mycoplasma pneumoniae* infection and Tourette's syndrome. *Psychiatry Research.* 2004;129(2):119–125

36. Ercan TE, Ercan G, Severge B, et al. *Mycoplasma pneumoniae* infection and obsessive-compulsive disease: a case report. *Journal of Child Neurology.* 2008;23(3):338–340

37. Nicolson, G. Pathogenic *Mycoplasma* Infections in chronic illnesses: general considerations in selecting conventional and integrative treatments. *International Journal of Clinical Medicine.* 2019;10:477–522

38. Barile MF. *Mycoplasma*-tissue cell interactions. In Tully JG and Whitcomb, editors. *Mycoplasmas II: Human and Animal Mycoplasmas.* Volume 2. Academic Press. New York, NY. 1979:425–474

39. Jacobs E, Bartl A, Oberle K, Schiltz E. Molecular mimicry by *Mycoplasma pneumoniae* to evade the induction of adherence inhibiting antibodies. *J Med Microbiol.* 1995;43(6):422–9

40. Waites KB, Talkington DF. *Mycoplasma pneumoniae* and its role as a human pathogen. *Clinical Microbiology Reviews.* 2004;17(4):697–728

41. Holzman RS, Simberkoff MS, Leaf HL. *Mycoplasma pneumoniae* and atypical pneumonia. In Bennet JE, Dolin R, Blaser MJ, editors. *Principles and Practice of Infectious Diseases.* Volume 2. 9th ed. Elsevier, Philadelphia, PA; 2020:2338

42. Fohner AE, Sparreboom A, Altman RB, et al. PharmGKB summary: macrolide antibiotic pathway, pharmacokinetics/pharmacodynamics. *Pharmacogenet Genomics.* 2017;27(4):164–167

43. Ray WA, Murray KT, Hall K, et al. Azithromycin and the risk of cardiovascular death. *N Engl J Med.* 2012;366(20):1881–90

44. Svanström H, Pasternak B, Hviid A. Use of azithromycin and death from cardiovascular causes. *N Engl J Med.* 2013;368(18):1704–12

45. Almalki ZS, Guo JJ. Cardiovascular events and safety outcomes associated with azithromycin therapy: a meta-analysis of randomized controlled trials. *Am Health Drug Benefits.* 2014;7(6):318–28

46. Hancox JC, Hasnain M, Vieweg WV, et al. Azithromycin, cardiovascular risks, QTc interval prolongation, torsade de pointes, and regulatory issues: a narrative review based on the study of case reports. *Ther Adv Infect Dis*. 2013;1(5):155–65

47. Ohara H, Nakamura Y, Watanabe Y, et al. Azithromycin can prolong QT Interval and suppress ventricular contraction, but will not induce torsade de pointes. *Cardiovasc Toxicol*. 2015;15(3):232–40

48. King GS, Goyal A, Grigorova Y, et al. Antiarrhythmic Medications. 2022 Aug 18. In *StatPearls* [Internet]. Treasure Island (FL): StatPearls Publishing; 2022 Jan

49. www.accessdata.fda.gov/drugsatfda_docs/label/2013/050710s039,050711s036,050784s023lbl.pdf, accessed 2/22/2023

50. Zarogoulidis P, Papanas N, Kioumis I, et al. Macrolides: from in vitro anti-inflammatory and immunomodulatory properties to clinical practice in respiratory diseases. *Eur J Clin Pharmacol*. 2012;68(5):479–503

51. Zheng X, Lee S, Selvarangan R, et al. Macrolide-resistant *Mycoplasma pneumoniae*, United States. *Emerging Infectious Diseases*. 2015;21(8):1470

52. Kim K, Jung S, Kim M, et al. Global trends in the proportion of macrolide-resistant *Mycoplasma pneumoniae* infections: a systematic review and meta-analysis. *JAMA network open*. 2022 Jul 1;5(7):e2220949:1–12

53. Lee H, Choi YY, Sohn YJ, et al. Clinical efficacy of doxycycline for treatment of macrolide-resistant *Mycoplasma pneumoniae* pneumonia in children. *Antibiotics*. 2021;10(2):192–203

54. Okada T, Morozumi M, Tajima T, et al. Rapid effectiveness of minocycline or doxycycline against macrolide-resistant *Mycoplasma pneumoniae* infection in a 2011 outbreak among Japanese children. *Clinical Infectious Diseases*. 2012;55(12):1642–9

55. Lung DC, Yip EK, Lam DS, et al. Rapid defervescence after doxycycline treatment of macrolide-resistant *Mycoplasma pneumoniae*–associated community-acquired pneumonia in children. *Pediatric Infectious Disease Journal*. 2013;32(12):1396–9

56. Sánchez AR, Rogers RS 3rd, Sheridan PJ. Tetracycline and other tetracycline-derivative staining of the teeth and oral cavity. *Int J Dermatol*. 2004;43(10):709–15

57. Cross R, Ling C, Day NP, et al. Revisiting doxycycline in pregnancy and early childhood—time to rebuild its reputation? *Expert Opinion on Drug Safety*. 2016;15(3):367–82

58. Volovitz B, Shkap R, Amir J, et al. Absence of tooth staining with doxycycline treatment in young children. *Clinical Pediatrics*. 2007;46(2):121–6

59. Pöyhönen H, Nurmi M, Peltola V, et al. Dental staining after doxycycline use in children. *Journal of Antimicrobial Chemotherapy*. 2017;72(10):2887–90

60. Todd SR, Dahlgren FS, Traeger MS, et al. No visible dental staining in children treated with doxycycline for suspected Rocky Mountain spotted fever. *J Pediatr*. 2015;166(5):1246–51

61. Ayaslioglu E, Erkek E, Oba AA, et al. Doxycycline-induced staining of permanent adult dentition. Aust Dent J. 2005;50(4):273–5

62. Wormser GP, Wormser RP, Strle F, et al. How safe is doxycycline for young children or for pregnant or breastfeeding women? *Diagnostic Microbiology and Infectious Disease*. 2019;93(3):238–42

63. Nelson ML, Levy SB. The history of the tetracyclines. *Annals of the New York Academy of Sciences*. 2011;1241(1):17–32

64. Sapadin AN, Fleischmajer R. Tetracyclines: nonantibiotic properties and their clinical implications. *Journal of the American Academy of Dermatology*. 2006;54(2):258–65

65. Greenwald RA, Golub LM, Lavietes B, et al. Tetracyclines inhibit human synovial collagenase in vivo and in vitro. *J Rheumatol*. 1987;14(1):28–32

66. Langevitz P, Bank I, Zemer D, et al. Treatment of resistant rheumatoid arthritis with minocycline: an open study. *J Rheumatol*. 1992;19(10):1502–4

67. Tilley BC, Alarcon GS, Heyse SP, et al. Minocycline in rheumatoid arthritis: a 48-week, double-blind, placebo-controlled trial. *Annals of Internal Medicine*. 1995;122:81–89

68. Griffin MO, Fricovsky E, Ceballos G, et al. Tetracyclines: a pleitropic family of compounds with promising therapeutic properties: review of the literature. *Am J Physiol Cell Physiol*. 2010 Sep;299(3):C539–48

69. Curci JA, Mao D, Bohner DG, et al. Preoperative treatment with doxycycline reduces aortic wall expression and activation of matrix metalloproteinases in patients with abdominal aortic aneurysms. *J Vasc Surg*. 2000;31(2):325–42

70. Tikka T, Fiebich BL, Goldsteins G, et al. Minocycline, a tetracycline derivative, is neuroprotective against excitotoxicity by inhibiting activation and proliferation of microglia. *J Neurosci*. 2001 Apr 15;21(8):2580–8

71. Nessler S, Dodel R, Bittner A, et al. Effect of minocycline in experimental autoimmune encephalomyelitis. *Ann Neurol*. 2002 Nov;52(5):689–90

72. Zabad RK, Metz LM, Todoruk TR, Zhang Y, Mitchell JR, Yeung M, Patry DG, Bell RB, Yong VW.et al. The clinical response to minocycline in multiple sclerosis is accompanied by beneficial immune changes: a pilot study. *Mult Scler*. 2007;13(4):517–26

73. Santa-Cecília FV, Socias B, Ouidja MO, et al. Doxycycline suppresses microglial activation by inhibiting the p38 MAPK and NF-kB signaling pathways. *Neurotoxicity Research*. 2016;29:447–59

74. Santa-Cecília FV, Leite CA, Del-Bel E, et al. The neuroprotective effect of doxycycline on neurodegenerative diseases. *Neurotoxicity Research*. 2019;35:981–6

75. Balducci C, Santamaria G, La Vitola P, et al. Doxycycline counteracts neuroinflammation restoring memory in Alzheimer's disease mouse models. *Neurobiology of Aging*. 2018;70:128–39

76. Buhner SH. *Healing Lyme Disease Coinfections: Complementary and Holistic Treatments for Bartonella and Mycoplasma*. Simon and Schuster. Rochester, VT. 2013

77. Krause I, Wu R, Sherer Y, et al. In vitro antiviral and antibacterial activity of commercial intravenous immunoglobulin preparations: a potential role for adjuvant intravenous immunoglobulin therapy in infectious diseases. *Transfus Med*. 2002;12(2):133–9

78. Balin BJ, Hammond CJ, Little CS, et al. Chlamydia pneumoniae: an etiologic agent for late-onset dementia. *Frontiers in Aging Neuroscience*. 2018;10:302

79. Brynska A, Tomaszewicz-Libudzic E, Wolanczyk T. Obsessive-compulsive disorder and acquired toxoplasmosis in two children. *Eur Child Adolesc Psychiatry*. 2001;10(3):200–4

TREATING TICK-BORNE INFECTIONS

What sense would it make or what would it benefit a physician if he discovered the origin of the diseases but could not cure or alleviate them?
~ **PARACELSUS**

KEY POINTS

▸ Tick-borne infections are best treated with a combination of prescription antimicrobials, herbs, and biofilm-disrupting agents

▸ Prolonged courses of antibiotics may be needed to eradicate persister organisms

The link between tick-borne illness (Lyme and coinfections) and PANS is detailed in Chapter 9. In this chapter, we will discuss effective antimicrobial strategies to REDUCE or eliminate tick-borne illnesses.

Lyme disease

The current CDC treatment guidelines[1] for Lyme disease are broken down into just four disease presentations:

1. Erythema migrans
2. Neurologic Lyme disease
3. Lyme carditis
4. Lyme arthritis

For erythema migrans, the options listed are either oral doxycycline or amoxicillin or cefuroxime for 10–14 days in children or adults. For neurologic Lyme disease (facial palsy, radiculoneuritis, or meningitis), the CDC recommends oral doxycycline or IV ceftriaxone for 14–21 days for adults or children. For Lyme carditis, oral doxycycline or amoxicillin or cefuroxime are recommended. Intravenous ceftriaxone is recommended for more severe cases such as patients with third-degree AV block. The treatment duration for Lyme carditis is also listed as 14–21 days for adults and children. Finally, for Lyme arthritis, the CDC recommends either oral doxycycline or amoxicillin or cefuroxime for twenty-eight days for adults and children. For recurrent Lyme arthritis after the initial course of antibiotics, IV ceftriaxone is recommended.

The problem with these limited guidelines is threefold. First, these four categories fail to account for other presentations of Lyme disease (including PANS). There is an extensive discussion of neuroborreliosis in Chapter 9 which outlines the multitude of neuropsychiatric signs and symptoms seen in this disorder, including encephalitis, myelitis, and cognitive impairment. MRI and SPECT scan lesions have been seen in patients with neuroborreliosis, which underscores the ability of *Borrelia* to affect the CNS. Presentations that mimic multiple sclerosis, ALS, or cerebral infarction have also been seen.

The second issue with current guidelines is that recommended antibiotic regimens are based upon treatments targeted at planktonic growth and fail to account for the fact that *Borrelia burgdorferi* is a biofilm producer.[2–4] As noted in Chapter 14, biofilms protect the organisms from host immune identification and clearance and also protect the

> 10–20% of patients with Lyme disease experience ongoing symptoms following the traditional 2–4 week treatment course.

organism from antibiotic therapy. Short courses of antibiotics *may* work for erythema migrans, but Lyme is seldom caught that early. Biofilm disruption is essential (see our approach in the following pages).

Finally, clinical experience with many patients in our practice and many of our colleagues' patients with tick-borne illnesses has shown that short courses of antibiotics (less than two months) are rarely successful in long-term erad-ication. This is likely responsible for the fact that 10–20% of patients with Lyme disease experi-ence ongoing symptoms following the traditional 2–4 week treatment course.[5,6] This leads to significantly increased healthcare expenditures.[7] Studies in nonhuman primates, dogs, and mice have shown that Lyme organisms can persist after antibiotic treatment.[8–10]

OUR APPROACH

Once we have educated the parents and/or patients on the natural history of Lyme disease as well as the pertinent medical literature concerning its proper diagnosis and treatment, we typically treat as follows.

Antibiotics

For confirmed cases of Lyme disease, we use an initial 2–3-month course of antibiotics. We prefer to use doxycycline or azithromycin. Alternatively, amoxicillin may be used. We have not had to use IV antibiotics for children with PANS due to Lyme disease. In addition, we seldom use more than one prescription antimicrobial agent concomitantly.

Herbals

Herbal medications have been used for thou-sands of years for various human maladies to help with symptoms and to cure disease. Many drugs we use every day are made from plants, including atropine, L-Dopa, digoxin, ephedrine, morphine, scopolamine, and several chemother-apeutic agents. In the field of integrative medi-cine, herbal medications and extracts are used for a wide range of indications.

There are many natural substances which have been anecdotally reported to improve symp-toms in patients with Lyme disease. In 2020,

Feng et al. published the results of an excellent in vitro study which investigated the efficacy of twelve natural compounds against both active and stationary forms of *Borrelia*.[11]

The study showed that *Cryptolepis sanguino-lenta*, *Juglans nigra* (black walnut), *Polygonum cuspidatum* (Japanese knotweed), *Artemisia annua* (sweet wormwood), *Uncaria tomentosa* (cat's claw), *Cistus incanus*, and *Scutellaria baicalensis* (Chinese skullcap) had good activity against stationary-phase *Borrelia*.

Further, *Cryptolepis sanguinolenta* and *Polygonum cuspidatum* had strong activity against both active and stationary forms. Unlike doxycycline, cefuroxime, and other active herbs, *Cryptolepis* resulted in complete eradication of the spirochete. The other herbs and antibiotics could not eradicate stationary *Borrelia*, and many spirochetes were seen after a twenty-one-day culture process. In this study, *Stevia rebaudiana*, *Andrographis paniculata*, grapefruit seed extract, colloidal silver, and monolaurin had little effect.

This article provides quite a bit of addi-tional basic science data concerning Lyme and immune/inflammation changes for each of the herbs discussed. Although this was an in vitro study, it is unlikely that a large in vivo study will ever be funded. For this reason, the findings of this study, coupled with our clinical experience, has allowed us to affirm the usefulness of herbs as an adjunctive therapy for patients with tick-borne illness (and a primary therapy in patients who may refuse antibiotics).

Master herbalist and physician Dr. Stephen Buhner recommends a similar group of herbs for Lyme disease, including *Cryptolepis sanguinolenta*, *Polygonum cuspidatum* (Japanese knotweed), and *Uncaria tomentosa* (cat's claw).[12] He also adds

Cordyceps, *Withania somnifera*, and *Eleutherococcus senticosus* for immune modulation.

We typically use *Cryptolepis* extract along with a combination product which includes *Uncaria tomentosa* (cat's claw), *Polygonum cuspidatum* (Japanese knotweed), and *Artemisia annua* (sweet wormwood). In younger children,

> Treatment failures in cases of *Bartonella* occur despite low MICs for antibiotics, suggesting persistence, likely due to both biofilms and the intracellular nature of this organism.

we often use Beyond Balance herbal products, particularly MC-BAR-2.

Biofilms

For biofilms, we use combination enzyme preparations (capsules or chewables) containing various proteases, bromelain, papain, lipase, and sometimes serrapeptase.

BORRELIA MIYAMOTOI

Borrelia miyamotoi and similar organisms from the relapsing fever group are susceptible to the same antibiotics and herbals as *Borrelia burgdorferi* but do seem to be more responsive to herbals than antibiotics alone. Herbal and biofilm treatments are identical to those used for Lyme.

BARTONELLA HENSELAE

The current recommendation for treatment of *Bartonella henselae* according to the CDC is just five days of azithromycin.[13] *Bartonella spp.*, however, are intracellular (intraerythrocytic) organisms and exist within a biofilm which helps them evade host cell immune responses.[14–17] Treatment failures in cases of *Bartonella* occur despite low MICs for antibiotics, suggesting persistence, likely due to both biofilms and the intracellular nature of this organism.[14]

This may be the reason that infections can be persistent despite prolonged courses of antibiotics. An in vitro study by Zheng et al. demonstrated that combinations of antibiotics were required to eliminate stationary-phase and biofilm *Bartonella*.[14] In this study, oral azithromycin plus oral methylene blue or oral rifampin plus oral methylene blue were effective at achieving these goals. Oral doxycycline and rifampin may also be effective. Oral methylene blue must be obtained from a compounding pharmacy.

Although combinations of antibiotics are sometimes required for adults, children typically respond well to a single antibiotic (azithromycin or doxycycline) plus herbals.

Herbals

A 2020 article out of Johns Hopkins found that *Cryptolepis sanguinolenta*, *Juglans nigra*, and *Polygonum cuspidatum* could eradicate all stationary-phase *B. henselae* cells in vitro and were also active against log-phase growing *Bartonella henselae*.[18] We typically use a combination product. For smaller children or those who cannot take the flavor of alcohol-based tinctures, we recommend MC-BAR2 from Beyond Balance.

Biofilms

For biofilms, we use combination enzyme preparations (capsules or chewables) containing various proteases, bromelain, papain, lipase, and sometimes serrapeptase.

BABESIA SPECIES

The CDC-recommended treatments for *Babesia* are either oral atovaquone (an antimalarial) and azithromycin or oral clindamycin and quinine.[19] The treatment duration for "ill patients" is

> **Patients with multiple tick-borne infections (which is increasingly common) may also require a longer course of therapy.**

listed as 7–10 days. The guideline also states that no treatment is needed if patients have no symptoms.

The issue is that *Babesia* species are intracellular malaria-like organisms. Asymptomatic parasitemia can persist without treatment for months to over two years while PCR may detect *Babesia* DNA for an average of eighty-two days.[20] Even in patients who receive appropriate antibiotic treatment, parasitemia can persist for over two years.[20] A case report from Spain describes a patient who had persistent severe anemia despite treatment with clindamycin and quinine and relapsed after eighteen days, requiring atovaquone/ proguanil and azithromycin.[21] *Babesia*

species also lead to worse outcomes in people who are immunocompromised.[22]

This is a concern in patients with PANS and PANDAS as they typically have immune dysregulation with a component of immune deficiency. An in vitro study of *Babesia duncani* showed low susceptibility to the four drugs recommended for treatment of human babesiosis, atovaquone, azithromycin, clindamycin, and quinine.[23] Patients with multiple tick-borne infections (which is increasingly common) may also require a longer course of therapy.[24]

In our practice, we use azithromycin (or doxycycline) and herbs for children with *Babesia microti* or *Babesia duncani*. In severe cases, we may use atovaquone with one of these other antibiotics, although this is not usually needed if herbs are used.

Herbals

A 2022 article out of Johns Hopkins found that *Cryptolepis sanguinolenta*, *Artemisia annua*, *Scuttelaria baicalensis*, *Alchornea cordifolia*, and *Polygonum cuspidatum* had good in vitro activity against *Babesia duncani*.[24] We typically use a combination product. For smaller children or those who cannot take the flavor of alcohol-based tinctures, we recommend MC-BAR2 from Beyond Balance.

Biofilms

For biofilms, we use combination enzyme preparations (capsules or chewables) containing various proteases, bromelain, papain, lipase, and sometimes serrapeptase.

EHRLICHIA AND *ANAPLASMA*

These two pathogens are rarely seen alone. They are usually coinfections with Lyme. They both respond to four weeks of doxycycline or rifampin. Herbs and biofilm treatments are similar to recommendations for *Bartonella*.

CHAPTER 16 REFERENCES

1. www.cdc.gov/lyme/treatment/index.html, accessed 3/6/2023

2. Di Domenico EG, Cavallo I, Bordignon V, et al. The emerging role of microbial biofilm in lyme neuroborreliosis. *Front Neurol.* 2018;9:1048:1–12

3. Sapi E, Bastian SL, Mpoy CM, et al. Characterization of biofilm formation by *Borrelia burgdorferi* in vitro. *PLoS One.* 2012;7(10):e48277:1–11

4. Feng J, Li T, Yee R, et al, et al. Stationary phase persister/biofilm microcolony of *Borrelia burgdorferi* causes more severe disease in a mouse model of Lyme arthritis: implications for understanding persistence, post-treatment Lyme disease syndrome (PTLDS), and treatment failure. *Discov Med.* 2019;27:125–38

5. Aucott JN. Posttreatment Lyme disease syndrome. *Infect Dis Clin North Am.* 2015;29(2):309–23

6. Marques A. Chronic Lyme disease: a review. *Infect Dis Clin North Am.* 2008;22(2):341–60

7. Adrion ER, Aucott J, Lemke KW, et al. Health care costs, utilization and patterns of care following Lyme disease. *PLoS One.* 2015;10:e0116767:1–9

8. Straubinger RK, Summers BA, Chang YF, et al. Persistence of *Borrelia burgdorferi* in experimentally infected dogs after antibiotic treatment. *J Clin Microbiol.* 1997;35:111–6

9. Hodzic E, Imai D, Feng S, et al. Resurgence of persisting non-cultivable *Borrelia burgdorferi* following antibiotic treatment in mice. *PLoS One.* 2014;9:e86907

10. Embers ME, Hasenkampf NR, Jacobs MB, et al. Variable manifestations, diverse seroreactivity and post-treatment persistence in non-human primates exposed to *Borrelia burgdorferi* by tick feeding. *PLoS One.* (2017) 12:e0189071

11. Feng J, Leone J, Schweig S, et al. Evaluation of natural and botanical medicines for activity against growing and non-growing forms of *B. burgdorferi*. *Front Med* (Lausanne). 2020;7:6:1–14

12. Buhner SH. *Healing Lyme: Natural Healing of Lyme Borreliosis and the Coinfections Chlamydia and Spotted Fever Rickettsioses*. Raven Press. Boulder, CO. 2015:208–237

13. www.cdc.gov/bartonella/bartonella-henselae/index.html, accessed 3/8/2023

14. Zheng X, Ma X, Li T, et al. Effect of different drugs and drug combinations on killing stationary phase and biofilms recovered cells of *Bartonella henselae* in vitro. *BMC Microbiol.* 2020;20(1):87:1–9

15. Schülein R, Seubert A, Gille C, et al. Invasion and persistent intracellular colonization of erythrocytes: a unique parasitic strategy of the emerging pathogen *Bartonella*. *J Exp Med.* 2001;193(9):1077–86

16. Seubert A, Schulein R, Dehio C. Bacterial persistence within erythrocytes: a unique pathogenic strategy of *Bartonella spp*. *Int J Med Microbiol.* 2002;291(6–7):555–60

17. Okaro U, George S, Anderson B. What is in a cat scratch? Growth of *Bartonella henselae* in a biofilm. *Microorganisms.* 2021;9(4):835:1–14

18. Ma X, Leone J, Schweig S, et al. Botanical medicines with activity against stationary phase *Bartonella henselae*. *bioRxiv*. 2020;08(19)256768:1–28

19. www.cdc.gov/parasites/babesiosis/health_professionals/index.html#tx, accessed 3/9/2023

20. Krause PJ, Spielman A, Telford SR 3rd, et al. Persistent parasitemia after acute babesiosis. *N Engl J Med*. 1998;339(3):160–5

21. Gonzalez LM, Rojo S, Gonzalez-Camacho F, et al. Severe babesiosis in immunocompetent man, Spain, 2011. *Emerg Infect Dis*. 2014;20(4):724–6

22. Vannier EG, Diuk-Wasser MA, Ben Mamoun C, et al. Babesiosis. *Infect Dis Clin North Am*. 2015;29(2):357–70

23. Abraham A, Brasov I, Thekkiniath J, et al. Establishment of a continuous *in vitro* culture of *Babesia duncani* in human erythrocytes reveals unusually high tolerance to recommended therapies. *J Biol Chem*. 2018;293(52):19974–19981

24. Zhang Y, Alvarez-Manzo H, Leone J, et al. Botanical Medicines *Cryptolepis sanguinolenta*, *Artemisia annua*, *Scutellaria baicalensis*, *Polygonum cuspidatum*, and *Alchornea cordifolia* demonstrate inhibitory activity against *Babesia duncani*. *Front Cell Infect Microbiol*. 2021;11:624745:1–15

OPTIMIZING DETOXIFICATION

Does it follow that because there are poisonous toadstools which resemble mushrooms, both are dangerous?
~ MARIANNE MOORE

KEY POINTS

▸ Individual genetic differences may affect biotransformation of drugs, toxins, toxicants, and natural metabolites in the body
▸ Some toxins can inhibit the removal of other toxins in the body
▸ Some natural agents can upregulate phase I and phase II biotransformation
▸ Glutathione and N-acetyl cysteine are important in the process of conjugation of toxins and toxicants
▸ Elimination of the end products of biotransformation is as important as phase I and phase II reactions
▸ Sequestrants and cholagogues improve elimination of toxins and toxicants
▸ Activated charcoal, zeolite, and fulvic and humic acids are examples of clinically useful sequestrants
▸ Photobiomodulation, infrared sauna, and lymphatic drainage are useful adjuncts to support elimination
▸ Maintenance of normal bowel movements is important to prevent enterohepatic reabsorption of toxins and toxicants

The third pillar of the Fully Functional process is OPTIMIZE detoxification. As physicians, when we hear the words *detox* or *detoxification,* we often think of drug and alcohol addiction. Those of us who work in emergency medicine and the critical care setting may also deal with iatrogenic poisonings (digoxin or lithium toxicity) or "voluntary toxicity" (alcohol and drug use or suicide attempts).

When we hear about detox in the context of everyday living, we may envision some type of green powder you can purchase on the internet and put in a drink. As physicians committed to science, this topic deserves a much closer look. Dismissing a topic or intervention solely because nonmedical people advocate for it may result in withholding potentially life-changing treatments from patients most in need.

As mentioned in Chapter 5, we are all exposed to toxins and toxicants every day through food, water, air, and skin. In addition, stress can best be thought of as a mental toxin. We are very fortu-

detoxification, as it is the preferred term in the published literature. Biotransformation occurs primarily in hepatocytes and has three phases. Although these phases are named phase I, phase II, and phase III, they don't always occur in numerical sequence. Occasionally they go in reverse order, the process occurs all at once, or steps may be skipped.

Phase I biotransformation occurs in the liver and takes place when compounds are converted to more polar, aqueous compounds. Many compounds are still active after phase I biotransformation. The chemical processes involved in

> If a CYP enzyme is inhibited, a drug or substance may be metabolized more slowly, and blood levels of a substance may be increased. If a phase I metabolite is an active toxic metabolite, induction could lead to increased toxicity.

nate that our bodies were designed with efficient and elegant mechanisms for detoxification. We are all natural detoxifiers as we sweat, urinate, and defecate to remove toxins from our bodies.

The conversion of substances (called substrates) in the body to intermediate forms to get them ready for elimination through sweat, feces, urine, and respiration is called *biotransformation.* This is, perhaps, a better term than

phase I biotransformation include reduction, hydrolysis, or most commonly oxidation via the cytochrome P450 (CYP450) enzyme system. There are many versions of CYP450 enzymes. Each of the different enzymes have different affinities for substrates and can be induced (to be more active) or inhibited (to be less active) by different chemicals, herbs, or drugs. If induction occurs, a drug or substance may be metabolized more quickly, and the blood levels of a substance may be decreased. This could result in subtherapeutic blood levels. If a CYP enzyme is inhibited, a drug or substance may be metabolized more slowly, and blood levels of a substance may be increased. If a phase I metabolite is an active toxic metabolite, induction could lead to increased toxicity.[1,2] This is particularly true for the wide array of man-made chemicals (toxicants) that we were never designed to metabolize.

The CYP enzymes have a particular nomenclature; they all start with the letters *CYP*, followed by letters and numbers. Examples are CYP1B1, CYP2A6, etc. The enzyme CYP3A4 is the most abundant enzyme, accounting for about half of all CYP enzyme reactions.[1] Some of the variation in enzyme activities can be explained by genetic mutations in the DNA which codes for the enzymes.

Phase II reactions also occur in the liver. In phase II, endogenous hydrophilic groups are added to either the original substance or to the intermediate compounds produced after phase I. This process is called *conjugation*. The conjugation processes are named according to what chemical groups are involved. The processes include sulfation, acetylation, glucuronidation (most common), methylation, conjugation with glutathione, and conjugation with amino acids (such as taurine, glycine, or glutamic acid). Phase II of biotransformation aims to produce a water-soluble compound that is ready for excretion from the body.

Phase III reactions involve transporter molecules and diffusion of compounds across membranes. It occurs both before phase I and after phase II. It is involved with transporting compounds into the blood or into the bile for elimination after phase II conjugation. The system involves hepatic efflux pumps. We will mainly discuss phase I and phase II biotransformation here.

> Many drugs can induce or inhibit CYP enzymes.

Drug interactions

Many drugs can induce or inhibit CYP enzymes. If this occurs to a significant degree, it can cause the levels of concomitantly administered drugs to either become supratherapeutic or subtherapeutic. It's always best to check for medication interactions when patients are on more than one prescription medication or when we are adding more than one medication to a treatment plan. This may change the treatment plan.

Programs like Epocrates (www.epocrates.com) enable physicians to enter patient medications and check for interactions. This site lists both serious and minor interactions. The program also has information on common dosage, pricing, available dosage forms, and pregnancy/lactation information.

Pharmacogenomic testing

In addition to genetic testing for interactions, more sophisticated testing has become available in the last ten years. This testing, known as *pharmacogenomics*, uses genetic testing for DNA differences called single nucleotide polymorphisms (also known as SNPs—pronounced "snips"). This information can help predict individual response to drugs and may help predict adverse drug effects. This testing is widely available and useful for warfarin, clopidogrel, statins, codeine, and some psychotropic drugs.[3]

In the right clinical context, these tests can be very helpful. The genomic testing may predict which drugs might accumulate at higher levels, which can then increase the chance of adverse effects.[3] There are also genomic tests that can predict better patient response to SSRIs in major depression.[4]

We don't currently use pharmacogenomic testing in our patients since we focus on discontinuing psychotropic medications as soon as possible. One drawback of pharmacogenomic testing is that some clinicians perform these tests and tell patients that the results can tell them which drugs are "bad for them." This is not an accurate representation of what the tests show. In addition, there can be factors which alter gene expression (the difference between genotype and phenotype). Genetic tests predict increased risk alone, so the results are not the end all and be all of prescribing. Finally, most drugs also undergo phase II biotransformation, which can be upregulated and downregulated by various factors or deficiencies. SNP testing does not provide any useful information about phase II biotransformation.

Some CYP genetic polymorphisms (SNPs) have been shown to be associated with increased cancer risk and poor response to environmental toxins.[5]

COMPOUNDS INHIBITING TOXIN EXCRETION

Just as medications may compete for biotransformation pathways and affect the absorption or efficacy of other drugs, toxins or toxic drug metabolites may do the same thing. This may lead to a buildup of drug metabolites, environmental toxins, or injurious endogenous compounds.

The classic example of this is acetaminophen toxicity. Acetaminophen is normally metabolized in the liver in phase II biotransformation through glucuronidation and sulfation. When the drug is taken in an acute overdose, these pathways are saturated, and more acetaminophen is subsequently metabolized by CYP450 enzymes to a compound called NAPQI.

NAPQI is a toxic substance that is safely reduced by glutathione to nontoxic compounds, which are then renally excreted. An acute over-

> Most drugs also undergo phase II biotransformation, which can be upregulated and downregulated by various factors or deficiencies.

dose depletes the stores of glutathione. The NAPQI levels then increase and subsequently bind to hepatic macromolecules, causing irreversible hepatic necrosis. Repletion of glutathione stores by giving IV N-acetylcysteine (one of the building blocks of glutathione) prevents this from happening. In addition to helping upregulate glutathione production, NAC may also bind directly to NAPQI to prevent damage. More on glutathione and NAC to come.

Studies have demonstrated that environmental toxins such as pesticides inhibit the metabolism of other environmental toxins.[6] The same studies have found that organophosphates are potent irreversible inhibitors of testosterone metabolism by cytochrome P3A4, and of estradiol metabolism by CYP3A4 and CYP1A2 enzymes.[6]

Mycotoxins also alter hepatic biotransformation pathways. An animal study showed that the mycotoxins T-2 (a trichothecene) and zearalenone inhibited drug biotransformation (in this case midazolam) by the CYP3A enzyme.[7] Hence pesticides and mycotoxins are toxic compounds which prohibit the removal of other toxic compounds or drug metabolites.

NUTRITIONAL REGULATION OF BIOTRANSFORMATION

Like medication, food can also alter drug biotransformation. The classic case most of us are familiar with is grapefruit juice. Grapefruit juice can block (or inhibit) phase I biotransformation of some drugs through the CYP3A4 pathway. This can lead to increased blood levels of statin drugs, calcium channel blockers, or warfarin. It can also block the transport of some drugs that can decrease blood levels, like fexofenadine.

> Organophosphates are potent irreversible inhibitors of testosterone metabolism by cytochrome P3A4, and of estradiol metabolism by CYP3A4 and CYP1A2 enzymes.

In addition to grapefruit juice, other foods and supplements can induce or inhibit CYP-driven metabolism.[8–11] Nutrients are important cofactors for phase II biotransformation. Each of the processes (glucuronidation, sulfation, glutathione conjugation) require specific nutrients or amino acids as fundamental building blocks by which to perform the conjugation.

An excellent review on modulation of metabolic detoxification pathways by foods and food-derived components was published by Hodges and Minich in 2015 in the *Journal of Nutrition and Metabolism*.[12] The article points out that there is quite a bit of basic science research and many in vitro cell studies on this topic, but wider clinical studies may need to be done to further clarify the effects of nutrients or supplements in vivo. Some nutrients/foods can exhibit biphasic, dose-dependent effects. With this caveat, it is worthwhile to provide examples of some of the authors' findings in relation to biotransformation pathway modulation. The salient points are:

- Some biotransformation reactions naturally produce reactive oxygen species, which may lead to oxidative stress if endogenous antioxidant stores are depleted.
- Some CYP enzymes are involved with biotransformation of mycotoxins, like the carcinogenic aflatoxin B1. SNPs here may affect proper biotransformation and elimination.
- Curcumin may upregulate CYP3A4 activity.
- Chronic exposures to high levels of toxins may overwhelm the CYP system. In this case, upregulating phase II biotransformation may help clear out toxins.
- Glutathione is not well absorbed from foods. N-acetylcysteine and curcumin can restore depleted levels.
- Nuclear factor erythroid 2 (NFE2)-related factor 2 (most often referred to as Nrf2) is key to regulating phase II detoxification and the antioxidant system within the body.

- Nrf2 deficient animals experience increased toxicity from environmental pollutants, drugs, carcinogens, and allergens.
- Nrf2 is protective against many chronic conditions, including neurologic diseases.
- In vivo evidence shows that Nrf2 activity can be increased by curcumin, broccoli, garlic, resveratrol, ginger, coffee, rosemary, blueberry, pomegranate, γ-tocopherol, fish oil, and lycopene.
- Metallothionein can be very helpful in heavy metal detoxification. It also scavenges free radicals and inhibits NFκB signaling.
- Studies have shown that zinc, sulforaphane, quercetin, and the mushroom cordyceps can upregulate metallothionein expression.
- Foods seem to be more effective than individual nutritional supplements.

> **For more information on oxidative stress, see Chapter 12. For information on testing glutathione levels, see Chapter 7.**

Although this is a very technical article, and keeping the inducing and inhibiting effects of the individual nutrients straight can be challenging, the clear takeaway point is that antioxidant-rich whole foods, including vegetables and fruits of all colors, are among the best agents to support healthy biotransformation.

If children are not eating a nutrient dense diet due to eating restriction or if gut absorption is impaired (as in cases of gut inflammation or increased intestinal permeability), supplements are helpful, as larger (concentrated) doses of the nutrients can be used to restore depletions which may affect biotransformation and other key processes within the body such as mitochondrial function.[13,14]

Specific nutraceuticals we use to help improve biotransformation include:

- Antioxidants such as vitamins A, E, and K, CoQ10, and alpha-lipoic acid. These are available in chewable, liquid, and capsule form as supplements. Gummy multivitamins are available, but we prefer to use these as a last resort as they typically contain a lot of sugar.
- Sulforaphane (from broccoli)
- Quercetin
- B vitamins (particularly B6, methyl-B12, and methyl-folate)
- Magnesium
- Milk thistle (*Silybum mariunum*, also called silymarin)—this compound, when taken as a supplement, has been shown to be very helpful at preventing liver injury, increasing antioxidant production, and decreasing lipid peroxidation.[15]

GLUTATHIONE AND N-ACETYLCYSTEINE (NAC)

As previously noted, glutathione (GSH) is a very important antioxidant in the body. Conjugation with glutathione in the liver helps inactivate fat-soluble biotransformation metabolites and endogenous oxidizing agents.[16] Deficiencies of GSH have been implicated in the pathogenesis of neurodegenerative conditions such as Alzheimer's disease and Parkinson's disease.[17–19].

For more information on oxidative stress, see Chapter 12. For information on testing glutathione levels, see Chapter 7.

NAC is one of the building blocks of glutathione. In acetaminophen overdose, IV NAC is given to help replete glutathione and rid the body of toxic metabolites.[20] Early IV NAC treatment of acetaminophen overdose saves patients from liver failure and death by increasing blood glutathione levels and acting as an independent free radical scavenger.

> **Glutathione has a vital role in maintenance of the blood-brain barrier.**

Just as mycotoxins have been shown to inhibit biotransformation through the CYP system,[7] they have also been shown to decrease cellular formation of glutathione.[21] Adequate glutathione stores have been shown to play a significant role in limiting toxicity from ochratoxin (OTX).[22] This toxicity is a result of oxidative stress and the formation of DNA adducts, which accounts for the carcinogenicity of OTX. OTX leads to decreased production of a rate-limiting enzyme in the production of glutathione and also an inhibition of Nrf2 expression, which subsequently reduces glutathione production through other pathways.[22]

As previously noted, mycotoxins are poisons which decrease their own excretion and the excretion of other toxins. Glutathione has a vital role in maintenance of the blood-brain barrier.[23–25] This may explain why mycotoxin exposure is seen almost universally in patients with PANS and PANDAS, during which anti-neuronal antibodies cross the blood-brain barrier. In vitro studies with human epithelial cells have shown that the administration of glutathione can protect cells from mycotoxin-induced injury.[26] Glutathione conjugation (phase II biotransformation) is the most important detoxification step for several mycotoxins, including aflatoxin and patulin.[27,28]

We use both oral liposomal glutathione gel (Tri-Fortify by Researched Nutritionals) and oral L-glutathione capsules (containing Setria glutathione) in children with PANS and PANDAS with mycotoxin exposures and/ or evidence of urine mycotoxins on provoked testing. Although oral glutathione is not well absorbed, these two formulations have been shown in studies to reliably increase serum glutathione levels.[29–30] At times we use oral NAC, which helps increase glutathione levels.[31]

Once phase I and phase II biotransformation have occurred, compounds to be eliminated hepatically are typically excreted in the bile.

ELIMINATION

Once endogenous substrates have undergone biotransformation, they must be eliminated from the body. This occurs via the processes of urination, defecation, and perspiration. If there are issues with any of these processes, the metabolites (which can still carry some toxicity) may build up and affect the health of the patient.

When discussing elimination, the first topic we discuss with parents or patients is the importance of having healthy bowel movements. People should have 1–2 bowel movements of normal size and consistency daily. Frequent bowel movements are necessary to prevent enterohepatic circulation (also called enterohepatic recycling).

When nutrients, medications, toxins, or toxicants are ingested orally, they are transported to the liver from the small intestine. After biotransformation occurs, some metabolites are excreted in the bile into the intestine. If those metabolites get reabsorbed and sent to the liver again, this is known as enterohepatic circulation. This can result in a second peak of the drug concentration and may result in re-exposure to the metabolite in the bloodstream. If the metabolite still carries toxicity, this can cause symptoms. Some toxicants known as persistent organic pollutants (POPs) due to their ability to persist in the environment (and the organism) undergo significant enterohepatic circulation. This is seen with per- and poly-fluoroalkyl substances (PFAS).[32] These toxicants are present in 97% of people tested and have been linked to cancers, obesity, and immune suppression.[33] Heavy metals such as mercury, lead, and cadmium are also subject to enterohepatic circulation.[34–36] Animal studies have shown that T-2 mycotoxins and ochratoxin undergo enterohepatic circulation.[37,38]

CHOLAGOGUES

For thousands of years, people have used plants, plant extracts, and nutrients to improve liver function and decrease digestive symptoms. In addition to potentiating phase I and phase II biotransformation, some of these substances also promote bile acid production. These are called *choloretics*. Other substances which promote bile acid excretion are known as *cholagogues*. In the small intestine, bile acids act as detergents, increase lipid absorption, and aid in nutrient absorption. They also act as natural laxatives.

Plants and plant extracts which have been found to have choleretic actions include *Artemisia*, turmeric, black pepper, chamomile, caffeine, rosemary, dandelion, olive oil, and silymarin.[39] Silibinin (from silymarin) prevents failure of the bile salt export pump.[40] *Artemisia*, a component of traditional bitters, has been found independently to improve digestion and increase vascular tone during digestion.[41]

We encourage the use of olive oil for our patients (while strongly discouraging inflammatory plant oils like canola oil). We use herbal preparations to treat infections that often contain *Artemisia*.

TUDCA

Tauroursodeoxycholic acid (TUDCA) is a taurine conjugate of a bile acid. It is FDA-approved for the treatment of some cholestatic hepatic disorders. It was first used for its choleretic action. TUDCA has been gaining increased interest as both a hepatic protective compound and as an agent which inhibits apoptosis in various tissues by interfering with the mitochondrial pathway of cell death. It does so by inhibiting free radical production and reducing caspase activation, which triggers inflammation and furthers cell death.[42]

There is substantial evidence both in vitro and in animal models showing that TUDCA may be helpful in preventing apoptosis and tissue damage in conditions such as Alzheimer's disease, Parkinson's disease, Huntington's disease, chemotherapy-induced neuropathy, retinitis pigmentosa, age-related macular degeneration, stroke, diabetes, cardiovascular disease, renal injury, glutamate-induced neuroexcitotoxicity, and microglial activation.[42]

TUDCA also helps maintain glutathione levels during periods of oxidative stress.[43] We do not routinely use TUDCA for children in our practice unless they are over twelve and can swallow pills, as there is no palatable liquid form. No risks following TUDCA administration are known. It is likely, however, that TUDCA will soon assume a more prominent role in the treatment of neuro-degenerative disorders.

PHOSPHATIDYLCHOLINE

Phosphatidylcholine (PC) is a phospholipid and is the most ubiquitous constituent of all cell membranes. Toxins and toxicants damage the liver by disrupting the membranes of the hepatic parenchymal cells. Many controlled studies in

the agents we have found to be useful in clinical practice.

Mycotoxins

When patients have had a significant mold exposure and/or elevated urine mycotoxin levels, we begin treatment. As mentioned previously, we start glutathione first. It helps us conjugate mycotoxins and pull them from tissues so that they can be excreted. It also helps increase the yield in urine mycotoxin testing. There are no studies on glutathione provocation and urine testing, but

> Sequestrants are nonabsorbable, orally administered compounds that bind toxins, toxicants, and chemicals which have undergone biotransformation.

animals and humans have shown that oral and IV administration of PC protects the liver against a wide range of toxins, toxicants, and infectious insults.[44] We use oral PC liquid and capsules to support and protect the liver and for their benefits to brain health, which is further discussed in Chapter 18.

SEQUESTRANTS

Sequestrants are nonabsorbable, orally administered compounds that bind toxins, toxicants, and chemicals which have undergone biotransformation. This prevents enterohepatic circulation and thus hastens removal from the body through defecation. Sequestrants are often referred to informally as binders.

In the sections immediately following, we discuss the removal of specific toxins and toxicants that we have found in our patients and

most physicians who order this testing will use glutathione for this purpose. Following glutathione, we add binders.

The first sequestrant compound (binder) noted in the literature was cholestyramine (CSM). CSM is a nonabsorbable, synthetic bile acid resin. It is available in a powder to add to water and was used in the past to lower cholesterol. Its use has largely been curtailed by statins for hypercholesterolemia, as they are much easier to take and associated with fewer GI side effects.

The first recorded use of CSM as a binder of toxic materials appeared in articles in 1978 in both the journal *Science*[45] and the *New England Journal of Medicine*.[46] At this time, it was being investigated as an intervention to help remove an organochlorine insecticide called chlordecone (brand name Kepone) from the body. As detailed in the *New England Journal of Medicine* article,[46] workers from a factory where chlordecone was manufactured were exposed to high levels of the chemical and developed neurologic, hepatic, and reproductive issues.

The neurologic issues noted in these patients were tremor, stuttering speech, opsoclonus, exaggerated startle reflex, visual and auditory hallucinations, anxiety, irritability, short-term memory loss, and headaches. Chlordecone is also carcinogenic. This compound has a long half-life and is excreted in the bile and into the stool. It undergoes significant enterohepatic recirculation, which prolongs toxicity. The study with the exposed workers noted that CSM bound to chlordecone effectively and significantly reduced levels in the body while increasing levels of the toxicant in the stool.

In the late 1980s and early 1990s, additional articles appeared which showed that CSM could bind to *E. coli* and *Vibrio* enterotoxins[47] and could be helpful in diarrhea from relapsing and remitting *C. difficile*.[48]

In 1992, a rat study showed that oral CSM can increase elimination of the mycotoxin ochratoxin A in the stool and significantly lower levels in the systemic circulation.[49] Over the next ten years, multiple animal studies confirmed the ability of CSM to enhance excretion of ochratoxin and prevent kidney injury.[50–52] CSM was also shown to be effective at binding another mycotoxin, zearalenone, in mice.[53] We do not use CSM in our pediatric patients since it is not pleasant to take, and it does not seem to help for all groups

> There are several articles discussing the use of nanotechnologies to prevent the absorption of mycotoxins.

of mycotoxins. It may also deplete the body of lipid-soluble vitamins.

In the late 1990s and early 2000s, articles were published which showed that activated charcoal (sometimes called activated carbon) was effective at binding several groups of mycotoxins in vitro.[54–56] These were animal studies and feed studies. Mycotoxin contamination of animal feed is a significant problem in agriculture. Activated charcoal is used in acute overdose situations in the emergency department.

Various forms of clay (mainly bentonite clay) have also been found to be effective in enhancing the excretion of multiple mycotoxins in vitro and in humans.[57–63] In these studies, the oral administration of clay did not deplete lipid-soluble vitamins in human subjects' serum.[64]

In recent years, articles have investigated the ability of zeolite clinoptilolite to bind toxins. Zeolites can be natural or man-made. They are aluminosilicate, microporous rocks with rigid anionic frameworks containing multiple channels and cavities. They contain metal cations, which are exchangeable. Most natural zeolites have a volcanic origin.

Zeolites have been used in both water and wastewater treatment. In vitro and in vivo animal studies have demonstrated the ability of zeolites to sequester mycotoxins including afla-toxin, zearalenone, ochratoxin, and T-2 toxin.[65] In these studies, zeolites did not affect mineral levels or fat-soluble vitamin levels in the blood. Like cholestyramine, zeolites may be used to treat diarrhea. Zeolites have also been shown to increase levels of glutathione.[66] Beneficial effects on the gut microbiome, including the removal of pathogenic bacteria, have been seen in animal studies.[67]

Humic substances arise from the decomposition of plant and animal tissues.[68] Two humic substances that have been well studied are humic acid and fulvic acid. Humic substances cannot be classified in any other chemical class of compounds (e.g., polysaccharides or proteins). Fulvic acids are soluble in water at all pH values. Humic acids are insoluble at acidic pH values (pH < 2) but are soluble at higher pH values.

Humic and fulvic acids bind metals and radionuclides in the environment, a property which can be used in water treatment facilities.[69] They improve the soil, increase crop yields, and promote the removal of pollutants. An in vitro study showed that humic acid binders resulted in the lowest zearalenone concentrations of the twenty-seven binders tested.[70] An in vivo animal study found that humic acid showed protective effects against liver damage, stomach and heart enlargement, and some of the hematological and serum biochemical changes associated with aflatoxin toxicity.[71] Another in vivo study in rats found that supplemental humic acid prevented oxidative stress due to the mycotoxin deoxynivalenol.[72]

Probiotic bacteria are a novel method by which to reduce mycotoxins. Some strains of *Lactobacillus rhamnosus* have been found to lower aflatoxin absorption in animal models.[73] Other probiotic strains have also been shown in vitro to lower concentrations of ochratoxin and aflatoxin.[74] The cell wall of *Saccharomyces cerevisiae* binds to the mycotoxin zearalenone via cell wall proteins.[75] Additional studies have confirmed the ability of *Saccharomyces* and lactic acid bacteria to bind to mycotoxins.[76–77] In poultry exposed to mycotoxins, the addition of *Saccharomyces* reduced mycotoxins and improved the immune status of the animals.[78]

In our practice, we use a binder with activated charcoal, zeolite, and shilajit, which is a mineral resin that contains humic acid and fulvic acid. It comes in a capsule, but the capsule can be opened to place the contents in food. We also use a probiotic containing *Saccharomyces boulardii*.

There are several articles discussing the use of nano-technologies to prevent the absorption of mycotoxins.[79] This will likely be a growing topic of interest in the future.

> Heavy metals such as arsenic, mercury, cadmium, and lead can produce significant neuropsychiatric symptoms.

Heavy metals

As noted in Chapter 5, heavy metals such as arsenic, mercury, cadmium, and lead can produce significant neuropsychiatric symptoms. These impairments can occur in patients even when blood levels are below what is considered "toxic." In fact, the US EPA, the CDC, and the World Health Organization agree that there is "no safe level of lead" in the blood.[80–81]

There are various sequestrants which remove metals from the body, including EDTA, DMSA, and DMPS. These chelating agents are typically recommended for severe intoxication with significant impairments and elevated blood levels from a conventional lab.

There are varied opinions on chelation in patients with chronic low-level elevations of metals (also called bioaccumulated toxic elements). We do not use prescription chelating agents at all in children.

The good news is that glutathione combined with a broad-spectrum binder (charcoal, humic acid, fulvic acid, and zeolite) is effective at reducing chronic mild elevations of heavy metals. In vivo human studies have shown that zeolite alone is effective at removing various heavy metals.[65]

Persistent organic pollutants

There are no specific chelating agents for persistent organic pollutants, but, as with heavy metals, glutathione and broad-spectrum binders remove these substances well.

MAINTAINING NORMAL BOWEL MOVEMENTS

Once biotransformation has taken place, processed toxins, toxicants, and other waste move through the small intestine and into the colon for evacuation. In the early part of the twentieth century, constipation was hypothesized to be the cause of various illnesses, including neurologic and mental disorders.[82]

This theory was subsequently abandoned until the late 1990s. At this time, evidence came to light which showed that decreased total intestinal transit time (as seen in constipation) resulted in increased

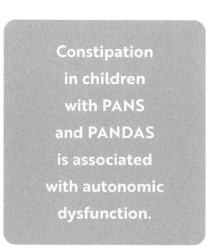

Constipation in children with PANS and PANDAS is associated with autonomic dysfunction.

enterohepatic circulation.[83] This can increase gallstone formation and can result in increased hormone and toxin reabsorption and decreased short-chain fatty acids, which are required for gut health and immune health.[83,84]

Water intake in euhydrated patients does not result in an increase in bowel movements if the patient is constipated.[85] However, dehydration is associated with constipation and increasing water intake in dehydrated children or adults helps increase frequency and quality of bowel movements.[85,86] Parents should make sure that children with PANS and PANDAS maintain adequate water intake to avoid dehydration. Higher fiber intake in the diet leads to more rapid stool transit time and less constipation.[85]

We commonly see constipation in children with PANS and PANDAS. It is not usually from frank dehydration. Rather, it is associated with autonomic dysfunction. These children are continually in sympathetic overdrive (fight or flight). In a study of patients with chronic refractory constipation using high-resolution colonic manometry and heart rate variability measurements, colonic dysmotility associated with autonomic dysfunction was noted.[87] In this study, the authors report that high sympathetic tone and reactivity was more prevalent than low parasympathetic activity, and suggested the possibility that sacral neuromodulation might be an effective treatment. The resolution of sympathetic overdrive and improvement on parasympathetic function is discussed in Chapter 20.

The most effective supplement we have found for constipation is magnesium citrate. It is available in capsule form and powder. Since it mostly remains in the gut, it is a very safe option if dosed properly. It is not addictive and there is no withdrawal associated with stopping this supplement once dietary changes, increased water intake, and reduction of sympathetic tone have been accomplished.

Various prescription and over-the-counter medications can lead to constipation. In addition to commonly used over-the-counter medications like antihistamines, some antidepressants and antipsychotic medications can cause significant constipation.[88]

Osteopathic manipulative therapy (OMT), when performed by a trained osteopathic physician, can be very helpful in patients with constipation.[89] Pelvic floor physical therapy by a specially trained abdominal and pelvic/floor physical therapist can also be helpful in children with constipation.[90]

Polyethylene glycol 3350 (available as MiraLAX and other brands) is commonly used in adults and children. It is available in powder form. We do not use polyethylene glycol or other stimulant laxatives in our practice.

SWEATING AND INFRARED SAUNA THERAPY

We may not commonly think about sweating as a method of detoxification, but the medical literature indicates that multiple toxins have been found in human sweat. Small studies in humans have demonstrated that toxins and toxicants,

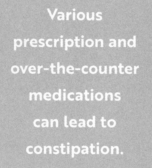

Various prescription and over-the-counter medications can lead to constipation.

including metals and persistent organic pollutants, are excreted in human sweat in significant amounts.[91–94] Metals and metalloids appear to be preferentially excreted in sweat; studies have shown that some patients have metals identified in their perspiration that are not seen in their serum or that are only seen there at lower levels.[91,92] Some small studies have shown that induced sweating (with exercise, stream sauna, or infrared sauna) is effective at removing persistent organic pollutants and heavy metals like mercury.[91,93]

There are no studies specifically on using sauna in children.

We usually recommend full-spectrum infrared sauna in our patients over the age of five, if tolerated. The sauna is usually set to about 130°F. As for the duration, we aim for one minute per year of age. We always have a parent accompany their child in the sauna. We use a Jacuzzi brand full-spectrum sauna (www.jacuzzi.com). Sunlighten (www.sunlighten.com) also makes saunas for professional use. It is widely believed that infrared saunas lead to greater toxin/toxicant excretion than traditional saunas, but we have not been able to find any studies to support this. We recommend infrared sauna as it is less oppressive to the respiratory system and various portable units are available.

PHOTOBIOMODULATION (RED-LIGHT THERAPY)

Photobiomodulation (PBM) involves the use of red and near-infrared light exposure as a therapeutic modality. An excellent review by Hamblin describes the mechanisms of action by which PBM improves mitochondrial function, decreases systemic inflammation, reduces oxidative stress, and reduces pro-inflammatory cytokines.[95] PBM has also been shown to improve muscular function in an animal model of multiple sclerosis and autoimmune encephalitis.[96] In other animal studies, PBM has been shown to inhibit microglial activation.[97]

The glymphatic system is a waste clearance pathway in the central nervous system which involves the glial cells. It rids the CNS of waste metabolic products and soluble proteins such as amyloid-beta. If the brain glymphatic system is not functioning normally, neuroinflammatory and neurodegenerative diseases may be potentiated. PBM can optimize effective clearance of waste products in the CNS. There are benefits of PBM therapy on glymphatic drainage and clearance.[98]

PBM is usually delivered by LED panels and is also known as red-light therapy. Red-light therapy is very safe. Children tolerate it well and red-light panels can be purchased for home use. One manufacturer that sells to consumers is Joovv (www.joovv.com). In our practice we use panels from Platinum LED Therapy Lights (www.platinumtherapylights.com).

LYMPHATIC DRAINAGE

The lymphatic system is a network of vessels, lymph nodes, and lymphatic tissues within the body. It is a passive system as it has no pump like the circulatory system. In addition to removing cellular debris and waste from tissues and aiding the resolution of inflammation, the lymphatic system plays an important role in immune modulation and tolerance to self-antigens.[99,100] Lymphatic system dysfunction with edema and lymphadenopathy occurs in patients with autoimmune diseases including lupus, systemic sclerosis, and rheumatoid arthritis.[101]

Lymphatic drainage massage or dry brushing is an ancient practice which has been shown to improve lymphedema in patients with filariasis.[102,103] We teach our parents of children with PANS and PANDAS to do dry brushing with a boar brush to aid lymphatic drainage.

> The lymphatic system plays an important role in immune modulation and tolerance to self-antigens.

CHAPTER 17 REFERENCES

1. Wrighton SA, VandenBranden M, Ring BJ. The human drug metabolizing cytochromes P450. *J Pharmacokinet Biopharm.* 1996;24(5):461–73

2. Zhou SF, Xue CC, Yu XQ, et al. Clinically important drug interactions potentially involving mechanism-based inhibition of cytochrome P450 3A4 and the role of therapeutic drug monitoring. *Ther Drug Monit.* 2007;29(6):687–710

3. Kitzmiller JP, Groen DK, Phelps MA, et al. Pharmacogenomic testing: relevance in medical practice: why drugs work in some patients but not in others. *Cleve Clin J Med*. 2011;78(4):243–57

4. Kato M, Serretti A. Review and meta-analysis of antidepressant pharmacogenetic findings in major depressive disorder. *Mol Psychiatry*. 2010;15:473–500

5. Hong JY, Yang CS. Genetic polymorphism of cytochrome P450 as a biomarker of susceptibility to environmental toxicity. *Environmental Health Perspectives*. 1997;105(suppl 4):759–62

6. Hodgson E, Rose RL. Human metabolic interactions of environmental chemicals. *J Biochem Mol Toxicol*. 2007;21(4):182–6

7. Schelstraete W, Devreese M, Croubels S. Impact of subacute exposure to T-2 toxin and zearalenone on the pharmacokinetics of Midazolam as CYP3A probe drug in a porcine animal model: a pilot study. *Front Pharmacol*. 2019;10:399:1–22

8. Tangjarukij C, Navasumrit P, Zelikoff JT, et al: The effects of pyridoxine deficiency and supplementation on hematological profiles, lymphocyte function, and hepatic cytochrome P450 in B6C3F1 mice. *J Immunotoxicol*. 2009;6(3):147–60

9. Gaudineau C, Auclair K. Inhibition of human P450 enzymes by nicotinic acid and nicotinamide. *Biochem Biophys Res Commun*. 2004;317(3):950–6

10. Kim JS, Yun CH. Inhibition of human cytochrome P450 3A4 activity by zinc(II) ion. *Toxicol Lett*. 2005;156(3):341–50

11. Guengerich FP. Influence of nutrients and other dietary materials on cytochrome P-450 enzymes. *Am J Clin Nutr*. 1995;61(3 Suppl):651S–658S

12. Hodges RE, Minich DM. Modulation of metabolic detoxification pathways using foods and food-derived components: a scientific review with clinical application. *J Nutr Metab*. 2015;2015:760689:1–23

13. Van der Hulst RR, von Meyenfeldt MF, van Kreel BK, et al. Gut permeability, intestinal morphology, and nutritional depletion. *Nutrition*. 1998;14(1):1–6

14. Teixeira TF, Collado MC, Ferreira CL, et al. Potential mechanisms for the emerging link between obesity and increased intestinal permeability. *Nutr Res*. 2012;32(9):637–47

15. Flora K, Hahn M, Rosen H, et al. Milk thistle (*Silybum marianum*) for the therapy of liver disease. *American Journal of Gastroenterology*. 1998;93(2):139–43

16. Ketterer B, Coles B, Meyer DJ. The role of glutathione in detoxication. *Environmental Health Perspectives*. 1983;49:59–69

17. Schulz JB, Lindenau J, Seyfried J, et al. Glutathione, oxidative stress and neurodegeneration. *Eur J Biochem*. 2000;267(16):4904–11

18. Jenner P, Dexter DT, Sian J, et al. Oxidative stress as a cause of nigral cell death in Parkinson's disease and incidental Lewy body disease. The Royal Kings and Queens Parkinson's Disease Research Group. *Ann Neurol*. 1992;32 Suppl:S82–7

19. Chinta SJ, Kumar MJ, Hsu M, et al. Inducible alterations of glutathione levels in adult dopaminergic midbrain neurons result in nigrostriatal degeneration. *Journal of Neuroscience*. 2007;27(51):13997–14006

20. Holmay MJ, Terpstra M, Coles LD, et al. N-acetylcysteine boosts brain and blood glutathione in Gaucher and Parkinson diseases. *Clin Neuropharmacol*. 2013;36(4):103–6

21. Guilford FT, Hope J. Deficient glutathione in the pathophysiology of mycotoxin-related illness. *Toxins*. 2014;6(2):608–23

22. Schaaf GJ, Nijmeijer SM, Maas RF, et al. The role of oxidative stress in the ochratoxin A-mediated toxicity in proximal tubular cells. *Biochim Biophys Acta*. 2002;1588(2):149–58

23. Agarwal R, Shukla GS. Potential role of cerebral glutathione in the maintenance of blood-brain barrier integrity in rat. *Neurochem Res*. 1999;24(12):1507–14

24. Ghersi-Egea JF, Strazielle N, Murat A, et al. Brain protection at the blood-cerebrospinal fluid interface involves a glutathione-dependent metabolic barrier mechanism. *J Cereb Blood Flow Metab*. 2006;26(9):1165–75

25. Muruganandam A, Smith C, Ball R, et al. Glutathione homeostasis and leukotriene-induced permeability in human blood-brain barrier endothelial cells subjected to in vitro ischemia. *Acta Neurochir Suppl*. 2000;76:29–34

26. Mahfoud R, Maresca M, Garmy N, et al. The mycotoxin patulin alters the barrier function of the intestinal epithelium: mechanism of action of the toxin and protective effects of glutathione. *Toxicology and Applied Pharmacology*. 2002;181(3):209–18

27. Fink-Grernmels J. Mycotoxins: their implications for human and animal health. *Veterinary Quarterly*. 1999;21(4):115–20

28. Berthiller F, Schuhmacher R, Adam G, et al. Formation, determination and significance of masked and other conjugated mycotoxins. *Analytical and Bioanalytical Chemistry*. 2009;395:1243–52

29. Richie JP Jr, Nichenametla S, Neidig W, et al Randomized controlled trial of oral glutathione supplementation on body stores of glutathione. *Eur J Nutr*. 2015;54(2):251–63

30. Sinha R, Sinha I, Calcagnotto A, et al. Oral supplementation with liposomal glutathione elevates body stores of glutathione and markers of immune function. *Eur J Clin Nutr*. 2018;72(1):105–111

31. Atkuri KR, Mantovani JJ, Herzenberg LA. N-acetylcysteine: a safe antidote for cysteine/glutathione deficiency. *Curr Opin Pharmacol*. 2007;7(4):355–9

32. Cao H, Zhou Z, Hu Z, et al. Effect of enterohepatic circulation on the accumulation of per- and polyfluoroalkyl substances: evidence from experimental and computational studies. *Environ Sci Technol*. 2022;56(5):3214–3224

33. www.niehs.nih.gov/health/topics/agents/pfc/index.cfm, accessed 3/17/2023

34. Zhai Q, Liu Y, Wang C, et al. Increased cadmium excretion due to oral administration of *Lactobacillus plantarum* strains by regulating enterohepatic circulation in mice. *J Agric Food Chem*. 2019;67(14):3956–3965

35. Liu W, Feng H, Zheng S, et al. Pb toxicity on gut physiology and microbiota. *Front Physiol*. 2021;12:574913:1–12

36. Cikrt M, Tichý M. Biliary excretion of phenyl- and methyl mercury chlorides and their enterohepatic circulation in rats. *Environ Res*. 1974;8(1):71–81

37. Roth A, Chakor K, Creppy EE, et al. Evidence for an enterohepatic circulation of ochratoxin A in mice. *Toxicology.*1988;48(3):293–308

38. Coddington KA, Swanson SP, Hassan AS, et al. Enterohepatic circulation of T-2 toxin metabolites in the rat. *Drug Metab Dispos*. 1989;17(6):600–5

39. Spiridonov NA. Mechanisms of action of herbal cholagogues. *Medicinal and Aromatic Plants*. 2012;1(5):1–4

40. Crocenzi FA, Basiglio CL, Pérez LM, et al. Silibinin prevents cholestasis-associated retrieval of the bile salt export pump, Bsep, in isolated rat hepatocyte couplets: possible involvement of cAMP. *Biochem Pharmacol.* 2005;69(7):1113–20

41. McMullen MK, Whitehouse JM, Towell A. Bitters: time for a new paradigm. *Evidence-Based Complementary and Alternative Medicine.* 2015;2015:670504:1–9

42. Vang S, Longley K, Steer CJ, et al. The unexpected uses of urso- and tauroursodeoxycholic acid in the treatment of non-liver diseases. *Glob Adv Health Med.* 2014;3(3):58–69

43. Castro-Caldas M, Carvalho AN, Rodrigues E, et al. Tauroursodeoxycholic acid prevents MPTP-induced dopaminergic cell death in a mouse model of Parkinson's disease. *Mol Neurobiol.* 2012;46(2):475–86

44. Kidd P. Phosphatidylcholine: a superior protectant against liver damage. *Altern Med Rev.* 1996;1(4):258–274

45. Boylan JJ, Egle JL, Guzelian PS. Cholestyramine: use as a new therapeutic approach for chlordecone (Kepone) poisoning. *Science.* 1978;199(4331):893–5

46. Cohn WJ, Boylan JJ, Blanke RV, et al. Treatment of chlordecone (Kepone) toxicity with cholestyramine: results of a controlled clinical trial. *N Engl J Med.* 1978;298(5):243–8

47. Brouillard MY, Rateau JG. Etude de l'aptitude de la cholestyramine à fixer les toxines d'Escherichia coli et de Vibrio cholerae [Ability of cholestyramine to bind Escherichia coli and Vibrio cholerae toxins. *Ann Gastroenterol Hepatol]* (Paris). 1988;24(3):133–8

48. Moncino MD, Falletta JM. Multiple relapses of Clostridium difficile-associated diarrhea in a cancer patient: successful control with long-term cholestyramine therapy. *Am J Pediatr Hematol Oncol.* 1992;14(4):361–4

49. Madhyastha MS, Frohlich AA, Marquardt RR. Effect of dietary cholestyramine on the elimination pattern of Ochratoxin A in rats. *Food and Chemical Toxicology.* 1992;30(8):709–714

50. Creppy EE, Baudrimont I, Betbeder AM. Prevention of nephrotoxicity of ochratoxin A, a food contaminant. *Toxicol Lett.* 1995;82/83:869–877

51. Kerkadi A, Barriault C, Tuchweber B, et al. Dietary cholestyramine reduces Ochratoxin A-induced nephrotoxicity in the rat by decreasing plasma levels and enhancing fecal excretion of the toxin. *Journal of Toxicology and Environmental Health Part A.* 1998;53(3):231–250

52. Kerkadi A, Barriault C, Marquardt RR, et al. Cholestyramine protection against ochratoxin A toxicity: role of ochratoxin absorption by the resin and bile acid enterohepatic circulation. *J. Food Prot.* 1999;62:1461–1465

53. Underhill KL, Totter BA, Thompson BK, et al. Effectiveness of cholestyramine in the detoxification of zearalenone as determined in mice. *Bull Environ Contam Toxicol.* 1995;54:128–134

54. Galvano F, Pietri A, Bertuzzi T, et al. Activated carbons: in vitro affinity for ochratoxin A and deoxynivalenol and relation of adsorption ability to physicochemical parameters. *J Food Prot.* 1998;61(4):469–75

55. Avantaggiato G, Havenaar R, Visconti A. Evaluation of the intestinal absorption of deoxynivalenol and nivalenol by an in vitro gastrointestinal model, and the binding efficacy of activated carbon and other adsorbent materials. *Food Chem Toxicol.* 2004;42(5):817–24

56. Döll S, Dänicke S, Valenta H, et al. In vitro studies on the evaluation of mycotoxin detoxifying agents for their efficacy on deoxynivalenol and zearalenone. *Arch Anim Nutr.* 2004;58(4):311–24

57. Kong C, Shin SY, Kim BG. Evaluation of mycotoxin sequestering agents for aflatoxin and deoxyniva-lenol: an in vitro approach. *Springerplus*. 2014;3:346:1–7

58. Ramos AJ, Fink-Gremmels J, Hernández E. Prevention of toxic effects of mycotoxins by means of nonnutritive adsorbent compounds. *J Food Prot*. 1996;59(6):631–641

59. Bhatti SA, Khan MZ, Hassan ZU, et al. Comparative efficacy of Bentonite clay, activated charcoal and *Trichosporon mycotoxinivorans* in regulating the feed-to-tissue transfer of mycotoxins. *J Sci Food Agric*. 2018;98(3):884–890

60. Moosavi M. Bentonite clay as a natural remedy: a brief review. *Iran J Public Health*. 2017;46(9):1176–1183

61. Phillips TD, Wang M, Elmore SE, et al. NovaSil clay for the protection of humans and animals from aflatoxins and other contaminants. *Clays Clay Miner*. 2019;67(1):99–110

62. Phillips TD, Afriyie-Gyawu E, Williams J, et al. Reducing human exposure to aflatoxin through the use of clay: a review. *Food Addit Contam Part A Chem Anal Control Expo Risk Assess*. 2008;25(2):134–45

63. Afriyie-Gyawu E, Ankrah NA, Huebner HJ, et al. NovaSil clay intervention in Ghanaians at high risk for aflatoxicosis. I. Study design and clinical outcomes. *Food Addit Contam Part A Chem Anal Control Expo Risk Assess*. 2008;25(1):76–87

64. Afriyie-Gyawu E, Wang Z, Ankrah NA, et al. NovaSil clay does not affect the concentrations of vitamins A and E and nutrient minerals in serum samples from Ghanaians at high risk for aflatoxicosis. *Food Addit Contam Part A Chem Anal Control Expo Risk Assess*. 2008;25(7):872–84

65. Kraljević Pavelić S, Simović Medica J, Gumbarević D, et al. Critical review on zeolite clinoptilolite safety and medical applications in vivo. *Front Pharmacol*. 2018;9:1350

66. Basha MP, Begum S, Mir BA. Neuroprotective actions of clinoptilolite and ethylenediaminetetraacetic acid against lead-induced toxicity in mice mus musculus. *Toxicol Int*. 2013;20(3):201–7

67. Rodríguez-Fuentes G, Barrios MA, Iraizoz A, et al. Enterex: anti-diarrheic drug based on purified natural clinoptilolite. *Zeolites* 1997;19:441–448

68. Gaffney JS, Marley NA, Clark SB. Humic and fulvic acids and organic colloidal materials in the environment. *ACS Symposium Series*. American Chemical Society. Washington, DC. 1996

69. Zhu X, Liu J, Li L, et al Prospects for humic acids treatment and recovery in wastewater: a review. *Chemosphere*. 2023;312(Pt 2):137193

70. De Mil T, Devreese M, De Baere S, et al. Characterization of 27 mycotoxin binders and the relation with in vitro zearalenone adsorption at a single concentration. *Toxins* (Basel). 2015;7(1):21–33

71. Jansen van Rensburg C, Van Rensburg CE, Van Ryssen JB, et al. In vitro and in vivo assessment of humic acid as an aflatoxin binder in broiler chickens. *Poult Sci*. 2006;85(9):1576–83

72. Haus M, Žatko D, Vašková J, et al. The effect of humic acid in chronic deoxynivalenol intoxication. *Environmental Science and Pollution Research*. 2021;28:1612–8

73. El-Nezami H, Mykanen H, Kankaanpää P, et al. Ability of *Lactobacillus* and *Propionibacterium* strains to remove aflatoxin B1 from the chicken duodenum. *J. Food Prot*. 2000;63:549–552

74. Kabak B, Brandon EF, Var I, et al. Effects of probiotic bacteria on the bioaccessibility of aflatoxin B(1) and ochratoxin A using an in vitro digestion model under fed conditions. *J Environ Sci Health B*. 2009;44(5):472–80

75. Jouany JP, Yiannikouris A, Bertin G. The chemical bonds between mycotoxins and cell wall components of *Saccharomyces cerevisiae* have been identified. *Arch. Zootech*. 2005;8(2650):4:1–25

76. Shetty PH, Jespersen L. *Saccharomyces cerevisiae* and lactic acid bacteria as potential mycotoxin decontaminating agents. *Trends in Food Science & Technology*. 2006;17(2):48–55

77. Alassane-Kpembi I, Pinton P, Oswald IP. Effects of mycotoxins on the intestine. *Toxins*. 2019;11(3):159:1–3

78. Arif M, Iram A, Bhutta MA, et al. The biodegradation role of *Saccharomyces cerevisiae* against harmful effects of mycotoxin contaminated diets on broiler performance, immunity status, and carcass characteristics. *Animals*. 2020;10(2):238:1–11

79. Horky P, Skalickova S, Baholet D, et al. Nanoparticles as a solution for eliminating the risk of mycotoxins. *Nanomaterials* (Basel). 2018;8(9):727

80. www.epa.gov/ground-water-and-drinking-water/basic-information-about-lead-drinking--water#:~:text=EPA%20and%20the%20Centers%20for,to%20health%2C%20especially%20for%20children, accessed 3/22/2023

81. www.who.int/news-room/fact-sheets/detail/lead-poisoning-and-health#:~:text=There%20is%20no%20known%20safe,symptoms%20and%20effects%20also%20increase, accessed 3/22/2023

82. Hertz A. *Constipation and Allied Intestinal Disorders*. Oxford. Oxford Medical Publications. 1909

83. Lewis SJ, Heaton KW. The metabolic consequences of slow colonic transit. *Am J Gastroenterol*. 1999;94(8):2010–6

84. Dowling RH, Veysey MJ, Pereira SP, et al. Role of intestinal transit in the pathogenesis of gallbladder stones. *Can J Gastroenterol*. 1997;11(1):57–64

85. Müller-Lissner SA, Kamm MA, Scarpignato C, et al. Myths and misconceptions about chronic constipation. *Official Journal of the American College of Gastroenterology*. 2005;100(1):232–42

86. Arnaud MJ. Mild dehydration: a risk factor of constipation? *European Journal of Clinical Nutrition*. 2003;57(2): S88–95

87. Liu L, Milkova N, Nirmalathasan S, et al. Diagnosis of colonic dysmotility associated with autonomic dysfunction in patients with chronic refractory constipation. *Scientific Reports*. 2022;12(1):12051:1–18

88. Branch RL, Butt TF. Drug-induced constipation. *Adverse Drug Reaction Bulletin*. 2009;(257):987–90

89. Erdrich LM, Reid D, Mason J. Does a manual therapy approach improve the symptoms of functional constipation? A systematic review of the literature. *International Journal of Osteopathic Medicine*. 2020;36:26–35

90. Zar-Kessler C, Kuo B, Cole E, et al. Benefit of pelvic floor physical therapy in pediatric patients with dyssynergic defecation constipation. *Digestive Diseases*. 2019;37(6):478–85

91. Sears ME, Kerr KJ, Bray RI. Arsenic, cadmium, lead, and mercury in sweat: a systematic review. *Journal of Environmental and Public Health*. 2012;2012: 184745:1–11

92. Genuis SJ, Birkholz D, Rodushkin I, et al. Blood, urine, and sweat (BUS) study: monitoring and elimination of bioaccumulated toxic elements. *Archives of Environmental Contamination and Toxicology*. 2011;61:344–57

93. Genuis SK, Birkholz D, Genuis SJ. Human excretion of polybrominated diphenyl ether flame retardants: blood, urine, and sweat study. *BioMed Research International*. 2017;2017: 3676089:1–15

94. Genuis SJ, Beesoon S, Birkholz D. Biomonitoring and elimination of perfluorinated compounds and polychlorinated biphenyls through perspiration: blood, urine, and sweat study. *International Scholarly Research Notices*. 2013;2013: 483832:1–7

95. Hamblin MR. Mechanisms and applications of the anti-inflammatory effects of photobiomodulation. *AIMS Biophys*. 2017;4(3):337–361

96. Muili KA, Gopalakrishnan S, Eells JT, et al. Photobiomodulation induced by 670 nm light ameliorates MOG35-55 induced EAE in female C57BL/6 mice: a role for remediation of nitrosative stress. *PLoS One*. 2013;8(6):e67358:1–16

97. Khuman J, Zhang J, Park J, et al. Low-level laser light therapy improves cognitive deficits and inhibits microglial activation after controlled cortical impact in mice. *J Neurotrauma*. 2012;29(2):408–17

98. Salehpour F, Khademi M, Bragin DE, et al. Photobiomodulation therapy and the glymphatic system: promising applications for augmenting the brain lymphatic drainage system. *International Journal of Molecular Sciences*. 2022;23(6):2975:1–18

99. Thomas SN, Rutkowski JM, Pasquier M, et al. Impaired humoral immunity and tolerance in K14-VEGFR-3-Ig mice that lack dermal lymphatic drainage. *J Immunol*. 2012;189:2181–90

100. Friedlaender MH, Baer H. Immunologic tolerance: role of the regional lymph node. *Science*. 1972;176:312–4

101. Schwartz N, Chalasani MLS, Li TM, et al. Lymphatic function in autoimmune diseases. *Front Immunol*. 2019;10:519:1–7

102. Narahari SR, Ryan TJ, Mahadevan PE, et al. Integrated management of filarial lymphedema for rural communities. *Lymphology*. 2007;40:3–13

103. Bongi SM, Del Rosso A, Passalacqua M, et al. Manual lymph drainage improving upper extremity edema and hand function in patients with systemic sclerosis in edematous phase. *Arthritis Care Res*. 2011;63:1134–41

SUPPORT

It's not enough to have lived. We should be determined to live for something. May I suggest that it be creating joy for others, sharing what we have for the betterment of personkind, bringing hope to the lost and love to the lonely.
~ LEO BUSCAGLIA

KEY POINTS

▸ The SUPPORT pillar has three main aspects
▸ Structural support addresses muscles, bones, cell membranes, mucous membranes, and the blood-brain barrier
▸ Biochemical support addresses the communication that happens in the body through chemical messengers, hormones, nutrients, and neurotransmitters
▸ Personal support addresses the need for community, communication, and guidance during the healing process

There are three areas we consider when discussing the SUPPORT pillar of the Fully Functional process:

1. Structural support
2. Support for biochemical system homeostasis
3. Personal support of the patient and the family during this journey to recovery

In this chapter, we speak about supplements to promote health and vital bodily processes.

We hear two myths in our practice concerning nutrient intake and supplements. The first is that people can get enough nutrients in their diet alone. The second is that, if you take supplements, you are just making expensive urine.

> Patients with PANS and PANDAS end up with nutrient deficiencies due to lack of healthy intake of nutrient-rich foods or to gut issues from toxin or toxicant exposures.

In regard to nutrients and food intake, we have seemingly healthy adult patients who come to us with balanced, organic diets and still have deficiencies on nutrient testing. After replacing nutrients, repeat testing shows adequate levels. Studies have demonstrated that the nutrient content of fruits and vegetables have declined over the past thirty years due to mineral soil depletion from overfarming.[1,2] Further, patients with PANS and PANDAS end up with nutrient deficiencies due to lack of healthy intake of nutrient-rich foods or to gut issues from toxin or toxicant exposures. Using the recommended daily allowance (RDA) does not usually help replace low total body stores and/or absorption impairments.

STRUCTURAL SUPPORT

Structural support has to do with the health of the muscles, bones, and cell membranes. Throughout Chapter 17, we focused on eliminating toxins and toxicants in our body. Now we focus on what we can do in the positive sense to build a healthy body and healthy cell membranes.

To support bone health, it is important to make sure that people get enough calcium. We often get questions about calcium and bone health since we advocate a trial of dairy elimination. Almond milk actually has more calcium than cow's milk. Fortified orange juice has about the same amount of calcium as cow's milk. There is also calcium in other fruits and vegetables. In addition to calcium, magnesium, vitamin D3, vitamin K, and boron are also important for bone health.[3,4]

Lean body mass is very important for general health and longevity. In older adults, higher muscle mass is inversely correlated with total mortality.[5] Quality protein intake is very important for muscle development. Unfortunately, the standard American diet is very high in carbohydrates and simple sugars and low in protein and healthy fats.

Membrane health is part of structural support since the cell membrane is responsible for our interface with our environment. This includes mucous membranes, the gut lining, the vascular epithelium, and the blood-brain barrier. Many of these barriers are compromised in children with PANS and PANDAS. Healthy fats are a vital component of cell membranes. Fats, though once demonized, are needed for most biochemical processes in the body.

One particularly important type of lipid is phosphatidylcholine (PC). Most cell membranes are made from PC. Numerous studies have shown that PC is important for normal neurologic function. It is also helpful in preventing and treating neurodegenerative disorders and decreasing neuroinflammation.[6-16] Phosphatidylcholine is manufactured as a supplement in both liquid and gel cap formulations. Liquid PC is often mixed with water using a small blender or mixer to make a liposomal formulation that may be better absorbed.

BIOCHEMICAL SYSTEMS HOMEOSTASIS

Homeostasis in biochemical systems is important for the maintenance of health and the prevention of disease. Many of the things we do in our practice focus on achieving this homeostasis in various organ systems.

The production of neurotransmitters depends on amino acid intake (from proteins) and also vitamins and minerals, which are required cofactors for the production of these chemical messengers.[17] There is some evidence that micronutrients can help resolve neuroinflammation.[18] Mitochondrial health and energy production also require various vitamins and minerals.

To maintain gastrointestinal health, we routinely use broad spectrum probiotics, *Saccharomyces*, and

> There is some evidence that micronutrients can help resolve neuroinflammation.

butyrate. Specific supplements used to help heal the gut include glutamine, humic and fulvic acid, omega 3 fats (fish oil), and vitamin D. Omega 3 fats increase butyrate-producing bacteria, reverse gut dysbiosis, reduce lipopolysaccharide-induced metabolic endotoxemia, and decrease intestinal inflammation.[19] Vitamin D deficiency increases intestinal permeability and vitamin D therapeutically decreases intestinal permeability.[20-21]

Probiotics (specifically *Saccharomyces*) have been shown to reduce antibiotic-associated diarrhea with a number needed-to-treat of six patients to prevent one case of diarrhea.[22-25]

Glutamine is the most abundant amino acid in the blood. Glutamine helps maintain gut integrity in health, sickness, and injury.[26] A randomized study of hospitalized patients demonstrated that glutamine maintained gut integrity while a control group developed increased intestinal permeability.[27] Oral glutamine reduces stomatitis in patients after cytotoxic chemotherapy.[28]

PERSONAL SUPPORT

As we have reiterated several times in this textbook, illness due to PANS or PANDAS is a difficult road for the patient and the family. It is a lonely time. It is a scary time. It is also a time when parents feel that they may lose their minds. Many physicians refuse to believe that PANS and PANDAS are real and blame parents for their child's behavior. Parents may be told what we were told when our daughter was sick: place your child in a facility and medicate them. We can do so much better for our patients, their families, and the profession of medicine. See Appendix D.

We assign each child (and their family) a health educator who supports them, guides them through our Fully Functional process, and provides a shoulder to cry on when needed. The health educators meet with the patients weekly for the first six weeks of the process while we are waiting for lab results and the initial response to treatment. The health educators make sure the patient is on track with supplements, antibiotics, other meds, and home testing. They are trained in nutritional health coaching and our Fully Functional process.

CHAPTER 18 REFERENCES

1. Davis DR, Epp MD, Riordan HD. Changes in USDA food composition data for 43 garden crops, 1950 to 1999. *J Am Coll Nutr*. 2004;23(6):669–82

2. Mayer, Anne-Marie. Historical changes in the mineral content of fruits and vegetables. *British Food Journal*. 1997;99(6):207–211

3. Ilich JZ, Kerstetter JE. Nutrition in bone health revisited: a story beyond calcium. *Journal of the American College of Nutrition*. 2000;19(6):715–37

4. Cashman KD. Diet, nutrition, and bone health. *The Journal of Nutrition*. 2007;137(11):2507S–12S

5. Srikanthan P, Karlamangla AS. Muscle mass index as a predictor of longevity in older adults. *Am J Med*. 2014;127(6):547–53

6. Ross RG, Hunter SK, Hoffman MC, et al. Perinatal phosphatidylcholine supplementation and early childhood behavior problems: evidence for CHRNA7 moderation. *American Journal of Psychiatry*. 2016;173(5):509–16

7. Qu MH, Yang X, Wang Y, et al. Docosahexaenoic acid-phosphatidylcholine improves cognitive deficits in an Aβ23-35-induced Alzheimer's disease rat model. *Current Topics in Medicinal Chemistry*. 2016;16(5):558–64

8. E Smith R, Rouchotas P, Fritz H. Lecithin (Phosphatidylcholine): healthy dietary supplement or dangerous toxin? *Natural Products Journal*. 2016;6(4):242–9

9. Tan W, Zhang Q, Dong Z, et al. Phosphatidylcholine ameliorates lps-induced systemic inflammation and cognitive impairments via mediating the gut-brain axis balance. *Journal of Agricultural and Food Chemistry*. 2020;68(50):14884–95

10. van der Veen JN, Kennelly JP, Wan S, et al. The critical role of phosphatidylcholine and phosphatidylethanolamine metabolism in health and disease. *Biochimica et Biophysica Acta (BBA)-Biomembranes*. 2017;1859(9):1558–72

11. Schaefer EJ, Bongard V, Beiser AS, et al. Plasma phosphatidylcholine docosahexaenoic acid content and risk of dementia and Alzheimer disease: the Framingham Heart Study. *Archives of Neurology*. 2006;63(11):1545–50

12. Chung SY, Moriyama T, Uezu E, et al. Administration of phosphatidylcholine increases brain acetylcholine concentration and improves memory in mice with dementia. *The Journal of Nutrition*. 1995;125(6):1484–9

13. Magaquian D, Delgado Ocaña S, Perez C, et al. Phosphatidylcholine restores neuronal plasticity of neural stem cells under inflammatory stress. *Scientific Reports*. 2021;11(1):22891:1–12

14. Tokés T, Eros G, Bebes A, et al. Protective effects of a phosphatidylcholine-enriched diet in lipopolysaccharide-induced experimental neuroinflammation in the rat. *Shock*. 2011;36(5):458–65

15. Blusztajn JK, Slack BE, Mellott TJ. Neuroprotective actions of dietary choline. *Nutrients*. 2017;9(8):815:1–23

16. Whiley L, Sen A, Heaton J, et al. AddNeuroMed Consortium. Evidence of altered phosphatidylcholine metabolism in Alzheimer's disease. *Neurobiol Aging*. 2014;35(2):271–8

17. Gibson GE, Blass JP. Nutrition and functional neurochemistry. In Siegel GJ, Agranoff BW, Albers RW, et al., editors. *Basic Neurochemistry: Molecular, Cellular and Medical Aspects*. 6th ed. Philadelphia, PA. Lippincott-Raven. 1999

18. Holton KF. Micronutrients may be a unique weapon against the neurotoxic triad of excitotoxicity, oxidative stress and neuroinflammation: a perspective. *Front Neurosci*. 2021;15:726457:1–11

19. Kaliannan K, Wang B, Li XY, et al. A host-microbiome interaction mediates the opposing effects of omega-6 and omega-3 fatty acids on metabolic endotoxemia. *Sci Rep*. 2015;5:11276:1–21

20. Lobo de Sá FD, Backert S, Nattramilarasu PK, et al. Vitamin D reverses disruption of gut epithelial barrier function caused by *Campylobacter jejuni*. *Int J Mol Sci*. 2021;22(16):8872:1–19

21. Yeung CY, Chiang Chiau JS, Cheng ML, et al. Effects of vitamin D-deficient diet on intestinal epithelial integrity and zonulin expression in a C57BL/6 mouse model. *Front Med* (Lausanne). 2021;8:649818:1–13

22. McFarland LV, Surawicz CM, Greenberg RN, et al. Prevention of beta-lactam-associated diarrhea by Saccharomyces boulardii compared with placebo. *Am J Gastroenterol*. 1995;90(3):439–48

23. Kotowska M, Albrecht P, Szajewska H. Saccharomyces boulardii in the prevention of antibiotic-associated diarrhoea in children: a randomized double-blind placebo-controlled trial. *Aliment Pharmacol Ther*. 2005;21(5):583–90

24. Szajewska H, Kołodziej M. Systematic review with meta-analysis: *Saccharomyces boulardii* in the prevention of antibiotic-associated diarrhoea. *Aliment Pharmacol Ther*. 2015;42(7):793–801

25. Guo Q, Goldenberg JZ, Humphrey C, et al. Probiotics for the prevention of pediatric antibiotic-associated diarrhea. *Cochrane Database Syst Rev*. 2019 Apr 30;4(4):CD004827:1–103

26. Souba WW, Klimberg VS, Plumley DA, et al. The role of glutamine in maintaining a healthy gut and supporting the metabolic response to injury and infection. *Journal of Surgical Research*. 1990;48(4):383–91

27. Van Der Hulst RR, Von Meyenfeldt MF, Deutz NE, et al. Glutamine and the preservation of gut integrity. *Lancet*. 1993;341(8857):1363–5

28. Anderson PM, Schroeder G, Skubitz KM. Oral glutamine reduces the duration and severity of stomatitis after cytotoxic cancer chemotherapy. *Cancer: Interdisciplinary International Journal of the American Cancer Society*. 1998;83(7):1433–9

CHAPTER 19

PERSONALIZE

It is much more important to know what sort of a patient has a disease than what sort of a disease a patient has.

~ UNKNOWN

KEY POINTS

- ▸ The Fully Functional process is personalized, beginning with the very first encounter with the patient
- ▸ This personalization is enhanced further once laboratory data is available
- ▸ Response to therapeutic interventions also helps enhance personalization
- ▸ Patients and parents must personalize (internalize) the process so that they can navigate their health journey differently in the future

Most medical trials, out of necessity, test one intervention at a time (versus a control intervention) and try to eliminate any other variables to maintain scientific rigor. If a medication or procedure is found to produce significantly positive results without harming the subject, it may become part of the clinical repertoire we use to treat the patient.

Although demographics are matched between intervention arms and control arms of trials, patients with significant comorbidities are often excluded from studies. Many drug studies are carried out on healthy individuals. The problem then becomes whether you can apply the results

> Personalized medicine considers the unique characteristics and desires of a patient along with their family dynamic and capabilities, and then uses all of these variables as a lens through which to make clinical decisions.

of a study of healthy people to a ninety-eight-year-old patient, or to a child, or to someone on multiple other medications.

The best medicine is personalized medicine. Personalized medicine considers the unique characteristics and desires of a patient along with their family dynamic and capabilities, and then uses all of these variables as a lens through which to make clinical decisions. As noted in

Chapter 2, this is the framework described in the original evidence-based medicine articles.

Although this textbook outlines the process we use in broad strokes, it is incapable of replacing the clinical expertise of a well-trained PANS and PANDAS physician. Algorithms can be helpful as a learning framework but should never be accepted as black-and-white rules for patient care. This undervalues the clinical experience of physicians and implies that anyone with a book of algorithms can treat patients.

We personalize our treatment plans from the very beginning of our patient encounters. There is a personalized aspect to the questions we ask, the medications and supplements we prescribe, the tests we perform, and the guidance we offer. As it should be.

At our six-week follow-up visit, we spend the first portion figuring out how the patient and the family have done. Next, we present a summary of the lab findings and provide the parents context for the results. This summary is presented within the framework of the Fully Functional process to help parents understand the interventions we will be recommending and any necessary adjustments to the initial plan. We also focus on infections, toxins, and the status of the immune system during this and subsequent appointments.

The lab results along with the parental report of the child's progress are then used to make a more personalized plan to achieve a long-term recovery.

In addition to providing a personalized plan, we also emphasize to our patients and their parents that we want them to personalize (or

> **The ideal situation for patients is that they view health as a positive vitality and not just the absence of disease.**

internalize) their health journey so that they can navigate it on their own in the future. The ideal situation for patients is that they view health as a positive vitality and not just the absence of disease. Health care that is purely transactional (take this pill for your chief complaint) is often devoid of relationship. Without a relationship, your patients are much less likely to do what you say.

Personalizing the patient experience is the best way, as physicians, that we will remain the captains of the ship in terms of patient care. Cookie-cutter, algorithmic care which is short on time and patience is what is leading far too many physicians to burnout and suicide. Trained integrative physician–led care teams can transform medicine for our patients and for us. We can do it. You can do it.

May we be bold enough.

CHAPTER 20

THERAPEUTIC APPROACHES TO AUTONOMIC NERVOUS SYSTEM DYSFUNCTION

"Playing nice" comes naturally when our neuroception detects safety and promotes physiological states that support social behavior. However, pro-social behavior will not occur when our neuroception misreads the environmental cues and triggers physiological states that support defensive strategies.

~ STEPHEN W. PORGES

KEY POINTS

▸ The autonomic nervous system is composed of two main parts: the sympathetic nervous system and the parasympathetic nervous system

▸ The parasympathetic nervous system may be further divided into the dorsal vagus response and the ventral vagus response

▸ The sympathetic nervous system is responsible for general wakefulness and the fight-or-flight response

▸ The dorsal vagus nerve is the "shutdown switch" and may foster social isolation, fainting, and feelings of hopelessness

▸ The ventral vagus nerve fosters peaceful feelings and a desire for social connection

▸ Simple exercises can be taught to patients which can help bring about a ventral vagus response when patients are caught in sympathetic activation or a dorsal vagus state

We decided to place information about autonomic nervous system regulation in a separate chapter since it is applicable to so many of the topics in this book (anxiety, depression, insomnia, constipation, diarrhea, urinary symptoms, irritability, etc).

The autonomic nervous system (ANS) is composed of the sympathetic nervous system and the parasympathetic nervous system. The sympathetic nervous system is made up of nerves which come from the spinal cord in the thoracic and lumbar region and is responsible for the fight-or-flight response. When activated, it increases heart rate and blood pressure,

> The dorsal vagus nerve is, in essence, the "shutdown switch."

increases the respiratory rate, dilates the pupils, and increases blood flow to the skeletal muscle. The brain is also put on alert—so activation of a strong sympathetic response often produces feelings of anxiousness or panic.

The second part of the ANS is the parasympathetic system, which is mainly responsible for digestion, rest, and social connection. Most (75%) of the parasympathetic nervous system is in the vagus nerve. The vagus nerve (cranial nerve 10 or CN X) comes from the brain stem and runs all the way to the abdominal cavity.

The vagus nerve has two portions.[1] The first is the ventral branch, which is responsible for digestive functions, social connection, and things like lowering the heart rate. We tell patients to think of the ventral vagus nerve as being activated while you are relaxing on the beach with someone you love, having a deep, intimate conversation.

The second part of the vagus nerve is the dorsal branch. The dorsal branch of the vagus nerve has some role in digestion and relaxation but is mainly of interest here because it is responsible for a primitive response to extreme stress. The dorsal vagus nerve is, in essence, the "shutdown switch."

If the dorsal part of the vagus nerve is activated by overwhelming stress, the response is disconnection from others and a feeling of being frozen for self-protection. It is typically triggered by extreme stress when the brain believes that significant injury or death is imminent (when fighting or fleeing may be futile).

This reaction is seen in animals when they "play dead" to avoid a predator. It is also seen at times when people freeze (or don't respond) in the midst of a trauma. Bystanders report that some people struck by trains when crossing the tracks will stop when they see the train coming and freeze. They don't even attempt to move out of the way. That is an extreme dorsal vagal shutdown response. A strong activation of the dorsal vagus nerve results in feelings of hopelessness or helplessness. Dissociation reactions in some rape survivors (who report that they felt absent from their body during the assault) is an example of a dorsal vagal response. A sudden strong activation of the dorsal vagal response may quickly drop your blood pressure and cause you to faint. This is the true origin of the vagal response we think of when people faint in response to pain or emotional upset. Whereas the sympathetic response to trauma is known as "fight or flight," the dorsal vagus response is sometimes referred to as "freeze or faint." Interestingly, a strong dorsal vagus response often occurs after an intense, excessively high sympathetic response has occurred.

Ideally, there should be a balance between the sympathetic and parasympathetic portions of the autonomic nervous system. The balance of the processes should change depending on which response is most appropriate at any given time. When imbalance occurs and problems arise, it is usually from overactivation of the sympathetic response or overactivation of the dorsal vagus nerve (social isolation, helplessness, fainting). The most problematic state exists when both the sympathetic response and dorsal vagal response get stuck in activation. This combination can leave patients feeling continually anxious (the sympathetic activation) and hopeless or disconnected from others (the dorsal vagal reaction).

Symptoms associated with overactivation of the sympathetic and/or dorsal vagal responses include anxiety, irritability, anger, emotional instability, difficulty sleeping, chest pain, high blood pressure, loss of appetite, trust issues, difficulty concentrating, memory issues, feelings of hopelessness or depression, high-risk behaviors, and many others. Imbalance of the different portions of the autonomic nervous system can also worsen menstrual pain and asthma.[2]

Traditionally, the symptoms above are treated as distinct problems or disorders. The problem is that treating any one symptom in isolation with medication may cause some improvements in the symptom being treated, but very rarely leave the patient feeling *balanced* or truly well. This is because imbalance of the autonomic nervous system impairs many distinct bodily processes.

The good news is that there are simple and effective exercises you can suggest that your

> **The most problematic state exists when both the sympathetic response and dorsal vagal response get stuck in activation.**

patients may perform at home to restore autonomic balance. These are mainly focused on reducing the exaggerated sympathetic and/or dorsal vagal responses and increasing the ventral vagal tone. There is also a strong association between vagal (parasympathetic) tone and emotional regulation.[3]

The best way to describe optimal autonomic nervous system balance is contentment and social connection, with the ability to defend against adversity when needed. Here are fourteen methods to restore healthy autonomic balance:

1. Deep breathing exercises[4]

We typically discuss breathing exercises with our patients for precisely this reason. It is especially helpful if slow breathing from the abdomen is performed. One simple technique is 4-7-8 breathing. To do this exercise, the patient finds a quiet spot where they will not be disturbed. They breathe in over a count of four, then hold the breath for a count of seven, and then exhale over a count of eight and repeat for at least three minutes.

If patients have never done this before, they may need to slowly work their way up to holding their breath for seven seconds to stay comfortable and avoid inadvertently raising stress levels.

> People who cultivate positive emotions (gratitude, joy, forgiveness of others) in themselves have improved health and increased vagal tone.

A good place to start if seven seconds seems too long initially is to do box breathing. Legend has it box breathing is used by Navy SEALs prior to missions to help them remain calm. To do this exercise, they breathe in for a count of four, hold for a count of four, breathe out for a count of four, hold for another count of four, and repeat for at least three minutes. If patients begin to feel dizzy, they can return to normal breathing until they feel better and then try again another day.

2. Singing, humming, or gargling

Most people learn to hum before they learn to talk. Small children often hum when they eat or play to self-soothe. The vagus nerve is connected to the larynx. The vibration produced with singing or humming stimulates the ventral portion of the vagus nerve. Since both of these activities are associated with prolonged exhalation, they also provide the benefits of deep breathing but in a more social and fun manner. Even if people can't sing, humming or using a kazoo can give them the same benefits. Repetitive chanting with meditation can help stimulate the ventral vagus. Gargling also stimulates the vagus nerve.

3. Exercise

Although exercise initially stimulates the sympathetic nervous system and increases heart rate and respiratory rate to supply blood to the muscles, the net effect after exercise is to stimulate a ventral vagal response. This is one of the reasons most people feel good after they finish exercising. Doing this with a partner also helps establish human connectedness. Studies have shown that exercise training modifies the autonomic nervous system response in patients with heart problems.[5]

4. Dancing

This is one of our favorite activities. It's a combination of exercise and increased breathing, and if patients also sing or hum while dancing, they have achieved the trifecta of vagus nerve stimulation. Like group exercise, dancing with others also adds connectedness to the mix.

5. Playing a musical instrument

Playing a musical instrument (or even just listening to music) stimulates the ventral vagus nerve. In musicians, a state of connectedness with the crowd and extreme peace or confidence while playing music masterfully is called the *flow state*. Several studies have examined the flow state and have found that this state positively affects heart rate variability (vagus tone).[6,7]

6. Cold water exposure

Placing cold water or ice on the face, taking a cold shower, or sitting in an ice bath can increase parasympathetic responses and lower sympathetic tone. This has been demonstrated in several studies.[8,9,10] The Wim Hof Method is a program designed to help induce a calm state and increase concentration. The three components of the method are focus, breathing, and cold exposure.

7. The valsalva maneuver

Patients can perform the valsalva maneuver while they are lying on their back. To perform this exercise, they tense the abdominal muscles and bear down as if having a bowel movement. They should hold their breath while doing this and continue for 5–10 seconds. This can be repeated 3–4 times with two-minute breaks in between. If they begin to feel dizzy or out of breath, they should stop the exercise and breathe normally. This exercise should not be done while sitting up or standing since it may cause fainting. Valsalva maneuvers are occasionally used in the emergency department when people come in with tachycardia, although antidysrhythmics are more effective.[11,12,13]

8. Prayer, meditation, or yoga

Prayer, meditation, and yoga are known as contemplative practices. There is evidence that these behaviors stimulate the vagus nerve.[14] Group prayer, meditation, yoga, support groups, and hobbies are also activities which can increase connectedness.

9. Positive emotions and attitude

People who cultivate positive emotions (gratitude, joy, forgiveness of others) in themselves have improved health and increased vagal tone.[15] There are various apps and programs available to help patients develop these strategies for themselves.

10. Journaling

One thing we encourage all our patients (and parents of our young patients) to do is to journal often. It does not have to be organized or fancy. Just a cheap notebook and a pen will do. We encourage people to write often about what they are thankful for or what good things they have.

Thankfulness can be hard to muster in the thick of the fight when a child is ill. But we almost always have something that we can name—air-conditioning on a hot day, heat when it's cold outside, food to eat, and clothes to wear.

Narrative expressive writing has been shown to lower heart rate and increase heart rate variability in adults following marital separation.[16] People write about an adverse event or condition, listing their deepest thoughts and feelings while trying to weave these emotions into a narrative story that tells them something about the meaning of the events. Expressive writing has also been shown to strengthen the immune system.[17]

> Expressive writing has been shown to strengthen the immune system.

11. Nutritional factors and the microbiome

Research from 2016 outlines a connection of the gut microbiome to post-traumatic stress disorder.[18] This connection relates to the development of PTSD and may serve as a potential target for treatment with specific probiotics. It has been proposed that the ability of oral probiotics to change behavior (which has previously been shown in mice) may be due to chemical signaling from the gut to the brain via the vagus nerve.[19,20] Omega 3 fats increase heart rate variability and may protect against abnormal heart rhythms.[21]

12. Vagus nerve exercises

Accessing the Healing Power of the Vagus Nerve by Stanley Rosenberg[2] contains several easy vagal nerve balancing exercises based upon the original work done by Dr. Stephen Porges. These exercises use the movements of eye muscles and head movements to balance the output of the sympathetic and parasympathetic nervous systems. The exercises can be done with a partner to facilitate personal connection.

13. Vagus nerve stimulators

Several surgically implantable devices are available which stimulate the vagus nerve. They have been used for years to help with intractable seizures, severe depression, and bipolar disorder.[22,23] Research has also shown that electrical vagus nerve stimulation can help with treatment-resistant anxiety.[24,25]

Recently, some good portable external devices to stimulate the vagus nerve have come to the market. Effective, FDA-cleared models require a physician's prescription and usually cost about $600 for a three-month course of treatment. Patients should be wary of cheap models online that promise vagal stimulation for a much lower price. We screen our patients carefully before recommending any device.

14. Stellate ganglion block

A stellate ganglion block is a minor surgical procedure which involves injection of a local anesthetic in the anterior portion of the neck by a specially trained physician. The procedure is conducted under ultrasound guidance, as the great vessels lie close to the injection site. Unlike the previous suggestions, which mostly involve increasing parasympathetic tone of the vagus nerve, a stellate ganglion block decreases sympathetic tone. Stellate ganglion blocks were originally used for sleep. Research has now shown that they can be useful for turning down the sympathetic response that seems to be stuck in the on position in patients with post-traumatic stress disorder.[26–28] These studies have primarily been conducted on military members with PTSD.

CHAPTER 20 REFERENCES

1. Porges SW. Orienting in a defensive world: mammalian modifications of our evolutionary heritage—a polyvagal theory. *Psychophysiology*. 1995;32:301–318
2. Rosenberg S. *Accessing the Healing Power of the Vagus Nerve: Self-Help Exercises for Anxiety, Depression, Trauma, and Autism*. North Atlantic Books. 2017
3. Porges SW, Doussard-Roosevelt JA, Maiti AK. Vagal tone and the physiological regulation of emotion. *Monogr Soc Res Child Dev*. 1994;59(2–3):167–186
4. Wang SZ, Li S, Xu XY, et al. Effect of slow abdominal breathing combined with biofeedback on blood pressure and heart rate variability in prehypertension. *J Altern Complement Med*. 2010;16(10):1039–1045

5. Besnier F, Labrunée M, Pathak A, et al. Exercise training-induced modification in autonomic nervous system: an update for cardiac patients. *Ann Phys Rehabil Med*. 2017;60(1):27–35

6. de Manzano O, Theorell T, Harmat L, et al. The psychophysiology of flow during piano playing. *Emotion*. 2010;10(3):301–311

7. Hamilton AK, Pernía DM, Puyol Wilson C, et al. What makes metalheads happy? A phenomenological analysis of flow experiences in metal musicians. *Qualitative Research in Psychology*. 2019;16(4):537–565

8. Kinoshita T, Nagata S, Baba R, et al. Cold-water face immersion per se elicits cardiac parasympathetic activity. *Circ J*. 2006;70(6):773–776

9. Hayashi N, Ishihara M, Tanaka A, et al. Face immersion increases vagal activity as assessed by heart rate variability. *Eur J Appl Physiol Occup Physiol*. 1997;76(5):394–399

10. Paulev PE, Pokorski M, Honda Y, et al. Facial cold receptors and the survival reflex "diving bradycardia" in man. *Jpn J Physiol*. 1990;40(5):701–712

11. Smith G. Management of supraventricular tachycardia using the Valsalva manoeuvre: a historical review and summary of published evidence. *European Journal of Emergency Medicine*. 2012;19(6), 346–352

12. Smith GD, Fry MM, Taylor D, Morgans A, Cantwell K. Effectiveness of the Valsalva manoeuvre for reversion of supraventricular tachycardia. *Cochrane Database of Systematic Reviews*. 2015;2:1–22

13. www.resources.acls.com/free-resources/knowledge-base/tachycardia/vagal-maneuvers, accessed 5/15/2022

14. Gerritsen RJS, Band GPH. Breath of life: the respiratory vagal stimulation model of contemplative activity. *Front Hum Neurosci*. 2018;12:397

15. Kok BE, Coffey KA, Cohn MA, et al. How positive emotions build physical health: perceived positive social connections account for the upward spiral between positive emotions and vagal tone. *Psychological Science*. 2013;24(7):1123–1132

16. Bourassa KJ, Allen JJB, Mehl MR, et al. Impact of narrative expressive writing on heart rate, heart rate variability, and blood pressure after marital separation. *Psychosom Med*. 2017;79(6):697–705

17. Pennebaker JW, Kiecolt-Glaser JK, Glaser R. Disclosure of traumas and immune function: health implications for psychotherapy. *J Consult Clin Psychol*. 1988;56(2):239–245

18. Leclercq S, Forsythe P, Bienenstock J. Posttraumatic stress disorder: does the gut microbiome hold the key? *Can J Psychiatry*. 2016;61(4):204–213

19. Grenham S, Clarke G, Cryan J, et al. Brain-gut microbe communication in health and disease. *Frontiers in Physiology*. 2011;2(94):1–15

20. Bonaz B, Bazin T, Pellissier S. The vagus nerve at the interface of the microbiota-gut-brain axis. *Front Neurosci*. 2018;12(49):1–9

21. Christensen JH. Omega-3 polyunsaturated fatty acids and heart rate variability. *Front Physiol*. 2011;2(84):1–9

22. Aaronson ST, Sears P, Ruvuna F, et al. A 5-year observational study of patients with treatment-resistant depression treated with vagus nerve stimulation or treatment as usual: comparison of response, remission, and suicidality. *American Journal of Psychiatry*. 2017;174(7):640–648

23. McAllister-Williams RH, Sousa S, Kumar, A. et al. The effects of vagus nerve stimulation on the course and outcomes of patients with bipolar disorder in a treatment-resistant depressive episode: a 5-year prospective registry. *Int J Bipolar Disord.* 2020;8(13):1–11

24. George MS, Ward HE, Ninan PT, et al. A pilot study of vagus nerve stimulation (VNS) for treatment-resistant anxiety disorders. *Brain Stimulation.* 2008;1(2):112–121

25. Klarer M, Arnold M, Günther L, et al. Gut vagal afferents differentially modulate innate anxiety and learned fear. *Journal of Neuroscience.* 2014;34(21):7067–7076

26. Alino J, Kosatka D, McLean B, et al. Efficacy of stellate ganglion block in the treatment of anxiety symptoms from combat-related post-traumatic stress disorder: a case series. *Mil Med.* 2013;178(4):e473–e476

27. Lynch JH, Muench PD, Okiishi JC, et al. Behavioral health clinicians endorse stellate ganglion block as a valuable intervention in the treatment of trauma-related disorders. *Journal of Investigative Medicine.* 2021;69:989–993

28. Rae Olmsted KL, Bartoszek M, Mulvaney S, et al. Effect of stellate ganglion block treatment on posttraumatic stress disorder symptoms: a randomized clinical trial. *JAMA Psychiatry.* 2020;77(2):130–138

CHAPTER 21

ADDITIONAL ADJUNCTIVE THERAPIES: NEUROLINGUISTIC PROGRAMMING AND HYPNOSIS

It is really amazing what people can do. Only they don't know what they can do.
~ MILTON ERICKSON

> ## KEY POINTS
>
> ▸ Neurolinguistic programming uses the power of specific language, self-perception, and the study of excellence to help patients overcome problems such as poor self-esteem, OCD, phobias, and negative self-talk
>
> ▸ Hypnosis is a valuable tool to help patients become aware of the capability they have to change their mind and find new abilities
>
> ▸ All hypnosis is self-hypnosis
>
> ▸ Hypnosis can be used to help pediatric patients react more favorably to painful or anxiety-producing procedures and may help them overcome fears, OCD, or habits such as bed-wetting

NEUROLINGUISTIC PROGRAMMING

Neurolinguistic programming (NLP) is a system of techniques and concepts that helps people break free from the pain of prior events and overcome fear and anxiety. To help people with anxiety, rather than studying anxious people looking for answers, NLP studied people who had significant anxiety and overcame it.

NLP then defined specific processes anxious patients used to heal, and developed a system to help others use these techniques to recover. NLP allows people to become "unstuck," find the posi-

> NLP allows people to become "unstuck," find the positive in a situation, and increase available choices. Increased choices equal increased freedom.

tive in a situation, and increase available choices. Increased choices equal increased freedom.

NLP is also very helpful in removing limiting beliefs, which are unhelpful internal stories people believe about themselves. When limiting beliefs are challenged and removed, people can achieve the true potential for which they were created.

NLP was developed in the 1970s by Dr. Richard Bandler (a psychologist and mathematician) and Dr. John Grinder (a linguist). It uses concepts based on mathematics, linguistics, psychology, and neurology. Several levels of certification are available in NLP, including NLP practitioner, NLP master practitioner, and NLP trainer.

Although we use our conscious mind to make decisions, our subconscious mind is responsible for most of our thoughts, which generate feelings and behaviors. Because NLP techniques operate on the subconscious part of our mind, they often provide success after other types of talk therapy have failed. The subconscious mind is very powerful.

NLP helps resolve anxiety, improves depressive thoughts, and helps children and their parents reframe situations.

How we use NLP in PANS and PANDAS

Some NLP techniques are difficult to use with children with PANS and PANDAS, especially if they are in a flare or are too young to participate. One of the NLP concepts we use universally with children involves establishing a positive identity. NLP describes different categories of influences on behavior that encourage or prevent change.

These categories are:
1. Environment
2. Habits
3. Capabilities
4. Beliefs and values
5. Personal identity
6. Sense of greater purpose or morality (that which is objectively right)

Of all the things that drive behavior, personal identity and the objective right are the most influential. One of things parents can do to subtly change behavior when children are not acting in an ideal manner is to create a positive family or personal identity and continually reinforce it with their child.

Since identity is such a strong driver of change or resistance to change, parents should always avoid calling their child bad or sick. They should not call them a baby and should especially not call them a *PANDAS patient*. Children readily accept labels and may hold these things as a reflection of their self-worth.

Instead, parents should say something like:

- "You are a member of the Jones family, and our family doesn't act like that."
- "I used to let you act like this when you were a baby, but you are ___ years old now so you have to act like an older child."
- "Come on, you are a better person than that."
- "Boy, I'm glad you are so much better now. I remember when you had problems with [handwashing, anxiety, or whatever] and now you are SO MUCH BETTER." (once a child overcomes a particular type of OCD or unwanted behavior)
- "This is a sign you are getting better and better every day."

Many children have a fear that their parents may leave due to their bad behavior. One good way for parents to ease this fear is for them to remind their children that they will always be there for them no matter how bad things get and they will always be a family.

Another NLP technique that can be very helpful with older children with PANS and PANDAS (and their parents) is positive kinesthetic anchoring. This technique takes about twenty minutes to properly teach the patient or parent.

To go from one emotional state (anxiety/anger) to another (peace/calm) your brain must dynamically remove the neurotransmitters from the agitated state (norepinephrine) and replace them with those from a calm state (oxytocin, serotonin, and dopamine). This can reliably be attained using NLP in a cooperative individual by establishing a kinesthetic anchor. This is best done in children over the age of ten. Younger

> **Since identity is such a strong driver of change or resistance to change, parents should always avoid calling their child bad or sick.**

children or children in a flare may not be able to cooperate. With a little patient cooperation, this technique can be very effective.

Here is a brief synopsis of the technique I use for establishing a positive kinesthetic anchor.

NOTE: This description is merely intended to familiarize physicians with the technique and is not meant to be instructional. The technique is best learned by observing a trained NLP practitioner perform the technique with patients.

Kinesthetic Anchor Exercise:

1. I initially have the patient assume a comfortable position in a chair or reclining.
2. I find out if the patient is left-handed or right-handed.
3. Before starting the technique, I have the patient touch their thumb to their small finger on their non-dominant hand and hold these fingers together.

4. I have the patient separate and put the fingers together several times, and then do it with their eyes closed.

5. I have the patient relax the hand (thumb and small finger apart).

6. Next, I ask the patient to tell me a story of a time when they were very happy and calm: common examples might be a vacation, their birthday, or a special time with a grandparent. I try to extract as much detail as we can about what the patient saw, heard, felt, etc. The more sensory detail the better.

7. I then let the patient know I will be telling them a story and have them close their eyes.

8. I have them put themselves in the place that they spoke about. I usually say, "I don't want you to just remember it; I want you to put yourself there as if you are back there right now." I give them prompts about what they are seeing, hearing, and feeling (sunshine on their face, the smell of the salt air at the beach, the blue sky in the summer, the smell of a holiday meal, etc.).

9. When their facial expression seems calm, I give them a prompt to touch their thumb to their small finger and hold it there.

10. When they do this, I suggest that they are experiencing a "certain pleasant sensation" in their body. Usually I will say, "In the chest or abdomen." I tell them that holding their small finger to their thumb will make the feeling even stronger.

11. After a minute or so, I tell them to separate their thumb from their small finger and feel the nice, warm feeling slowly melt away. (I usually say it is "emptying out through the bottom of their feet into the ground.")

12. I then have them open their eyes. When they do, I ask them a left-brained (analytical question) like a simple math problem or their address or birthday. This is called "clearing the state." It helps strengthen the technique.

13. I then have them close their eyes again and repeat the anchoring process. I usually do this 2–3 times and clear the state between each.

14. At the end of the technique, I have them open their eyes and, without concentrating on the place we spoke about I have them touch their thumb to their small finger and I say, "Do you feel that?"

15. Without fail, the patients smile and say "yes." I ask what the feeling is, and they usually say calm, relaxed, content, or happy.

16. I then instruct them to do this several times at home to strengthen the anchor.

17. Next, I tell them to think of other times or places when they were very happy and relaxed, and to repeat this process at home as they did in the office. This is called "stacking anchors" and makes the calming action of the anchor (touching the thumb to the small finger) stronger and shortens the onset.

The reason this technique works is because we continually encode positive experiences as sensory experiences. A song that was popular when we were in high school may give us a nice feeling when we hear it twenty years later. The same thing happens when we smell or taste a food that reminds us of something a grandparent made for us when we were younger. This can happen with smells, sights, sounds, tastes, or feelings.

Kinesthetic anchoring helps establish a strong touch anchor that gives the patient a calming sensation. This allows a rapid change in state from anxiety or fear to calmness and connection. The opposite can happen if we are suddenly scared (for example, when a car pulls out suddenly in front of us when we are driving). That sudden rush of sympathetic activity and norepinephrine release almost instantly increases our heart rate and respiratory rate, causes mydriasis, and causes us to grip the wheel and tense up. Just as that sudden rush can change our state very quickly, a strong kinesthetic anchor can do the same thing in reverse.

Wouldn't it be great if we all knew about this technique in medical school before final exams!

Establishing a positive identity and installing a positive kinesthetic anchor are the most commonly used elements of NLP in our PANS and PANDAS cases. There are over three hundred recognized NLP techniques or patterns; NLP prides itself on being adaptable to any situation or struggle.

Training in NLP is available through these professional organizations:

www.purenlp.com

www.nlpco.com

www.inlpcenter.org

FURTHER STUDY ON NLP

Andreas S, Faulkner C, editors. *NLP: The New Technology of Achievement*, Harper Collins, 1996

Bandler R, Grinder J. *The Structure of Magic I: A Book About Language and Therapy*, Science & Behavior Books, 1975

Dilts RB, DeLozier JA. *Encyclopaedia of Systemic Neuro-Linguistic Programming and NLP New Coding*, NLP University Press, 2000

Grinder John, Bandler R. *The Structure of Magic II: A Book About Communication and Change*, Science & Behavior Books, 1975

O'Connor J, McDermott I. *Principles of NLP*, Thorsons, 1996

O'Connor J, Seymour J. *Introducing Neuro-Linguistic Programming: Psychological Skills for Understanding and Influencing People*, Thorsons, 1993

Gibson BP. *The Complete Guide to Understanding and using NLP: Neuro-Linguistic Programming Explained Simply*, Atlantic Publishing, 2011

Hoobyar T, Dotz T, Sanders S. *NLP: The Essential Guide to Neuro-linguistic Programming*, Morrow, 2013

Vaknin S, *The Big Book of NLP Expanded*, Shlomo Vaknin, 12th ed., 2022

Alexander R, Aragón OR, Bookwala J, et al. The neuroscience of positive emotions and affect: Implications for cultivating happiness and wellbeing. *Neuroscience & Biobehavioral Reviews*. 2021;121:220–249

HYPNOSIS

In PANS and PANDAS, OCD and severe anxiety create a state of disorganized, repetitive, and intrusive thinking which prevents reasoning with these patients and makes direct suggestions for behavioral change very difficult. Hypnosis is an effective method of managing anxiety and rendering the mind amenable to healing suggestions. As you will see, hypnosis can also help reduce or eliminate tics and painful sensations.

Popular culture often portrays hypnosis as a strange party trick whereby the hypnotist places someone under a spell, makes them act like a chicken, and then causes them to forget what happened when they were in a trance. Unfortunately, this misconception has caused many people (especially physicians) to shy away from considering hypnosis as an effective treatment option. They view it as some sort of unproven hocus-pocus, but nothing could be further from the truth.

Hypnosis is basically an exercise where a hypnotist assists a participant's entrance into a state of relaxation in which the person becomes more receptive to helpful suggestions. During hypnosis, the relaxed state (known as the *trance state*) allows one to bypass the normal critical

> **Hypnosis is basically an exercise where a hypnotist assists a participant's entrance into a state of relaxation in which the person becomes more receptive to helpful suggestions.**

faculty or skeptical nature of the mind. Once induction of the trance has taken place, the hypnotist gives the patient one or a series of suggestions to support positive change, to help remove unwanted feelings, or to help manage pain perception.

Although hypnotists may sometimes use language which implies that hypnosis is synonymous with sleep, it is an awake but relaxed state. Most patients will remember everything that was said during a session. Trance is a normal state that people enter when they are daydreaming, watching an engaging movie, concentrating on a task on the computer, or reading an interesting

book. At these times, subconscious activities such as hearing continue, but the ability to respond is often affected. At the end of the hypnosis session, the hypnotist brings the patient out of trance and back to a normal state of consciousness (although they are not really in an abnormal state during hypnosis).

Hypnosis is not mind control. There is no way to effectively provide suggestions to a person which go against their moral standards. If this is attempted, participants will emerge from the trance state quickly and lose trust in the hypnotist. In stage hypnosis, participants are usually volunteers who want to be hypnotized and don't mind doing something outrageous. These are the folks who dance on tables in a college bar or loudly sing karaoke regardless of who is watching. That is not to say that there is no hypnosis going on in stage shows, but the suggestibility is very much heightened by the desire of the participants to be demonstrative.

Hypnosis in medicine

Although hypnosis in some form has been recognized for several thousand years, the modern era of hypnosis began in the late 1700s. Controversy and doubt kept hypnosis from mainstream medicine until the nineteenth century, when surgeons John Elliotson and James Esdaile used hypnosis for surgical anesthesia in hundreds of cases before the modern era of chemical anesthesia.[1]

In the twentieth century, hypnosis using stories, metaphors, and indirect suggestions was popularized by a psychiatrist, Dr. Milton H. Erickson. In the period between 1955 and 1961, the American Medical Association, the British Medical Association, and the American Psychiatric Association each affirmed the benefits of hypnosis in medical and dental care.[2–4]

Is hypnosis real?

Like many effective integrative therapies, hypnosis carries a certain mysterious quality. There is no doubt that it is effective, as noted in the numerous adult and pediatric studies cited below. However, some skeptics hold the position that patients who have claimed success from hypnosis may be lying, just following commands voluntarily, or simply experiencing positive effects due to the placebo effect.

One study used functional MRI technology to investigate brain responses to painful thermal stimuli.[5] The study compared patients who were hypnotized at the time of a painful stimulus to those who were not, using functional MRI scanning. The hypnosis group showed less activation in the primary sensory cortex and increased activity in the basal ganglia and the left anterior cingulate cortex during the painful stimulus. These changes were not seen in the control group.

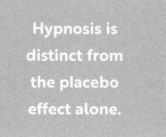

Hypnosis is distinct from the placebo effect alone.

Similarly, multiple studies using PET scans have demonstrated changes in regional cerebral blood flow (rCBF) in distinct areas of the brain while patients were hypnotized and subjected to painful stimuli.[6–9] Another PET scan study showed patients either colored or grayscale pictures while hypnotized.[10] Suggestions were given that patients were seeing color, and the area of the brain that processes color imagery became more active, even if the subject was looking at a grayscale image. The color activation areas were less active when it was suggested that they see grayscale images, even if they were looking at color images. One of the PET scan studies also

incorporated EEG monitoring, which demonstrated increased delta wave EEG activity in hypnotized patients.[6] Delta wave activity is typically seen in periods of deep sleep or meditation.

Hypnosis is not deception or placebo effect

Studies have shown that patients in hypnotic trance are not simply complying or deceiving the examiner to gain favor or pretending that the techniques are effective.[11,12] Hypnosis is distinct from the placebo effect alone.[13,14]

Is hypnosis effective?

The central questions with any treatment modality are whether it works and whether it is reproducible in clinical practice. Once relegated to smaller clinical settings due to controversy, hypnosis has now gained the respect and support of larger, more mainstream medical societies and organizations. In addition to evidence for the efficacy of hypnosis for specific symptoms or disease states (as referenced below), several well-done reviews supporting the use of hypnosis have appeared in the anesthesia literature,[9] the pediatric literature,[15,16] and the Mayo Clinic proceedings.[4]

There is a wealth of literature (including randomized trials) supporting the use of hypnosis in pain control and as an adjunct in painful medical procedures in children and adults.[4,15–22] Hypnosis is also effective for chronic pain.[23] A Cochrane review analyzing fifty-nine trials and over 5,000 patient encounters reported that hypnosis is effective at reducing needle-related pain and distress.[24] Another meta-analysis of eighty-five trials with

3,632 participants found beneficial effects of hypnosis for all pain outcomes.[25] Hypnosis has been shown to be effective for pediatric fracture reduction in a small case series[26] in an emergency department in Mexico where general anesthesia, regional anesthesia, and hematoma blocks were not available.

Needle phobia is a significant barrier to pediatric venipuncture. There are several case reports demonstrating the effectiveness of brief hypnotic suggestions in easing or eliminating needle phobia.[27-29]

Gut-focused hypnotherapy has been shown to be effective in 88% of children and adolescents with IBS in one study.[30] Hypnosis outperformed propranolol and placebo for pain control in a study in pediatric migraine patients.[31] Hypnotherapy is effective in treating children with dysphagia and food aversion,[32] childhood habit disorders such as trichotillomania,[33,34] Tourette syndrome,[35,36] and sleep terrors.[37]

Group hypnosis is also an effective treatment format for patients with chronic pain.[38]

In the very well-referenced reviews already cited, hypnosis is noted to be effective for modulation of the immune system, surgical anesthesia (usually as an adjunct to medications), dermatologic conditions, accelerating healing from surgery, lowering blood pressure, reducing pain, decreasing complications and shortening hospital stays in the obstetrical setting, decreasing post-chemotherapy nausea in children, better asthmatic control, reduction of anxiety, improvement of enuresis, and improvement in impotence.[4,16]

I am a certified clinical hypnotherapist and have successfully used hypnotherapy as a treatment modality to help PANS and PANDAS patients overcome selective mutism, needle phobia, and contamination OCD in our office.

Are there risks to hypnosis?

There are no significant risks to hypnosis. Very rarely, periods of agitation may be evoked while the patient is in trance. These are called *abreactions*; they are very rare and easily managed by breaking the state, bringing the patient out of trance, and then practicing relaxation techniques. In our practice, we have never had a patient have an abreaction during or after hypnosis.

A simple hypnosis technique you can use for children prior to a blood draw (this works best with children between five and twelve):

1. First and foremost, establish rapport with the child. Be silly. Take off your shoes spontaneously. Make faces. Don't wear a lab coat. Talk to the child and not about the child.
2. Say, "I would like to see you do a magic trick. I can help you make it work."
3. Then have them sit down and put their hands on their lap.
4. Ask them if they know what will happen if you push down a light switch on the wall. They usually will tell you the light will go off.
5. Explain that that is because the switch turns off the power through a wire and then the light cannot work. You can actually flip the switch on and off in the room while talking.
6. Then tell them you have studied the brain and that it works the same way. Tell them to think of the switches in their brain and that there are colored wires from those brain switches to their arms and legs. Ask them what color the wire is that goes from

their brain to their left arm. Then their right arm. Then their left leg. Finally, their right leg. Tell them you are about to teach them how to do the trick.

7. Have them close their eyes and imagine finding the switch from their brain to their left arm. (Use the color they assigned to this wire.)

8. Ask them to flip that switch so their arm "does not work." Suggest that the arm does not feel normal, but is really heavy or asleep. Grab the arm and drop it and affirm that that is the case (even if they don't respond). Let them know that this arm will not feel anything, and you are going to test their magic.

9. Lightly pinch or touch this arm and then their other arm and say, "See, your magic works and you DID IT!" Tell them they did a great job and to remember how different this arm feels.

10. Then have them "turn the power back on" and suggest that the arm now feels normal, and they can move it whenever they want.

11. Then do a leg. Then do the other leg.

12. Lastly, repeat the process with the other arm.

13. Then let them know that you are going to tell everyone you see that day that you saw a patient do some great magic.

14. Finally, suggest that they turn the power off to the arm that blood is being drawn from and tell them to "not tell the person drawing blood until they are finished." The idea that

they are playing a trick on the phlebotomist will make them even more susceptible and will increase the chance of success.

15. When it's over, have them let the phlebotomist know they tricked them and could not feel the blood draw.

Breathing exercises can help too. We sometimes do these together. The key to this working is to be confident and have great rapport.

FINDING A CLINICAL HYPNOTHERAPIST

The American Society of Clinical Hypnosis (ASCH) was founded by Dr. Milton Erickson in 1957. The society is unique in that members must hold a professional license in a field of health care, such as a doctorate. The website is www.asch.net and there is a provider finder here: www.asch.net/aws/ASCH/pt/sp/find-member. The society also conducts hypnosis training programs.

FOR FURTHER READING

Lynn SJ, Rhue JW, Kirsch I. *Handbook of Clinical Hypnosis, 2nd ed.*, American Psychological Association, 2010

Bandler R, Grinder J. *Patterns of the Hypnotic Techniques of Milton H. Erickson, M.D., Volume 1*, Meta Publications, 1975

Kohen DP, Olness K. *Hypnosis with Children, 5th ed.*, Routledge, 2023

Old G. *Revisiting Hypnosis: The Principles and Practice of Post-Hypnotic Re-induction Training*, Plastic Spoon, 2016

Hand K. *Magic Words and Language Patterns*, ReMind Publishing, 2017

CHAPTER 21 REFERENCES

1. Forrest DW. *Hypnotism: A History*. London. Penguin. 1999

2. Medical use of hypnotism: report of a subcommittee appointed by the Psychological Medicine Group Committee of the British Medical Association. *Supplement to the BMJ* April 23, 1955: 190–193, Appendix X

3. Council on Mental Health. Medical use of hypnosis. *JAMA*, Sep 13, 1958: 186–189

4. Stewart JH. Hypnosis in contemporary medicine. *Mayo Clin Proc*. 2005;80(4):511–24

5. Schulz-Stübner S, Krings T, Meister IG, et al. Clinical hypnosis modulates functional magnetic resonance imaging signal intensities and pain perception in a thermal stimulation paradigm. *Reg Anesth Pain Med*. 2004;29(6):549–56

6. Rainville P, Hofbauer RK, Paus T, et al. Cerebral mechanisms of hypnotic induction and suggestion. *Journal of Cognitive Neuroscience*. 1999;11(1):110–25

7. Rainville P, Hofbauer RK, Bushnell MC, et al. Hypnosis modulates activity in brain structures involved in the regulation of consciousness. *Journal of Cognitive Neuroscience*. 2002;14(6):887–901

8. Wik G, Fischer H, Bragée B, et al. Functional anatomy of hypnotic analgesia: a PET study of patients with fibromyalgia. *European Journal of Pain*. 1999;3(1):7–12

9. Faymonville ME, Laureys S, Degueldre C, et al. Neural mechanisms of antinociceptive effects of hypnosis. *Anesthesiology*. 2000;92(5):1257–67

10. Kosslyn SM, Thompson WL, Costantini-Ferrando MF, et al. Hypnotic visual illusion alters color processing in the brain. *Am J Psychiatry*. 2000 Aug;157(8):1279–84

11. Kinnunen T, Zamansky HS, Block ML. Is the hypnotized subject lying? *J Abnorm Psychol*. 1994;103(2):184–91

12. Kinnunen T, Zamansky HS, Nordstrom BL. Is the hypnotized subject complying? *Int J Clin Exp Hypn*. 2001;49(2):83–94

13. Spiegel D, Bierre P, Rootenberg J. Hypnotic alteration of somatosensory perception. *Am J Psychiatry*. 1989;146(6):749–54

14. McGlashan TH, Evans FJ, Orne MT. The nature of hypnotic analgesia and placebo response to experimental pain. *Psychosom Med*. 1969;31(3):227–46

15. Saadat H, Kain ZN. Hypnosis as a therapeutic tool in pediatrics. *Pediatrics*. 2007;120(1):179–81

16. Kohen DP, Kaiser P. Clinical hypnosis with children and adolescents: What? Why? How? Origins, applications, and efficacy. *Children* (Basel). 2014;1(2):74–98

17. Liossi C, White P, Hatira P. A randomized clinical trial of a brief hypnosis intervention to control venipuncture-related pain of paediatric cancer patients. *Pain*. 2009;142(3):255–263

18. Butler LD, Symons BK, Henderson SL, et al. Hypnosis reduces distress and duration of an invasive medical procedure for children. *Pediatrics*. 2005;115(1):e77–85

19. Geagea D, Tyack Z, Kimble R, et al. Hypnotherapy for procedural pain and distress in children: a scoping review protocol. *Pain Med*. 2021;22(12):2818–2826

20. Richardson J, Smith JE, McCall G, et al. Hypnosis for procedure-related pain and distress in pediatric cancer patients: a systematic review of effectiveness and methodology related to hypnosis interventions. *J Pain Symptom Manage*. 2006;31(1):70–84

21. Lang EV, Benotsch EG, Fick LJ, et al. Adjunctive non-pharmacological analgesia for invasive medical procedures: a randomised trial. *Lancet*. 2000;355(9214):1486–90

22. Wood C, Bioy A. Hypnosis and pain in children. *Journal of Pain and Symptom Management*. 2008;35(4):437–446

23. Jensen MP, Patterson DR. Hypnotic approaches for chronic pain management: clinical implications of recent research findings. *Am Psychol*. 2014;69(2):167–77

24. Uman LS, Birnie KA, Noel M, et al. Psychological interventions for needle-related procedural pain and distress in children and adolescents. *Cochrane Database Syst Rev*. 2013;(10):CD005179:1–100

25. Thompson T, Terhune DB, Oram C, et al. The effectiveness of hypnosis for pain relief: a systematic review and meta-analysis of 85 controlled experimental trials. *Neurosci Biobehav Rev*. 2019;99:298–310

26. Iserson KV. Hypnosis for pediatric fracture reduction. *J Emerg Med*. 1999;17(1):53–6

27. Cyna AM, Tomkins D, Maddock T, et al. Brief hypnosis for severe needle phobia using switch-wire imagery in a 5-year-old. *Paediatr Anaesth*. 2007;17(8):800–4

28. Dash J. Rapid hypno-behavioral treatment of a needle phobia in a five-year-old cardiac patient. *Journal of Pediatric Psychology*. 1981;6(1):37–42

29. Weigold C. The use of hypnosis in the management of needle phobia. *Australian Journal of Clinical & Experimental Hypnosis*. 2011;39(2):1–8

30. Vasant DH, Hasan SS, Cruickshanks P, et al. Gut-focused hypnotherapy for children and adolescents with irritable bowel syndrome. *Frontline Gastroenterol*. 2020;12(7):570–577

31. Olness K, MacDonald JT, Uden DL. Comparison of self-hypnosis and propranolol in the treatment of juvenile classic migraine. *Pediatrics*. 1987;79(4):593–7

32. Culbert TP, Kajander RL, Kohen DP, Reaney JB. Hypnobehavioral approaches for school-age children with dysphagia and food aversion: a case series. *J Dev Behav Pediatr*. 1996;17: 335–341

33. Kohen DP. Hypnotherapeutic management of pediatric and adolescent trichotillomania. *J Dev Behav Pediatr*. 1996;17:328–334

34. Gardner GG. Hypnotherapy in the management of childhood habit disorders. *J Pediatr*. 1978;92(5):838–40

35. Kohen DP, Botts P. Relaxation-imagery (self-hypnosis) in Tourette syndrome: experience with four children. *Am J Clin Hypn*. 1987;29:227–237

36. Lazarus JE, Klein SK. Nonpharmacological treatment of tics in Tourette syndrome adding videotape training to self-hypnosis. *Journal of Developmental & Behavioral Pediatrics*. 2010 Jul 1;31(6):498–504

37. Kohen DP, Mahowald MW, Rosen GM. Sleep-terror disorder in children: the role of self-hypnosis in management. *Am J Clin Hypn*. 1992;34:233–244

38. McKernan LC, Finn MTM, Crofford LJ, et al. Delivery of a group hypnosis protocol for managing chronic pain in outpatient integrative medicine. *Int J Clin Exp Hypn*. 2022;70(3):227–250

LABORATORY AND RADIOLOGY TESTS

NOTE: *This appendix is for informational purposes only and is not meant to function as a protocol for evaluation or care. Physicians need to use their own good judgment when ordering tests to make sure the tests ordered are appropriate for the unique patient in front of them. As noted in Chapter 1, there is no lab test or radiology study that is required to diagnose PANS or PANDAS. They are both clinical diagnoses. Testing helps rule out other diagnoses and helps provide an initial direction of therapy. Physicians should know the safe volume limits for blood draws since testing can be extensive. We sometimes split the initial labs over two visits. Safe phlebotomy volume guidelines have been published by the World Health Organization.[1] Items with an asterisk (*) are part of our usual initial panel. Items with a (#) may be available conventionally but are ideally ordered through specialty labs. Normal values are defined by the individual test reference ranges unless otherwise noted.*

CONVENTIONAL LABS

LabCorp: (www.labcorp.com) **Quest Diagnostics:** (www.questdiagnostics.com)

Laboratory Test	LabCorp Test Number	Quest Test Number
CBC with diff/plt*	005009	6399
Comprehensive metabolic panel (CMP)*	322000	10231
hs-CRP	120766	10124
Celiac antibody panel*	164010	19955
Celiac disease HLA (DQ2/DQ8)*	167082	1735
Ferritin*	004598	457
Iron/TIBC*	001321	7573
Vitamin D, 25-OH*	081950	17306
TSH*	004259	899

Laboratory Test	LabCorp Test Number	Quest Test Number
Free T4*	001974	866
Free T3	010389	34429
TPO antibodies	006676	5081
Anti-Thyroglobulin AB	006685	267
Reverse T3 (rT3)	070104	90963
ANA with reflex*	340897	249
Copper	001586	35378
Ceruloplasmin	001560	326
Homocysteine* (optimal = 7)	706994	31789
Folate#	002014	466
Methylmalonic acid#	706961	34879
Lipid panel	303756	14852
MTHFR#	511238	17911
IgA, IgG, IgM quant*	001768	7083
IgG subclasses 1–4*	209601	7903
IgA subclasses*	123049	34188
Rheumatoid factor	006502	19705
Anti-CCP ab (IgA/IgG)	164914	11173
Complement C4a*	004330	19956
Human TGFβ-1*	821342	91238
Anti-DNase B Strep ab*	096289	256
ASO Strep ab*	006031	265
Strep culture (throat or anal)	008169	14541
Rapid Strep antigen test	180800	11479
Chlamydia pneum IgG/IgM/IgA*	130317	37111
EBV antibody profile*	240610	6421
EBV early antigen*	096248	15447

Laboratory Test	LabCorp Test Number	Quest Test Number
Glutathione#	007700	——----
Mycoplasma pneumoniae IgG/IgM*	163758	34127
Toxoplasma gondii IgG*	006478	3679
Toxoplasma gondii IgM*	096651	37207
Area 5 environmental allergies (IgE)	602632	7905
Mold allergies (IgE)	062448	92170
Pneumococcal ab titers (23)*	812166	16963
Tetanus/diph ab titers*	163253	34042
Autoimmune encephalitis antibodies*	505535	93890
Tryptase	004280	34484
Prostaglandin D2	505530	——----
RBC magnesium#	080283	623
RBC Zinc#	070029	6354
B6#	004655	926
Serum heavy metals profile 2, whole blood#	706200	7655

SPECIALTY LABS

Genova Diagnostics: (www.gdx.net)

Test	Elements of the Test
Genovations MTHFR*	MTHFR 677 and 1298 genotypes
Genovations COMT	COMT genotype
Metabolomix*	Nutrients (antioxidants, all B vitamins, magnesium, manganese, zinc), organic acids (yeast markers, malabsorption, histamine metabolites, Krebs cycle intermediates), oxidative stress markers, omega fatty acids, metals (20 toxic metals), amino acids.

Alletess: (www.foodallergy.com)

Test	Elements of the Test
184 IgG test*	IgG antibody test for 184 foods
14 IgE panel*	IgG antibody test for 14 foods
IgE 12 or 25 environmental allergy panel	IgE antibodies to 12 or 25 env allergens

Doctor's Data: (www.doctorsdata.com)

Test	Elements of the Test
CSA+P (comprehensive stool analysis plus parasitology)*	Bacterial speciation and quantification (through culture), yeast culture, complete parasite evaluation (viruses, bacteria, worms, flukes, protozoa), absorption markers, pancreatic elastase, inflammatory markers (lysozyme, calprotectin, lactoferrin), occult blood, short-chain fatty acids, fat stain, carbohydrates, occult blood
Heavy metals test (urine)	20 toxic metals

Realtime Laboratories: (www.realtimelab.com)

Test	Elements of the Test
Urine mycotoxin test*	16 different mycotoxins from the following families: ochratoxin group, aflatoxin group, macrocyclic tricothecenes, gliotoxin-derivatives, zearalenone
Environmental mycotoxin test and EMMA	16 different mycotoxins from the following families: ochratoxin group, aflatoxin group, macrocyclic tricothecenes, gliotoxin-derivatives, zearalenone. EMMA tests for mold DNA from 10 different molds including *Stachybotrys*

IGeneX Incorporated: (www.igenex.com)

Test	Elements of the Test
Babesia species	ImmunoBlot IgG and IgM, IFA, FiSH, PCR screen. We order *B. duncani* ImmunoBlot*. Testing can identify *B. microti* and *B. duncani*.

Test	Elements of the Test
Borrelia burdorferi	ImmunoBlot (most sensitive), PCR, WB IgM ab, WB IgG ab, IFA, ELISA IgG and IgM, *Borrelia* speciation, IgX Spot (ELISPOT T-cell test). Testing can identify *B. burgdorferi sensu stricto, B. afzelii, B. garinii, B. californiensis, B. mayonii, B. spielmanii,* and *B. valaisiana.*
Bartonella species	ImmunoBlot IgG and IgM, IFA, IgX Spot (ELISPOT T-cell test), PCR, FiSH. Testing can identify *B. henselae, B. quintana, B. elizabethae,* and *B. vinsonii.*
Tick-borne relapsing fever tests	Broad coverage antibody test, PCR, ImmunoBlots (IgM and IgG). Testing can identify *B. turicatae, B. miyamotoi, B. parkeri, B. coriaceae,* and *B.recurrentis.*
Various combination panels are available	—————

Medical Diagnostic Laboratories: (www.mdlab.com)

Test	Elements of the Test
Vector-borne testing	Lyme WB IgG and IgM, *Babesia microti* IgG and IgM ab, *Babesia duncani* (WA-1) PCR, tick-borne relapsing fever group PCR testing (*B. turicatae, B. miyamotoi, B. parkeri, B. hermsii),* *Anaplasma* IgG and IGM IFA, *Ehrlichia* PCR, *Rickettsia* species PCR

Infectolab: (www.infectolab-americas.com)

Test	Elements of the Test
IFN-γ and IL-2 T-cell responses	*Borrelia burgdorferi**, *Borrelia miyamotoi**, *Babesia microti**, *Bartonella henselae**, *Ehrlichia, Rickettsia,* CMV, Epstein-Barr virus, *Chlamydia pneumoniae,* COVID, *Mycoplasma pneumoniae**, *Candida albicans,* HHV-6, HSV 1 and 2
Various combination panels are available	—————

Galaxy Diagnostics: (www.galaxydx.com)

Test	Elements of the Test
Bartonella digital single or triple-draw ePCR	PCR ELISA, IgG, fresh/frozen tissue analysis
Borrelia and *Bartonella* serology	WB, IgG, and IGM

Moleculera Labs: (www.moleculeralabs.com)

Test	Elements of the Test
Cunningham panel	Anti-dopamine D1 receptor, anti-dopamine D2L receptor, anti-lysoganglioside GM-1, anti-tubulin, CaMKII stimulation assay

MicrobiologyDX: (www.microbiologydx.com)

Test	Elements of the Test
Nasal swab	Nasal bacterial culture, nasal fungal culture, biofilm analysis

Mycometrics: (www.mycometrics.com/ermi.html)

Test	Elements of the Test
ERMI or HERTSMI testing	DNA PCR for various molds

RADIOLOGY TESTING

Test	Test notes
MRI of the brain without gadolinium	This is not part of the typical workup unless the child has an atypical presentation, severe headaches, memory issues, or another concerning neurologic symptom. If needed, this can be ordered with sedation at a children's hospital. Gadolinium is not typically used for these children unless some other clinical indication exists.

OTHER TESTING

Test	Test notes
EEG	This can be ordered if a clinical indication exists, but is not part of the typical workup.

APPENDIX A REFERENCES

1. Howie SR. Blood sample volumes in child health research: review of safe limits. *Bull World Health Organ*. 2011;89(1):46–53

MEDICATION AND SUPPLEMENT DOSAGES

NOTE: *This textbook is for physicians and is intended to help them understand PANS and PANDAS through our unique clinical experience in these cases. The information in this text is for educational use only and is not intended to be medical advice. Patients should always consult their personal physician before starting any new medications or supplements, or before implementing any lifestyle changes. Physicians must make decisions about patient care based upon the history and in-person physical examination findings they obtain from their patients. They must also base treatment decisions upon their own medical experience and understanding of the disease process they are treating. Nothing in this text is intended to diagnose, treat, cure, or prevent any condition or disease.*

PRESCRIPTION ANTIMICROBIALS

NOTE: *Maximum pediatric doses should not exceed adult doses. Pediatric doses in our practice are for children age five and older. If behavior worsens, dosages may need to be reduced or spaced out or the agent may need to be stopped.*

Drug	Dosage forms	Dose
Amoxicillin	**Liquid:** 400 mg/5 mL, 200 mg/5 mL, 250 mg/5 mL. **Capsules/tablets:** 250 mg, 500 mg, 875 mg. **Chewable:** 250 mg and 500 mg	**Children:** 50 mg/kg daily divided q12. Maximum 1,000 mg/day **Adults:** 500 mg BID
Amoxicillin/clavulanate	**Liquid:** 125 mg/31.25 mg per 5 mL, 200 mg/28.5 mg per 5 mL, 250 mg/62.5 mg per 5 mL, 400 mg/57 mg per 5 mL. **Tablets:** 250 mg/125 mg, 500 mg/125 mg, 875 mg/125 mg; **ER tablet:** 1000 mg/62.5 mg.	**Children:** 45 mg/kg/day divided q12 (based upon amoxicillin component) **Adults:** 500 mg/125 mg or 875 mg/125 mg q12

Drug	Dosage forms	Dose
Cephalexin	**Liquid:** 125 mg/5 mL, 250 mg/5 mL **Capsules:** 250 mg, 500 mg, 750 mg. **Tablets:** 250 mg, 500 mg.	**Children:** 40 mg/kg/day divided q12 **Adults:** 500 mg q12
Cefdinir	**Liquid:** 125 mg/5 mL, 250 mg/5 mL **Capsules:** 300 mg	**Children:** 14 mg/kg q24 or divided q12 **Adults:** 300 mg q12
Azithromycin	**Liquid:** 100 mg/5 mL, 200 mg/5 mL. **Tablets:** 250 mg, 500 mg, 600 mg.	**Children:** 5–7.5 mg/kg once daily **Adults:** 250 mg daily
Clarithromycin	**Liquid:** 125 mg/5 mL, 250 mg/5 mL. **Tablets:** 250 mg, 500 mg.	**Children:** 15 mg/kg/day divided q12 **Adults:** 250 mg q12
Doxycycline monohydrate	**Liquid:** 25 mg/5 mL. **Capsules:** 50 mg, 75 mg, 100 mg, 150 mg	**Children:** 2.2 mg/kg q12-q24 **Adults:** 100 mg BID
Atovaquone	**Liquid:** 750 mg/5 mL	**Children:** 20 mg/kg dose q12 **Adults:** 750 mg BID
Nystatin	**Liquid:** 100,000 units/mL **Tablets:** 500,000 units	**Children:** 500,000 units BID **Adults:** 500,000 – 1 million units BID

STEROIDS

Drug	Dosage forms	Dose
Prednisone	**Tablets:** 5 mg, 10 mg, 20 mg	1 mg/kg daily for 5 days

LOW-DOSE NALTREXONE

Drug	Dosage forms	Dose
Low-dose naltrexone	(Compounded) Liquid, Capsules, Topical cream	**Children:** 0.05–0.1 mg/kg qHS (titrate up and customize dose; max 4.5 mg) **Adults:** 3–4.5 mg qHS (titrate up and customize dose)

IBUPROFEN

Drug	Dosage forms	Dose
Ibuprofen	**Liquid:** 100 mg/5 mL **Tablets/gelcaps:** 200 mg **Chewable:** 50 mg, 100 mg	**Children:** 10 mg/kg q6–8 **Adults:** 400 mg q6–8

SUPPLEMENTS AND HERBALS

NOTE: *All supplements should be GMP certified and organic with no added preservatives or fillers as much as possible. We use pharmaceutical-grade supplements which are third-party tested. Dosages are approximate and based upon our clinical experience. If patients experience side effects from supplements, the dose can be reduced, or the supplement may need to be discontinued. Patients and parents can get overwhelmed if too many supplements are used at once, and it may also increase the risk of side effects. Supplements below marked with ** are a part of our initial treatment approach while waiting for lab results. As with the medications previously noted, the information in this text is for educational use only and is not intended to be medical advice. Patients should always consult their personal physician before starting any new medications or supplements, or before implementing any lifestyle changes. Nothing in this text is intended to diagnose, treat, cure, or prevent, any condition or disease. Combination supplements are our own Fully Functional Health products unless the brand is otherwise noted.*

Supplement	Dosage forms	Dose
Fish oil EPA and DHA	**Liquid** **Capsules** **Gummies**	**Children (5–15 years):** 500–1000 mg **Age 16 and older:** 2,000–3,000 mg (total) EPA+DHA
SPM omegas**	**Gel caps:** 300 mg	**Children (5–12 years):** 1 capsule daily **Age 13 and older:** 2 capsules daily
Vitamin D3/K2**	**Liquid:** various strengths **Capsules:** various strengths	**Children (5–15 years):** start with 1,000–2,000 IU daily and titrate based upon lab values **Age 16 and older:** start with 5,000 IU daily and titrate based upon lab values
Curcumin (with phospholipid or piperine)	**Chewables** **Liquid** **Capsules**	**Children (5–12 years):** 500 mg daily **Age 13 and older:** 1,000–2,000 mg daily

Supplement	Dosage forms	Dose
Digestive enzymes (should contain multiple types of proteolytic enzymes, papain, bromelain)**	**Chewables** **Capsules**	**Children (5–13 years):** 1 BID daily with meals **Age 14 and older:** 1 TID with meals
Serrapeptase	**Capsules**	**Children (8–15 years):** 1,000–2,000 SPU **Age 16 and older:** 60,000–130,000 units daily
Tauroursodeoxycholic acid (TUDCA) - (BodyBio brand)	**Capsules:** 500 mg	**Children (8–16 years):** 1 daily with food **Age 17 and older:** 2 capsules daily with food
Probiotics (multi-strain, at least 20 billion CFU)**	**Liquid, Capsules, Chewables, Powder**	**Children and Adults:** 20–100 billion CFU daily
*Saccharomyces boulardii***	**Powder** **Capsules**	**Children and Adults:** 250–500 mg daily
Spore-based probiotics	**Capsules**	**Children and Adults:** 50–100 billion CFUs
Strep salivarius K12 (BLIS Probiotics brand)	**Lozenges**	**Children** (*older than 7 to avoid choking hazard*) **and adults:** 1 lozenge daily (2.5 billion CFU)
Humic and fulvic acid (Ion Gut Health brand)	**Liquid**	**Children (5–15 years):** 1 tsp BID **Age 16 and older:** 1 tsp TID
Liposomal glutathione (Tri-Fortify brand by Researched Nutritionals)**	**Gel:** 450 mg/5 mL	**Children (5–13 years):** ½ tsp daily **Age 14 and older:** 1 tsp daily
L-Glutathione capsules (should be Setria formulation)	**Capsules:** 250 mg	**Children (5–14 years):** 1 capsule daily **Age 15 and older:** 1 capsule BID
N-acetyl cysteine (NAC)	**Powder** **Capsules** **Effervescent tablets**	**Children (5–12 years):** 500–900 mg BID **Age 12 and older:** 900 mg BID-TID Titrate to tolerance
Inositol (*do not use in ADHD*)	**Powder** **Capsules**	**Children (5–14 years):** 1,400 mg twice daily **Age 15 and older:** 4100 mg BID
Magnesium glycinate chelate (Albion formulation)	**Capsules** **Liquid** **Powder**	**Children aged 5–15 years:** 125 mg daily **Age 16 and older:** 250 mg daily

Supplement	Dosage forms	Dose
Magnesium citrate	**Powder** **Capsules** **Gummies**	**Children (5–12 years):** 80–150 mg daily **Age 13 and older:** 300 mg daily
L-theanine	**Capsules**	**Children (5–12 years):** 200 mg once daily **Age 13 and older:** 200 mg BID-TID
Cryptolepis	**Liquid 1:5 dilution** **Capsules**	**Children 5–8 years:** 0.35 mL once daily of the 1:5 dilution mixed in 4 ounces of fluid **Ages 9 and older:** 0.7 mL of the 1:5 dilution once daily (1 dropper) in 4 ounces of liquid. Slowly work up to these doses.
GABA	**Liquid (tincture)** **Capsules**	**Children (5–10 years):** 70 mg q8h **Age 11 and older:** 125–250 mg q8h
Phosphatidylserine	**Capsules**	**Children (5–14 years):** 100 mg qHS **Age 15 and older:** 200 mg qHS
Phosphatidylcholine	**Gelcaps** **Liquid**	**Children (age 5–12):** 1,000–2,000 mg daily **Age 13 and older:** 3,000 mg daily
Butyrate	**Gelcaps**	**Age 6 and older:** 300 mg daily

COMBINATION SUPPLEMENT PREPARATIONS

NOTE: *Combination supplements are our own Fully Functional Health products unless the brand is otherwise noted.*

Supplement	Dosage forms	Dose
Beyond Balance (*brand*) products: www.beyondbalanceinc.com (need a physician account)	MC-BAR2 MC-BAB2 Pro-Myco Myco-Regen IMN-VII ENL-MC IMN Calm MAST Ease **(All tinctures with dropper)**	**Children and adults:** Begin with 1 drop in 1 tablespoon of liquid. Slowly increase to 10 drops twice daily and take this dose for 2 months.
Myc-P (Researched Nutritionals *brand*)	**Tincture with dropper:** contains *Isatis, Cordyceps, Houttuynia, Scuttelaria baicalensis, Cat's claw, Sida acuta, Stillingia, uva-ursi*	**Children 5–8 years:** slowly work up to 20 drops daily in 4 ounces of liquid **Age 9 and older:** slowly work up to 40 drops (1 full dropper) once daily in 4 ounces of liquid
Fully Functional Health *brand* Magnesium Powder	**Powder: 1 scoop =** 200 mg magnesium chelate and 1,000 mg Magnesium-L-threonate (*Note: Mag-L-threonate has 144 mg elemental magnesium per 2 grams*)	**Children (5–10 years):** ½ tsp in 4 ounces liquid qHS **Age 11 and older:** 1 tsp in 4 ounces liquid qHS
Fully Functional Health *brand* Relaxation Powder **	**Powder: 1 scoop =** 75 mg Di-magnesium malate , 2000 mg myo-Inositol, 100 mg GABA, 500 mg Taurine, 50 mg L-theanine	**Children (5–10 years):** ½ scoop in 4 ounces liquid qHS **Age 11 and older:** 1 scoop in 4 ounces liquid qHS
Fully Functional Health *brand* Detox Binder**	**Capsules: 2 caps =** 400 mg Zeolite 100 mg activated charcoal, 100 mg Shilajit, 50 mg Fulvic acid, 5 mg Humic acid	**Children (5–10 years):** 1 capsule daily 2 hours away from other supplements or medicines **Age 11 and older:** 2 capsules daily 2 hours away from other supplements or medicines

SAMPLE PANS/PANDAS FLARE PROTOCOL

NOTE: *This textbook is for physicians and is intended to help them understand PANS and PANDAS through our unique clinical experience in these cases. The information in this text is for educational use only and is not intended to be medical advice. Patients should always consult their personal physician before starting any new medications or supplements, or before implementing any lifestyle changes. Physicians must make decisions about patient care based upon the history and in-person physical examination findings they obtain from their patients. They must also base treatment decisions upon their own medical experience and understanding of the disease process they are treating. Nothing in this text is intended to diagnose, treat, cure, or prevent, any condition or disease.*

This is a sample flare protocol that we give our parents in case their child has a sudden change in behavior. It is designed for parents to use with their children. Flares always seem to happen at night and on the weekend.

A well-constructed flare protocol can help parents avoid an unneeded trip to the ER for purely behavioral reasons. We encourage physicians who see children with PANS and PANDAS to develop their own protocol based on their experience and the needs of their particular patient population.

During a flare, we encourage parents to:
1. Remain calm
The first thing parents should remember is that a flare of PANS is out of their child's control. We tend to think of neuropsychiatric symptoms differently from physical illnesses, but there is really no distinction. These children are scared and suffering during a flare. No matter the behavior, it is much better for the parent-child relationship (and the parents' mental health) to remain curious and empathetic. If parents ask questions during the episode rather than becoming critical, it will help diffuse the situation. Curiosity will help the parents think of unique solutions as well. It also models calmness in the face of the storm for the child. If both the parents and the child are spun up and anxious, conflict is inevitable.

2. Pay no attention to the opinions of other parents who do not know the situation

Although outsiders may view the parents' care and concern for their child as "permissive parenting" or enabling, a flare is not the time for strict discipline. Violent or self-injurious behavior cannot be tolerated, however, and this must be communicated to the child in a kind, peaceful manner (preferably before the flare occurs).

3. Identify triggers

Parents should continue journaling foods, activities, where they spend time during the day, and mood/behaviors/tics. They should also journal about what helped in a flare so they can use successful strategies in the future if needed. One of the reasons we have parents do symptom journals with possible triggers is both to identify patterns and also to document how far the child has come as they recover.

4. Reduce inflammation

Parents should reduce inflammatory foods (sugars, preservatives, nonorganic foods, gluten) unless the child has food restrictive behaviors. If behavior is unmanageable and removal of foods makes things worse, they can skip this step.

Parents can administer:

    A. *DYE-FREE* ibuprofen
    B. Curcumin
    C. SPM omegas

Dosages we have found helpful are in Appendix B. Parents should document responses in their journal.

5. Optimize detoxification

This can be accomplished by:

A. Exercise: Taking the child to an open gym or trampoline (with safety measures) can be helpful. Swimming is a great option as well since it has some vagus nerve calming properties due to the cold water on the face. Even a brisk walk outside can help. Parents should be creative and try to find a new activity the child will get excited about. Pleasurable and exciting experiences can help balance neurotransmitters.

B. Infrared sauna: If available and agreeable to the child. See details about infrared sauna in Chapter 17.

C. Maintaining good bowel movements: Magnesium powder or capsules can be efficacious. Fresh fruits and fiber can help as well. Dosages we have found helpful are in Appendix B. Parents should document responses in their journal.

D. Avoiding mold exposures or spending time in water-damaged buildings: Often, taking the child out of a suspicious environment and staying in a clean setting (some hotels or homes of relatives) for as little as a week can help improve behavior. This works best if glutathione and binders (such as activated charcoal) are used during this time. Dosages we have found helpful are in Appendix B. Parents should document responses in their journal.

6. Support

It is important for parents to establish a care plan before it is actually needed. Getting a list of family or close friend caretakers in place to help during a flare can be life-changing. Just having a close adult friend nearby who can stop by to offer encouragement or spend time in the chaos is extremely comforting. A friend or family member who can watch and manage the child at this time so the parent can take some time for self-care (even if just having time in another room to take a bath or converse with their spouse) is truly a blessing. Parents should be encouraged to ask for help.

7. Additional interventions

A. Weighted blankets: These can be helpful to children but may not be tolerated if sensory issues are present.

B. Magnesium baths (or foot baths): Children must be supervised in a bath at all times. Note: Plug-in ionic foot baths are not required and provide no additional benefit.

C. Vagal exercises: Details about therapeutic interventions for sympathetic overactivation can be found in Chapter 20.

D. Positive klnesthetic anchors: This is a neurolinguistic programming (NLP) technique which can be very helpful for older children and adolescents. For details on NLP and a description of kinesthetic anchors, see Chapter 21.

    E. L-theanine

    F. Magnesium threonate, malate, or glycinate

    G. GABA

    H. Inositol

    I. Cognitive behavioral therapy (CBT): CBT is very helpful at breaking what we call "neural loop behaviors." We also recommend organized CBT as part of an ongoing counseling program.

From a physician standpoint, we always go back to looking for an infection or a toxin or toxicant exposure (including a stressful event) as the trigger for the flare. We may start antibiotics, even if there are no signs or symptoms of an infection. Children with PANS and PANDAS may have infections without discernible signs or symptoms (other than behavioral changes).

PARENT RESOURCES

This appendix contains the type of information that is not commonly found in a medical textbook. The rest of this textbook is dedicated to healing the patient. I have written this appendix to help heal the parents and the family. We have found it very helpful in clinical practice.

UNDERSTANDING WHAT IT'S LIKE TO PARENT CHILDREN WITH PANS AND PANDAS

Beyond the sea of tests and treatments, parents battle with the fear and frustration of watching their little one suffer. No parent would wish for a sick child, and yet the parents of PANDAS patients face additional pain as they are often told that PANS and PANDAS don't exist.

Loneliness comes with being the parent of a child with PANS or PANDAS. Other diagnoses, like cancer, are very hard to deal with, but people know what to do: they come over, pray fervently, and bring gifts. Family and friends band together, creating meal train sign-ups, tackling laundry, and cleaning the house. If the battle is long, they take the other kids out so the parents can have a break or get a haircut or a cup of coffee. People let the parents cry on their shoulders. They encourage the parents and help them fight loneliness.

Parents of children with PANS and PANDAS often do not receive this level of support. On a particularly bad day, they're fighting through the judgmental comments of other parents and friends. They may hear:

"Gosh, control your kid. Don't you have any parenting skills?"

"What is wrong with your child? Can't they just behave?"

These parents are also the subject of hurtful gossip, as PANDAS can look different in different settings. Since the child may not "seem sick" in public, parents may be accused of exaggeration or attention-seeking. Our daughter's psychologist said she did not have a medical illness but was just "manipulative." It was easy to feel like we were drowning in criticism.

Then there are the dreaded suggestions: "If you would just _____, your child would be fine." Suddenly, everyone is an armchair expert, suggesting things they are sure will work. When things go wrong, it's human nature to step into a problem-solving role. No one wants to see a child they care about hurting. Although these suggestions may come from a good place, when parents are struggling to get through each day, the endless recommendations from their loved ones may feel hurtful and insulting.

We asked a large cohort of parents of children with PANS and PANDAS two questions:

1. What is the one thing you wish friends and family would do to support you?

2. What do you wish they would understand?

Their answers may surprise you, and possibly even break your heart. In their own words, they said:

- "I look stronger on the outside than I feel on the inside."
- "I'm not canceling or flaking; I'm burned out and need to retreat."
- "We aren't comfortable asking for support. I wish they would just offer it to us."
- "I wish they knew how incredibly hard this is and how I worry that she will never be 100% independent."
- "Anxiety and OCD are mentally and physically exhausting and we need breaks for our own mental health. I wish they would offer us those breaks without us having to ask."
- "Stop judging our decisions for our child. We didn't make these decisions on a whim. A lot of agonizing goes into making our choices. Please don't try to make him a 'normal' child and stop asking me 'what's wrong with him' when he's melting down."
- "I'm doing everything I can. There is no need to ask if I've tried 'XYZ.' I'm doing my best. And when I vent, minimizing hurts. Saying things like, 'They will grow out of it; and this is totally normal' is really hard, because it doesn't work that way."

- "I wish they would help me and stand up for my child in public if they are melting down instead of being embarrassed and telling me people are staring at us."
- "I'm doing my best. I don't need judgment. My kids will not grow out of this. Every day is exhausting, and I wish you cared to listen to my challenges, because it's so isolating and lonely."
- "I wish they understood how serious this is and just because a person can function in some areas doesn't mean they have a full life."
- "My child is gifted. I wish they would acknowledge his struggles even though he doesn't have a learning disorder."
- "I wish everyone understood my daughter is not rude or lacking manners. But socializing and giving hugs make her very uncomfortable."
- "I wish my family would stop talking to me like I haven't done enough research about medication."
- "I think people oversimplify and need black and white. We live in a gray area that requires a different way of parenting."
- "Your rules don't apply to us. This illness is unique, and she is suffering enough just living in her own body. Please don't judge."
- "We cannot punish the anxiety out of our kids. Please understand this illness requires a more compassionate, tolerant approach."
- "I wish they understood that PANS/PANDAS and OCD are very real and very hard. Saying 'everyone has OCD and anxiety' is so hurtful. If people only knew how hard this all is and did not throw those terms around lightly . . . "

- "Just because my daughter holds in her anxiety around you doesn't mean she doesn't have it. She unleashes when she gets home, and it is VERY real and heartbreaking."

- "After choosing to not attend a family function because my daughter's sensory processing was flared, I received this message from my mother: 'If you love us, don't shut us out. Don't segregate yourselves from your family when we celebrated together for years. I don't understand. Your daughter needs her cousins.' She just doesn't get it and doesn't try to."

- "I wish they would ask for reading material instead of assuming they know it all. Then maybe that would help their understanding and we can meet in the middle."

- "I wish they would trust our choices, research, and doctors instead of trying to fix it for us."

One response was particularly striking: "I wish they could just love us through it."

Parents long for someone to be a friend, not a fixer. They need breaks from desperately trying to heal their children. We share the list above with parents and let them know they should share it with their family and friends.

Parents often wonder how they can explain PANS and PANDAS to family and friends, so we offer them this language:

Your immune system has the job of fighting off infections and even toxins using proteins it makes called *antibodies*. Antibodies attack infectious organisms (like bacteria and viruses) and toxins to help your body get rid of them. In PANS (or PANDAS) these antibodies not only attack the infection or toxin but also attack a very specific part of the child's brain and produce scary symptoms like sudden onset OCD (obsessive-compulsive disorder) or trouble eating as well as severe anxiety, bladder issues, defiance, and terrible insomnia. It is a type of autoimmune encephalitis. Although effective treatments are available, recovery can take some time and not every doctor understands PANS (or PANDAS) enough to help. For that reason, we must see a specialist in these disorders.

SELF-CARE FOR THE CAREGIVER

Having a sick child often leads to some serious neglect of parents' own self-care. It goes without saying that caring for a sick family member is exhausting physically, emotionally, and mentally due to the chronic stress and physical demands.

The effects of caregiving on health and well-being are well-documented. If not managed well, these stressors can cause some serious health consequences. The pressures and chronic stress a caregiver feels may lead to irritability, insomnia, weight gain, exhaustion, anxiety, depression, digestive issues, reduced immune function, brain fog, and social isolation.

Caretakers may feel burned-out and unable to cope. They often suffer from feelings of guilt. While it may not be their first instinct, we, as physicians, have to let them know that they simply can't afford to put themselves last and risk the breakdown of their physical and mental well-being. We need to communicate to them that it is not selfish to care for their own needs.

Making time to nourish themselves and creating the space to attend to their own needs makes them more centered, stronger, and better able to support others.

We give patients the following information to help them practice the crucial self-care needed as a caregiver:

1. Make eating well a priority. It's easy to let nutrition fall by the wayside when life is complicated and busy. It's also tempting to skip meals altogether. But nourishing your body is more important now than ever. You have to eat, so eat well! Eat nutrient-dense, anti-inflammatory, regularly scheduled meals to fuel the energy you need for caregiving. Chronic stress leads to inflammation, so it's important to avoid inflammatory foods, such as highly refined, processed, and fast foods and foods high in sugar. These foods will also zap your energy and lead to mood swings and blood sugar issues, all of which will work against you, not for you!

2. Optimize sleep. It's vital to maintain adequate sleep habits, especially during times of stress. Sleep affects every aspect of our mental, emotional, and physical performance. It's crucial for the restoration of your body and gives you the leverage and resilience you need to face and overcome daily challenges. Consider creating a short and simple evening ritual that promotes relaxation such as some deep-breathing exercises, a calming bath, meditation, journaling or light stretching, and restorative yoga poses. Create a sleep sanctuary with an environment that encourages rest! This is your time off. Make the most of it.

3. Engage your "relaxation response" with mind-body practices. Your relaxation response is your body's natural way to combat stress and is regulated through the parasympathetic nervous system. You have the means to activate this response in the body through mind-body practices and deep relaxation techniques such as meditation, prayer, yoga, and deep breathing. Try this simple breathing technique to reset your parasympathetic nervous system in times of acute stress or proactively throughout the day:

Breathe in through the nose for a count of four.

Hold for a count of seven.

Slowly release the breath through the mouth for a count of eight.

Repeat five times or for several minutes until you feel a deeper sense of calm.

If these counts are too challenging, you can shorten the counts or simplify the breath even more by just breathing deeply for four counts in and four counts out, slowly, deeply, and intentionally.

4. Practice grace and self-compassion. Have grace for yourself (and your other family members!). There is a ripple effect on the whole family when one member is suffering with chronic illness. The stress can cause tensions to run high. You won't manage this perfectly and neither will your family. Everybody deserves some grace, but especially you if you are the main caregiver. Quiet the harsh inner voice that is critical of self. Practice self-compassion by giving yourself credit for the challenging and complex work of caregiving and grace for your mistakes. This is the foundation of self-care!

5. Feed your spirit and nurture your soul. Practice simple acts of kindness for yourself. This includes those practices that lift your spirit and keep you functioning optimally. What feeds your soul? What makes you feel stronger, more energized, more relaxed? Make room for creativity and commit to aligning at least a small part of your day to participate in activities that light you up and fuel your inspiration.

6. Maintain social connection. Your social connections can be a great support for you during this time of caregiving. Find someone to help with the caregiving from time to time to allow you to get out and reconnect with friends. It can also be tempting to reject help that is offered, not wanting to "inconvenience" your friends, thinking you can do it all on your own. Take the help! Allow your friends to support you.

7. Cultivate gratitude. Even in the face of massive challenges, we can always find things to be grateful for. Tapping into this gratitude forces a mindset shift toward the positive and helps us to be more resilient when dealing with challenges. Life has thrown you a curveball, but you have the strength to handle it when you make your own self-care a priority! When you replenish your physical, mental, and emotional well-being, you will have more to give. It also makes you less vulnerable to self-sabotage and sets a good example for those you care about.

SCHOOL RESOURCES TO PROTECT AND ACCOMMODATE THE CHILD'S ILLNESS

Federal statutes define a disabled student as "a student who has a physical or mental impairment that substantially limits one or more major life activities, has a record of such an impairment, or is regarded as having such an impairment." The most common federal laws that guarantee the rights of students with disabilities include a 504 Plan and an IEP (individualized education plan).

The difference between a 504 plan and an IEP

504 Plan: This is for children with physical or intellectual impairments that substantially limit their ability to function but who do not meet the requirements of an IEP. It is meant to ensure that the child has access to the same learning environment as their non-impaired peers so that they aren't discriminated against. Parental consent is necessary for an evaluation of the child, but accommodations can be provided without a formal evaluation or parental consent.

IEP: The child must meet one or more of the following criteria

    Autism

    Deaf-blindness

    Deafness

    Developmental delay (ages 3–7 years)

    Emotional disturbance

    Hearing impairment

    Intellectual disability

    Multiple disabilities

    Orthopedic impairment

    Other health impairment

    Specific learning disability

    Speech or language impairment

    Traumatic brain injury

    Visual impairment

The purpose of an IEP is to ensure that the child is able to make meaningful educational progress and the school receives funding in order to meet the needs of the child. An IEP requires a parent to consent and must be completed within 120 days of the parent's request.

Which does the child need?

If simple accommodations (such as extra time to take a test) will be helpful for the child so they will not be discriminated against because of their disability, then a 504 plan might suffice. If the child requires additional help (such as extra time to take a test and additional resources to learn the material) and they meet one of the medical requirements, then an IEP would be more appropriate. For children with PANS and PANDAS, "other health impairment" is the medical requirement criterion they meet most commonly. In order to determine what is best for the child, the school will require several evaluations. A medical evaluation and letter stating what their "other health impairment" is, as well as other testing performed by behavioral health specialists, and in some cases occupational and/or speech therapy (OT and PT).

Getting the process started
This is the list of action items
we give to the parents:

- Get a letter from your treating doctor.
- Keep a portfolio of your child's school-work. Show the difference in what they were able to do before they became ill and after. This comparison can be quite helpful in getting what your child needs.
- Ask for an evaluation by PT and OT or get these done on your own.
- Emphasize "other health impairment" as the primary disability condition.
- Reach out to the school immediately and request an evaluation for an IEP—once you do this, they have 120 days to organize a formal meeting.
- Use this language when speaking with the school: "These are the things that are getting in the way of my child keeping up with their regular school curriculum and ability to learn."
  - Fine motor skills
  - Visual processing—tracking, speed, visual acuity, etc.
  - Auditory and language processing—receptive language, expressive language

  - Memory concerns/skills
  - Gross motor skills (learning in PE or on the playground is also important)
  - Social/emotional impairment
  - Need for assistive technology—having a computer or headphones to hear the teacher more clearly, etc.
  - Psychiatric issues—OCD, anxiety, etc.

This is a list of the reasonable accommodations that parents can ask for:

- Organizational support—someone to help them organize papers, their backpack, their locker, their schedule, etc.
- Preferential seating
- Extra time for tests—perhaps in a separate and quiet room
- Questions for tests may be read to them by an aide rather than relying on them having to read it themselves—this allows them to get up and walk during the quiz/test
- Ability to present oral speech in private with the teacher
- An assignment notebook with lists of what is needed
- Detailed instructions for projects with the steps essentially spelled out
- Extra set of books and supplies at home
- Ability to leave the classroom to use the restroom frequently
- Ability to leave the classroom and get a "walking break" or other opportunities to exercise/move to mitigate hyperactivity or agitation
- A system of regular communication with teachers and administrators
- Ability to stand up in the back of the classroom or have fidgets at their desk

- Expectation of the teacher to provide discrete cues/prompts to keep on track
- An aide (discrete) if necessary in order for your child to ask questions or be escorted to the bathroom/hall breaks
- Earphones to block out noise/distractions
- Specific auditory devices for sound amplification of the teacher
- Positive reinforcement when they are doing what is expected
- Ability to wear sunglasses or close the blinds if they are visually overloaded
- Ability to use a calculator, graph paper, have lists, etc.
- Assistance on field trips to ensure safety with additional support if needed
- Social skills groups
- Speech or occupational therapy if needed
- Shortened assignments
- Eliminate homework and/or unnecessary busy work
- Summary charts and checklists

- Assistive technology for dictation if writing is an issue or there is a need for books to be read to the child
- Allow dictated responses rather than written responses for tests/quizzes
- A written plan to involve the nurse and to otherwise address health concerns/ emergencies
- Create peer assistance if needed/helpful to work on projects/assignments
- Allow child to leave class a little early to get to next class, particularly if walking in the busy hallway is overwhelming for them
- Have a system in place for home assignments to be received when the child is unable to attend school/class
- Modify attendance policy if needed (this may be one of the most essential needs)
- Make sure every teacher/staff member is aware of the health concerns of the child and is prepared to offer the appropriate accommodations

SAMPLE IVIG ORDERS AND HELPFUL TIPS

NOTE: *The ordering and administration of IVIG should only be done by or in consultation with a physician experienced in the administration of IVIG in children. The orders and tips that follow are for informational purposes only and are not intended to diagnose, treat, cure, or prevent any condition or disease. IVIG is the last modality listed in this book since most children in our practice recover before it is needed.*

The IVIG orders on the next page are based on the orders that we use for our patients. They represent what we feel are the current best practices for ordering IVIG for patients with PANS and PANDAS. Before ordering, the physician must document all medications, supplements, and medication allergies and obtain proper informed consent from a parent or guardian. Orders are typically sent to an infusion pharmacy or hospital with demographic information, insurance information, and clinical notes.

_____

SAMPLE IVIG TEMPLATE ORDERS

1. Demographic information with contact information and parents' names

2. Medication allergies

3. Diagnoses (with ICD-10 code) for the infusion.
   NOTE: *If more than one diagnosis is listed, it will not increase the chance of insurance approval since the reviewers typically only consider the first listed diagnosis. Common diagnoses include G04.81 (autoimmune encephalitis / other encephalitis or encephalomyelitis) or B95.5 (PANDAS). There is no ICD-10 code currently for PANS.*

4. First infusion is to be given at an infusion center with trained personnel and emergency equipment present. If the patient tolerates the infusion well, subsequent infusions may be administered in the home by a trained infusion nurse.

5. The infusion pharmacy should supply all equipment, pumps, poles, monitoring devices, and medications.

6. Skilled nursing services will be required for all infusions to establish IV access, administer medications, and assess the patient's condition during infusions.

7. IVIG therapy is to be administered over two days every four weeks for ___ weeks. *(We usually use twelve weeks as the initial period. Occasionally, insurance will only approve a single infusion. I count this as a victory—it is better than nothing. Orders may be written in advance of when they are needed. The approval and appeal process takes time. Parents may be counseled that they don't have to have the infusion if the child improves while they are waiting for approval. There are no charges from the pharmacy unless the patient receives the medication.)*

8. Before beginning, the RN will verify patient identity, medication allergies, dose and expiration dates of medications, and concentration and volume of IVIG. The RN will also ensure that emergency medications and equipment are present.

9. Weight and vital signs are to be obtained by the RN. If vital signs are outside age expected norms, the ordering physician will be notified before the infusion is started.

10. Diet: NPO after midnight and for the first 2 hours of the infusion, then as tolerated. The importance of frequent oral hydration should be emphasized.

11. Activity: Bed rest or quiet play while infusing, with bathroom privileges.

12. Pre-medications (to be given 1 hour prior to IVIG initiation by RN or parents)
    a. Acetaminophen 15 mg/kg/dose PO x 1 (not more than 650 mg total dose) **or** ibuprofen 10 mg/kg/dose PO x 1 (not more than 600 mg total dose)
    b. Decadron 3 mg IV slow push or mix in 50 cc of NaCL 0.9% and infuse over 20 minutes.
    c. Benadryl 1.25 mg/kg PO x 1 (max dose 25 mg)
    d. Lidocaine 2.5% / Prilocaine 2.5%, 2 mL to each antecubital fossa and cover with Tegaderm or a small amount of plastic wrap.

13. RN to maintain peripheral IV catheter during infusion. Flush with 3–5 mL of sterile saline flush PRN.

14. IV normal saline bolus to be given before IVIG. Dose is _____ mL (typically 150 mL).

15. IVIG: **NOTE:** *This is a 2 g/kg dose of IVIG to be split over 2 days (1 g/kg/day). Maximum dose of 100 g/day. See below for specific dosing instructions.*

e. Brand of IVIG.

NOTE: *Brands are largely interchangeable, and the infusion pharmacies will often tell you what will be covered by the patient's specific insurance. Brands are not in order of preference. Other brands not listed may be preferred by the patient's insurance or may qualify for patient assistance programs.*

○ Gammunex C, 10% solution. 2 g/kg = _____ TOTAL grams = 1 g/kg/day for 2 days. Max dose 100 g/day

○ Privigen 10% solution. 2 g/kg = _____ TOTAL grams = 1 g/kg/day for 2 days. Max dose 100 g/day

○ Octagam 10% solution. 2 g/kg = _____ TOTAL grams = 1 g/kg/day for 2 days. Max dose 100 g/day

○ Gammagard SD 5% solution. 2 g/kg = _____ TOTAL grams = 1 g/kg/day for 2 days. Max dose 100 g/day

NOTE: *this is an IgA-poor preparation which is used if patients have a low serum IgA level to prevent reactions, as some patients with low IgA levels have IgA antibodies.*

○ OTHER _____. 2 g/kg = _____ TOTAL grams = 1 g/kg/day for 2 days. Max dose 100 g/day

16. Infusion rates. All rates are to be followed exactly as written.

Infuse slowly over 5–7 hours depending on total volume as follows:	
Infusion rates (DAY 1):	Infusion rates (DAY 2):
15 mL/hr for 30 minutes	15 mL/hr for 30 minutes
30 mL/hr for 30 minutes	30 mL/hr for 30 minutes
60 mL/hr for 30 minutes	60 mL/hr for 30 minutes
100 mL/hr until completed	100 mL/hr until complete.

17. Monitoring guidelines during the infusion:

a. Vital signs will be measured and recorded every 15 minutes (pulse, blood pressure, respiratory rate, and temperature) from baseline until final IVIG rate escalation. Thereafter, vital signs will be measured every 15 minutes times 2, and then every 30 minutes, and more often as indicated until the end of the infusion, and then at the end of the infusion.

b. If any of the following occur, the infusion rate should be immediately decreased by 50% and a call should be placed to the ordering physician:

i. Temperature increase more than one degree Celsius from baseline or chills

ii. Nausea or vomiting

iii. Pain in joints, muscles, or back

  iv. Palpitations or dizziness

  v. Diaphoresis

  vi. Itching or rash

  vii. Flushing

  viii. Headache (if present, administer dexamethasone 0.5 mg/kg slow IV push (max 30 mg) and 150 mL saline bolus should be given once)

c. The following will dictate immediate cessation of infusion and a call to the ordering physician:

  i. Fall in systolic blood pressure to less than 70 mm plus (2X age) of subject, or to less than 90 mm if subject is greater than or equal to ten years old

  ii. Tachypnea (without respiratory distress)

  iii. Chest tightness or tachycardia (heart rate more than 25% over baseline)

d. For acute anaphylaxis (shortness of breath, respiratory distress, edema of the lips or tongue, persistent hypotension, altered mental status):

  i. Stop the infusion

  ii. Activate EMS/call 911 immediately

  iii. Initiate BLS/CPR as needed and do not leave patient unattended

  iv. Administer rescue medications as needed (see chart below)

  v. Change IV fluids to 0.9% saline and give an initial bolus of 20 mL/kg and then put rate at 50 mL/hour maintenance. Additional 20 mL/kg boluses as required for hypotension.

Rescue Medications				
Ordered	Weight	Epinephrine 1/1,000 amp (IM only)	Decadron (unless previously given)	Diphenhydramine injection
☐	< 15 kg	0.01 mg/kg IM May repeat x1 in 3–5 min PRN	3 mg IV slow push x1	12.5 mg by slow IV push (30 sec) or IM x 1
☐	15–30 kg	0.15 mg IM May repeat x 1 in 3–5 min PRN	5 mg IV slow push x1	12.5 mg by slow IV push (30 sec) or IM x 1
☐	>30 kg	0.3 mg IM May repeat x 1 in 3–5 min PRN	10 mg IV slow push x1	25 mg by slow IV push (30 sec) or IM x 18

18. Upon completion of the IVIG infusion,
    give IV fluids NaCl 0.9% _____ mL *(usually 150 mL)* over 30 minutes.

Observe for another 30 minutes with IV in place. Recheck VS and if stable discontinue (or flush and cap) IV for discharge.

19. Provide verbal and written discharge instructions.
20. Physician's attestation: *I certify/recertify that the patient is under my care and in need of the ordered medical services listed above.*
21. Physician signature/Date

POST-IVIG COURSE

Most children have an uneventful recovery from IVIG. Some patients, however, may develop a significant headache with nausea (with or without vomiting). The headache is positional and resembles that of a postdural puncture headache. The best thing to do is prevent this headache before it starts by making sure the patient stays very well hydrated during and after the infusion. Patients tend to urinate frequently during the infusion and if they get dehydrated, the chance of this headache and nausea is much higher. For this reason, we tell parents to give the child their favorite drink during the infusion to make sure they consume enough fluid.

This post-IVIG headache is referred to as "aseptic meningitis" in some places in the professional medical literature. We don't use this term with parents as they become alarmed when they hear "meningitis," and it may alarm other clinicians reviewing office notes.

We urge parents to continue aggressive hydration between infusions and after. We send our IVIG patients home with prescriptions for steroids (usually prednisone, 1 mg/kg PO daily for 3 days) and ondansetron ODT 4 mg to take one every 6 hours if needed. We tell parents to fill these medications and hold them in case they are needed, as symptoms may crop up in the middle of the night. We don't use them prophylactically. For unknown reasons, some children get a headache even if they stay hydrated. A post-IVIG headache may motivate the child to drink more during subsequent infusions or may make the child less cooperative in the future.

Rarely, a post-IVIG headache with vomiting is refractory to oral medications and the child must be sent to the pediatric ED for IV anti-emetics and IV fluids. The ordering PANS/PANDAS physician should always call and speak with the ED physician on duty to let them know that the patient has had IVIG and let them know what is desired from the ED encounter. Parents cannot be relied upon to accurately communicate what is needed.

IVIG INSURANCE APPROVAL TIPS

Since IVIG is, on average, $25,000 per two-day course, insurance plans are very selective with the indications for which they will approve IVIG. In the case of PANS and PANDAS, requests for IVIG are almost always denied initially. It is important to pay attention to the reason for denial, which will be on the letter that is issued by the insurer.

The first-level appeal is usually a letter from the ordering physician. The most common reason for denial in children with PANS and PANDAS is that the "treatment is experimental or has not been shown to be effective for this diagnosis." I will send an appeal letter back (see the next section for a sample letter) with references from the peer-reviewed medical literature that outline the effectiveness of IVIG for PANS and PANDAS. I have a section in the appeal letter that calls attention to the fact that denials on the grounds that it is "unproven" in the face of the literature I am citing constitutes non-evidence-based medicine. This has resulted in the denial being overturned several times.

The reason that it is important to pay attention to the reason listed in the denial letter is that the insurance company may deny three infusions if ordered that way but may be willing to approve one infusion. One is better than none, so I may resubmit orders for a single infusion. If the child experiences a benefit from the infusion, I will then submit a second request afterward as a "continuation of therapy." Continuation of therapy with documented improvements are usually easier to secure.

If the letter is unsuccessful, you can usually request a peer-to-peer conference by phone with a clinician from the insurance company. Calling this meeting a "peer-to-peer" conference is a bit misleading at times as you may be speaking with a pharmacist, a nurse, or a physician from a nonclinical or unrelated medical specialty. Often, the insurance company will have an administrative person call and schedule the peer-to-peer at their convenience, which may occur right in the middle of the day during office hours. Some infusion pharmacies will write the letter of appeal and may even have a physician on staff who does the peer-to-peer conferences for you.

Considering both levels of appeal, I have an overall success rate of about 85% at getting denials overturned. There is a bit of an art to it, and I have summarized my best tips below.

To be most successful in a peer-to-peer meeting:

1. Establish rapport early. Figure out where the person is calling you from. Make small talk. Be pleasant. Find commonality. Match their tone of voice and tempo of speech (without mimicking them). This is known as mirroring and is very effective at helping establish rapport early, as mentioned in Chapter 6. Humans tend to like people who are like them.

2. Remain calm. If you start the call angry (as you have a right to be) and are rude or imply that the insurance company is harming patients, just in it for money, or practicing medicine without a license, the person on the other end of the line will be less likely to help you. It's human nature.

3. Start the call by grouping the company representative *with* you and not against you. Say something like, "Let's talk about this case and see if *we* can get the therapy covered for this sick child who needs it. Can you help me get what *our* patient needs?" By bringing them in with you, you have a better chance at activating their identity as a caretaker and clinician rather than just an administrator.

4. If the reviewer still denies coverage based upon effectiveness, speak about some of the studies listed in Chapter 13. Point out that a denial on this basis is not evidence based medicine and say something like, "I know your company wants to practice evidence-based medicine to help its subscribers." You can also ask them about "other approved diagnoses that may fit."

It may require resubmitting orders with a new diagnosis or new clinical information to meet their criteria. My experience is that the insurance reviewers don't enjoy denials. They have a book of criteria, and if the case does not fit the criteria, they may not have the ability to overturn it. Leave the morality of the denial or what they do for a living out of the discussion. This is neither the time nor the place for that conversation, and it will alienate the reviewer. Give them case details and outline how sick the child is and how hard it is for the parents. That may stimulate their parental instincts if they have their own children. It is best if you can get the reviewer *curious* about the case. Everyone wants to solve problems and think of themselves as a detective. That's why mystery shows and crime podcasts do so well. Just like us, it's likely that the reviewer wants to feel good when they put their head down on the pillow at night. If they overturn the denial, I usually say something like, "We did something good here today. I'll let the parents know how helpful you were." It's a small world, and I have spoken to the same reviewers on more than one occasion. These little bits of hypnotic language can set the stage for better interactions in the future.

5. If the denial stands, the patient's parents will get another letter, which may have additional levels of appeal or may state that the peer-to-peer conference was the final level of appeal. If it was the final level and the orders were not approved, there may be no recourse.

6. Most companies have instructions on post peer-to-peer denials that list an option for an independent third-party review. I have not been successful in making this happen. The process is clunky, and I have never been contacted back when I inquired on this type of appeal.

7. One golden nugget which has helped in the past is something called a "pharmacy benefit." Usually, when a medication is ordered, it goes to the main insurance coverage. Several infusion pharmacies have suggested resubmitting orders under the pharmacy benefit of the policy. This has been successful on several occasions. It seems to be a separate pile of money with less restrictive criteria. Some policies don't have this benefit.

8. Finally, Indiana and ten other states at the time of this writing have passed laws which prevent insurance companies from denying coverage for IVIG based on a diagnosis of PANS or PANDAS. This has been a great benefit to families. Unfortunately, the insurance companies have found two counterarguments to sidestep these laws. The first is to send a denial letter which says that they will approve the IVIG for PANS or PANDAS only if the child has failed therapy for one year. They then go on to list their criterial for "therapy." One company's letter required consultations with neurology, rheumatology, and psychiatry. The company also required a yearlong trial of antibiotics with steroids and psychiatric medications. This is meant to be onerous. I have successfully argued against this type of denial by pointing out that I have peer-reviewed evidence for IVIG in

PANS and PANDAS and that their required protocol was not evidence-based and may be harmful for some children. The second strategy some insurance companies are starting to use involves their location and some semantics. In Indiana, for example, the companies are denying coverage if the insurance office processing the claim (listed on the back of the insurance card) is in a state which does not have a coverage law. My guess is that this will only stop when state legislatures or state insurance commissions are notified. The spirit of the law in Indiana (and other states, I'm sure) is to provide coverage for residents of these states, not to benefit out-of-state insurance companies.

————————

SAMPLE IVIG APPEAL LETTER

DATE

Insurance Company

Address

RE: Patient Name, DOB, subscriber number (should be on the denial), reference number (may be on the denial)

To Whom It May Concern,

I am the treating physician for XXXXXXXXX. XXXXX is a/an X-year-old (fe)male patient who presented for treatment on XXXXXX. He/She presented with severe OCD and anxiety following an illness and was diagnosed with pediatric autoimmune neuropsychiatric disorder associated with *Strep* infection (PANDAS), which is a form of autoimmune encephalitis due to anti-neuronal antibodies.[1,2] This diagnosis was made in accordance with published criteria from peer-reviewed medical literature from the National Institute of Mental Health.[3,4]

XXXXX was started on appropriate antibiotics and initially showed some improvement with symptoms, as is common in this disorder.[5] However, s/he soon worsened and began to have disabling OCD, intrusive thoughts, and developed severe anxiety. S/he was unable to attend school. At this point, it was clear that IVIG was indicated in accordance with published criteria from peer-reviewed medical literature from the National Institute of Mental Health.[6]

1 Swedo, SE, Leonard HL, Kiessling LS. Speculations on antineuronal antibody-mediated neuropsychiatric disorders of childhood. *Pediatrics*. 1994;93(2):323–326.

2 Swedo, Susan E., et al. Identification of children with pediatric autoimmune neuropsychiatric disorders associated with streptococcal infections by a marker associated with rheumatic fever. *American Journal of Psychiatry*. 1997;154(1):110–112.

3 Wald, E. A Pediatric Infectious Disease Perspective on Pediatric Autoimmune Neuropsychiatric Disorder Associated With Streptococcal Infection and Pediatric Acute- onset Neuropsychiatric Syndrome. *The Pediatric Infectious Disease Journal*. 2019;38(7):706–709.

4 Swedo SE, Leonard HL, Garvey M, et al. Pediatric Autoimmune neuropsychiatric disorders associated with streptococcal infections: clinical description of the first 50 cases. *American Journal of Psychiatry*. 1998;155:264–271.

5 Cooperstock M, et al. Clinical management of pediatric acute-onset neuropsychiatric syndrome: Part III—Treatment and prevention of infections. *Journal of Child and Adolescent Psychopharmacology*. 2017;27(7):594–606.

6 Frankovich J, et al. Clinical management of pediatric acute-onset neuropsychiatric syndrome: part II—use of immunomodulatory therapies. *Journal of child and adolescent psychopharmacology* 2017;27(7):574–593.

The peer-reviewed literature previously cited (reference 6) as well as an excellent article from the peer-reviewed journal the *Lancet*[7] firmly establish the effectiveness of IVIG for this condition. The denial in the case is not supported by the weight of the published medical evidence or the experience of hundreds of physicians treating children with this devastating disorder across the country. Denying IVIG in the case would not be evidence-based medicine.

There is a law that we were successful in passing in Indiana which does not allow insurers to refuse coverage for IVIG in cases of PANDAS in the state. This law is located in 2020 Indiana Code, Title 27. Insurance Article 13. Health Maintenance Organizations, Chapter 7. Requirements for Group Contracts, Individual Contracts, and Evidence of Coverage 27-13-7-26. Coverage for Pediatric Neuro-psychiatric Disorders.

It reads as follows: IN Code § 27-13-7-26 (2020)

Sec. 26. (a) An individual contract and a group contract must provide coverage for treatment of:

(1) pediatric autoimmune neuropsychiatric disorders associated with streptococcal infections (PANDAS); and

(2) pediatric acute-onset neuropsychiatric syndrome (PANS);

including treatment with intravenous immunoglobulin therapy.

(b) The coverage required by this section may not be subject to annual or lifetime limitation, deductible, copayment, or coinsurance provisions that are more restrictive than the annual or life-time limitation, deductible, copayment, or coinsurance provisions that apply generally under the individual contract or group contract.

As the denial letter presented no peer-reviewed published evidence to support the denial, and because we know the entire aim of your company is to provide the very best evidence-driven care, we ask that you reverse this denial and provide coverage for this life-changing care. In these cases, parents feel like their child has been taken away from them. Please make this right by providing coverage for this much needed treatment.

Thank you,
Signature
Printed name

Contact information

7 Perlmutter S, et al. Therapeutic plasma exchange and intravenous immunoglobulin for obsessive--compulsive disorder and tic disorders in childhood. *Lancet*. 1999;354(9185):1153–1158.

ABOUT THE AUTHOR

Dr. Scott Antoine completed his undergraduate training at the University of Scranton in Scranton, Pennsylvania, after which he completed his doctorate at the Philadelphia College of Osteopathic Medicine.

He completed an emergency medicine residency and an emergency medical services fellowship at Albert Einstein Medical Center in Philadelphia. He then served seven years of active duty with the United States Army as an emergency physician and as an emergency physician in Indianapolis, Indiana, for fifteen years. He served as teaching faculty at the Indiana University School of Medicine. He has also trained family medicine residents and PA students.

In addition to his board certification in emergency medicine, he achieved board certification in integrative medicine through the newly formed American Board of Integrative Medicine in 2016. He also holds certifications in functional medicine through the Institute for Functional Medicine and A4M.

In 2019, he successfully lobbied the Indiana legislature and helped pass a law which prohibits insurance companies in Indiana from denying coverage for medical care (including IVIG) for children with PANS and PANDAS.

He is the co-owner of the Center for Fully Functional Health with Dr. Ellen Antoine, who first developed the revolutionary Fully Functional process. This process has helped thousands of children and adults live their happiest, most productive, most joy-filled lives.

When the doctors' daughter, Emma, was twelve, she became ill with PANS. The doctors then modified the Fully Functional process, which helped bring their daughter back to a fully healthy state by re-regulating her immune response and removing the infections and toxins responsible for her PANS presentation.

Since then, Dr. Scott Antoine has further refined this process and has helped hundreds of children recover from PANS and PANDAS.

The doctors enjoy time with their children, their dogs, and each other.